Appleton & Lange's Review of
ANATOMY FOR THE USMLE STEP 1

Appleton & Lange's Review of
ANATOMY FOR THE USMLE STEP 1

Royce L. Montgomery, PhD
Associate Professor of Anatomy
School of Medicine
University of North Carolina
Chapel Hill, North Carolina

Gerald A. Montgomery, MD
Adjunct Professor of Anatomy
School of Medicine
University of North Carolina
Chapel Hill, North Carolina

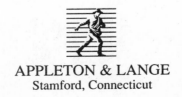

APPLETON & LANGE
Stamford, Connecticut

Copyright © 1995 by Appleton & Lange
A Division of Simon and Schuster
Copyright © 1989 by Appleton & Lange
A Publishing Division of Prentice Hall
Copyright © 1974, 1978, 1982 by Arco Publishing, Inc.

95 96 97 98 99 / 10 9 8 7 6 5 4 3 2

Prentice Hall International (UK) Limited, *London*
Prentice Hall of Australia Pty. Limited, *Sydney*
Prentice Hall Canada, Inc., *Toronto*
Prentice Hall Hispanoamericana, S.A., *Mexico*
Prentice Hall of India Private Limited, *New Delhi*
Prentice Hall of Japan, Inc., *Tokyo*
Simon and Schuster Asia Pte. Ltd., *Singapore*
Editora Prentice Hall do Brasil Ltda., *Rio de Janeiro*
Prentice Hall, *Englewood Cliffs, New Jersey*

Library of Congress Cataloging-in-Publication Data

Montgomery, Royce L.
    Appleton & Lange's review of anatomy for the USMLE Step 1, / Royce L. Montgomery.
        p.   cm.
    Includes bibliographical references.
    ISBN 0–8385–0246–6
    1. Human anatomy—Examinations, questions, etc.   I. Title.
II. Title: Appleton and Lange's review of anatomy.   III. Title:
Review of anatomy.   IV. Title: Anatomy.
    [DNLM: 1. Anatomy—examination questions.   QS 18 M788h 1995]
    QM32.M65   1995
    611—dc20
    DNLM/DLC
    for Library of Congress   94–31509
                                                                        CIP

Aquisitions Editor: Jamie Kircher
Production Editor: Sondra Greenfield
Production Services: Rainbow Graphics, Inc.

ISBN   0-8385-0246-6

9 780838 502464

90000

PRINTED IN THE UNITED STATES OF AMERICA

Contents

Introduction

If you are planning to prepare for the United States Medical Licensing Examination (USMLE) Step 1, then this book is designed for you. Here, in one package, is a comprehensive review resource with 1,000 examination type Anatomy multiple-choice questions with referenced, paragraph-length explanations of each answer.

This introduction provides specific information on the USMLE Step 1, information on question types, question-answering strategies, and various ways to use this review.

THE UNITED STATES MEDICAL LICENSING EXAMINATION STEP 1

The United States Medical Licensing Examination Step 1 is a two-day examination consisting of approximately 800 questions to test your knowledge in the basic sciences. It contains multiple-choice questions organized within three dimensions. Each dimension is weighted; however the projected percentages for these dimensions are subject to change from exam to exam. The three dimensions are: (1) System, (2) Process, and (3) Organizational Level. The application materials illustrate the percentage breakout, and offer you a detailed content outline to aid you in your review.

Question Formats

The style and presentation of the questions have been fully revised to conform with the United States Medical Licensing Examinations. This will enable you to familiarize yourself with the types of questions to be expected, and provide practice in recalling your knowledge in each format. Following the answer to each question, a reference to a particular and easily available text is provided for further reference and reading.

Each of the chapters contains multiple-choice questions (or "items" in testing parlance). Most of these are "one best answer–single item" questions, some are "one best answer–matching sets," and some are "extended one best answer–matching set" questions. In some cases, a group of two or three questions may be related to a situational theme. In addition, some questions have illustrative material (eg, x-rays and line illustrations of anatomy) that require understanding and interpretation on your part. Moreover, questions may be of three levels of difficulty: rote memory, memory question that requires more understanding of the problem, and a question that requires both understanding and judgment. In view of the fact that the USMLE Step 1 is moving toward the judgment, critical-thinking type question, we have attempted to write this review with this emphasis. Finally, some of the items are stated in the negative. In such instances, we have printed the negative word in capital letters (eg, "All of the following are correct EXCEPT," "Which of the following choices is NOT correct," and "Which of the following is LEAST correct").

One Best Answer–Single Item Question. The majority of the questions are posed in the A-type, or "one best answer–single item" format. This is the most popular question format in most exams. It generally contains a brief statement, followed by five options of which only ONE is entirely correct. The options on the USMLE are lettered A, B, C, D, and E. Although the format for this question type is straightforward, the questions can be difficult because some of the distractors may be partially right. The instructions you will see for this type of question will generally appear as below:

DIRECTIONS (Question 1): Each of the numbered items or incomplete statements in this section is followed by answers or by completions of the statement. Select the ONE lettered answer or completion that is BEST in each case.

An example of this question type is:

1. An obese 21-year-old woman complains of increased growth of coarse hair on her lip, chin, chest, and abdomen. She also notes menstrual irregularity with periods of amenorrhea. The most likely cause is

   (A) polycystic ovary disease
   (B) an ovarian tumor
   (C) an adrenal tumor
   (D) Cushing's disease
   (E) familial hirsutism

In the question above, the key word is "most." Although ovarian tumors, adrenal tumors, and Cushing's disease are causes of hirsutism (described in the stem of the question), polycystic ovary disease is a much more common cause. Familial hirsutism is not associated with the menstrual irregularities mentioned. Thus, the most likely cause of the manifestations described can only be "(A) polycystic ovary disease."

STRATEGIES FOR ANSWERING ONE BEST ANSWER–SINGLE ITEM QUESTIONS

1. Remember that only one choice can be the correct answer.
2. Read the question carefully to be sure that you understand what is being asked. Pay attention to key words like "most" or "least."
3. Quickly read each choice for familiarity. (This important step is often not done by test takers.)
4. Go back and consider each choice individually.
5. If a choice is partially correct, tentatively consider it to be incorrect. (This step will help you eliminate choices and increase your odds of choosing the correct answer.)
6. Consider the remaining choices and select the one you think is the answer. At this point, you may want to quickly scan the stem to be sure you understand the question and your answer.
7. Fill in the appropriate circle on the answer sheet.
8. If you do not know the answer, make an educated guess. Your score is based on the number of correct answers, not the number you get incorrect. **Do not leave any blanks.**
9. The actual examination is timed for an average of 50 seconds per question. It is important to be thorough to understand the question, but it is equally important for you to keep moving.

One Best Answer–Matching Sets. This format presents lettered options followed by several items generally related to a common topic. The directions you will generally see for this question type are as follows:

DIRECTIONS (Questions 2 through 4): Each set of matching questions in this section consists of a list of up to twenty-six lettered options followed by several numbered items. For each item, select the ONE lettered option that is most closely associated with it. Each lettered heading may be selected once, more than once, or not at all.

Below is an example of this type of question:

For each adverse drug reaction listed below, select the antibiotic with which it is most closely associated.

   (A) tetracycline
   (B) chloramphenicol
   (C) clindamycin
   (D) cefotaxime
   (E) gentamicin

2. Bone marrow suppression

3. Pseudomembranous enterocolitis

4. Acute fatty necrosis of liver

Note that, unlike the single item questions, the lettered choices in the matching sets PRECEDE the numbered questions. However, as with the single item questions, only one choice can be correct for a given question.

STRATEGIES FOR ANSWERING ONE BEST ANSWER–MATCHING QUESTIONS

1. Remember that the lettered choices are followed by the numbered questions.
2. As with single item questions, only one answer will be correct for each item.
3. Quickly read each choice for familiarity.
4. Read the question carefully to be sure that you understand what is being asked. Pay attention to key words like "most" or "least."
5. Go back and consider each choice individually.
6. If a choice is partially correct for a particular item, tentatively consider it to be incorrect. (This step will help you eliminate choices and increase your odds of choosing the correct answer.)
7. Consider the remaining choices and select the one you think is the answer.
8. Fill in the appropriate circle on the answer sheet.
9. If you do not know the answer, make an educated guess. Your score is based on the number of correct answers, not the number you get incorrect. **Do not leave any blanks.**
10. Again, the actual examination allows an average of 50 seconds per question.

Extended One Best Answer–Matching Questions. The United States Licensing Examination Step 1 utilizes a new type of matching question that is similar to the one above, but can contain up to 26 lettered options followed by several items. The directions you will see for this type of question will generally read the same as the one listed for the one best answer–matching sets since this is a version of the same type. An example of this type of question is:

(A) sarcoidosis

(B) tuberculosis

(C) histoplasmosis

(D) coccidiomycosis

(E) amyloidosis

(F) bacterial pneumonia

(G) mesothelioma

(H) carcinoma

(I) fibrosing alveolitis

(J) silicosis

627. A right lower lobectomy specimen contains a solitary 1.2 cm diameter solid nodule. The center of the nodule is fibrous. The periphery has granulomatous inflammation. With special stains, multiple 2 to 5 μm budding yeasts are evident within the nodule. Acid-fast stains are negative.

628. A left upper lobectomy specimen is received containing a 4.6 cm nodule with central cystic degeneration. Microscopically, the nodule is composed of anaplastic squamous cells. Similar abnormal cells are seen in a concomitant biopsy of a hilar lymph node.

629. After a long history of multiple myeloma, a 67-year-old male is noted to have abundant acellular eosinophilic deposits around the pulmonary microvasculature at autopsy. A congo red special stain demonstrates apple green birefringence.

630. A large, pleural-based lesion is found on chest x-ray of an asbestos worker. Electron microscopy of the biopsy shows abundant long microvilli.

Note that, like other matching sets, the lettered options are listed first.

STRATEGIES FOR ANSWERING EXTENDED ONE BEST ANSWER–MATCHING SET QUESTIONS

1. Read the lettered options through first.
2. Work with one item at a time.
3. Read the item through, then go back to the options and consider each choice individually.
4. As with the other question types, if the choice is partially correct, tentatively consider it to be incorrect.
5. Consider the remaining choices and select the answer.
6. Fill in the appropriate circle on the answer sheet.
7. Remember to make a selection for each item.
8. Again, the test allows for 50 seconds per item.

Answers, Explanations, and References

In each of the sections of this book, the question sections are followed by a section containing the answers, explanations, and references to the questions. This section (1) tells you the answer to each question; (2) gives you an explanation/review of why the answer is correct, background information on the subject matter, and why the other answers are incorrect; and (3) tells you where you can find more in-depth information on the subject matter in other books and/or journals. We encourage you to use this section as a basis for further study and understanding.

If you choose the correct answer to a question, you can then read the explanation (1) for reinforcement and (2) to add to your knowledge about the subject matter (remember that the explanations usually tell not only why the answer is correct, but also why the other choices are incorrect). **If you choose the wrong answer** to a question, you can read the explanation for a learning/reviewing discussion of the material in the question. Furthermore, you can note the reference cited (e.g., "Joklik et al, pp 103-114"), look up the full source in the bibliography at the end of the section (e.g., "Joklik WK, Willett HP, Amos DB. *Zinsser's Microbiology.* 20th ed. Norwalk, Conn: Appleton & Lange; 1992), and refer to the pages cited for a more in-depth discussion.

SPECIFIC INFORMATION ON THE STEP 1 EXAMINATION

The official source of all information with respect to the United States Medical Licensing Examination Step 1 is the National Board of Medical Examiners (NBME), 3930 Chestnut Street, Philadelphia, PA 19104. Established in 1915, the NBME is a voluntary, nonprofit, independent organization whose sole function is the design, implementation, distribution, and processing of a vast bank of question items, certifying examinations, and evaluative services in the professional medical field.

In order to sit for the Step 1 examination, a person must be either an officially enrolled medical student or a graduate of an accredited medical school. It is not necessary to complete any particular year of medical school in order to be a candidate for Step 1. Neither is it required to take Step 1 before Step 2.

In applying for Step 1, you must use forms supplied by NBME. Remember that registration closes *ten weeks* before the scheduled examination date. Some United States and Canadian medical schools require their students to take Step 1 even if they are noncandidates. Such students can register as noncandidates at the request of their school. A person who takes Step 1 as a noncandidate can later change to candidate status and, after payment of a fee, receive certification credit.

Scoring

You will receive two scores after completing Step 1. According to the information booklet provided by the National Board of Medical Examiners, a minimum score of 176 is recommended to pass Step 1, and 167 is recommended to pass Step 2. These two scores (from three digit scale) equate to a score of 75 on the two digit scale. Keep in mind that the passing score for all three steps is determined on your proficiency of the examination content. Although the number of correct items to obtain these passing scores may change, the percentage of correct responses necessary to achieve them will fall between 55 and 65 percent.

Remember, there is no deduction for wrong answers, so even if you are unsure, you should answer every question.

Physical Conditions

The NBME is very concerned that all their exams be administered under uniform conditions in the numerous centers that are used. Except for several No. 2 pencils and an eraser, you are not permitted to bring anything (books, notes, calculators, etc.) into the test room. All examinees receive the same questions at the same session. However, the questions are printed in different sequences in several different booklets, and the booklets are randomly distributed. In addition, examinees are moved to different seats at least once during the test. And, of course, each test is policed by at least one proctor. The object of these maneuvers is to frustrate cheating or even the temptation to cheat.

Appleton & Lange's Review of
ANATOMY FOR
THE USMLE STEP 1

CHAPTER 1

The Thorax
Thoracic Region
Questions

DIRECTIONS (Questions 1 through 98): Each of the numbered items or incomplete statements in this section is followed by answers or by completions of the statement. Select the ONE lettered answer or completion that is BEST in each case.

1. All the following statements concerning the inferior thoracic aperture are correct EXCEPT

   (A) it is closed by the diaphragm
   (B) it is bounded behind by the 12th thoracic vertebra and the 12th ribs
   (C) it is bounded at the sides by the cartilages of ribs 12 to 7
   (D) it is bounded in front by the xiphosternal junction
   (E) it is small and kidney-shaped

2. All the following statements concerning the xiphosternal junction are correct EXCEPT

   (A) it is a landmark in the median line for the upper surface of the liver
   (B) it is a landmark for the diaphragm
   (C) it is a landmark for the lower border of the heart
   (D) it is located at the vertebral level of T9
   (E) it is located at the level of the cartilage of the 5th rib

3. Which of the following statements concerning the first rib is correct?

   (A) it has a costal groove
   (B) it is attached to the sternal angle by its costal cartilage
   (C) its head has two facets for articulation with the first thoracic vertebra
   (D) it contains a tuberosity for the serratus anterior
   (E) it has a scalene tubercle

4. All the following statements concerning the costal cartilages are correct EXCEPT

   (A) the costal cartilages are bars of hyaline cartilage
   (B) the upper eight cartilages join the sternum
   (C) the cartilage of the first rib joins the manubrium
   (D) costal cartilages two to seven join the sternum
   (E) the costal cartilages contribute materially to the elasticity of the wall of the chest

5. Which of the following muscles is located on the inner surface of the sternochondral portion of the chest?

   (A) subcostal
   (B) external intercostal
   (C) internal intercostal
   (D) transversus thoracis
   (E) subclavius

6. The parietal thoracic fascia has continuity through the openings of the diaphragm with which of the following fasciae?

   (A) prevertebral
   (B) transversalis
   (C) scalene
   (D) infrahyoid
   (E) investing

7. The thoracoabdominal intercostal nerves are the ventral rami of which of the following nerves?

   (A) T1–T12
   (B) T7–T11
   (C) T4–T8
   (D) T2–T6
   (E) C5–T2

8. All the following statements concerning intercostal veins are correct EXCEPT

(A) they accompany the intercostal arteries and nerves
(B) there are 12 intercostal veins
(C) they contain valves
(D) they anastomose with anterior intercostal veins
(E) of the intercostal vessels and nerves in the costal groove, they are located highest

9. All the following statements concerning the pericardiacophrenic artery are correct EXCEPT

(A) it gives rise to the musculophrenic artery
(B) it accompanies the phrenic nerve to the diaphragm
(C) it gives branches to the pleura and the pericardium
(D) it supplies the upper surface of the diaphragm
(E) it is a branch of the internal thoracic artery

10. All the following structures are located in the superior mediastinum EXCEPT the

(A) great vessels related to the heart
(B) arch of the aorta
(C) vagus nerve
(D) thoracic duct
(E) arch of the azygos vein

11. All the following structures are located in the posterior mediastinum EXCEPT the

(A) thoracic portion of the descending aorta
(B) azygos vein
(C) hemiazygos vein
(D) bronchi
(E) thoracic splanchnic nerves

12. Which of the following statements concerning the cervical dome of the pleura is correct?

(A) it projects through the superior thoracic aperture
(B) it arises above the neck of the first rib
(C) it projects into the superior mediastinum
(D) it is visceral pleura
(E) it projects into the middle mediastinum

13. The cervical pleura is maintained in position by the

(A) pulmonary ligament
(B) sternopericardial ligament
(C) transversus thoracis muscle
(D) internal intercostal membrane
(E) Sibson's fascia

14. The upper portion of the pericardium is separated from the sternum by the

(A) internal thoracic vessels
(B) phrenic nerves
(C) anterior portions of the pleurae and the lungs
(D) vagus nerves
(E) superior epigastric artery

15. The space between the arterial and venous mesocardia is known as the

(A) oblique sinus of the pericardium
(B) transverse sinus of the pericardium
(C) superior sternopericardial ligament
(D) inferior sternopericardial ligament
(E) coronary sinus

16. The posterior interventricular sulcus lodges the

(A) great cardiac vein
(B) small cardiac vein
(C) coronary sinus
(D) middle cardiac vein
(E) left coronary artery

17. The underside of the arch of the aorta is located at the level of the

(A) suprasternal notch
(B) sternal angle
(C) xiphosternal junction
(D) sternoclavicular joint
(E) fourth intercostal space

18. All the following statements concerning the right pulmonary artery are correct EXCEPT

(A) it passes under the arch of the aorta
(B) it passes behind the ascending aorta
(C) it passes behind the superior vena cava
(D) it passes in front of the right bronchus
(E) it is connected to the underside of the aortic arch

19. Which of the following statements concerning the right vagus nerve is correct?

(A) it enters the chest on the right side posterior to brachiocephalic arterial trunk and the brachiocephalic vein
(B) it crosses the aortic arch
(C) it passes the ligamentum arteriosum
(D) it is a branch of the cervical plexus
(E) it passes to the root of the right lung, where it forms the posterior pulmonary plexus

20. All the following statements concerning the phrenic nerves are correct EXCEPT

   (A) they are branches of the cervical plexus *C3–C5*
   (B) they overlie the anterior scalene muscles at the base of the neck
   (C) they are located beneath the prevertebral fascia
   (D) they enter the chest by passing deep to the subclavian arteries *subcl. is behind middle scalene*
   (E) they cross the origin of the internal thoracic artery

21. The right coronary artery provides which of the following branches?

   (A) anterior interventricular
   (B) posterior interventricular
   (C) circumflex
   (D) marginal branch to the left ventricle
   (E) posterior artery of the left ventricle

22. The tributaries of the coronary sinus include all the following veins EXCEPT the

   (A) great cardiac
   (B) small cardiac
   (C) middle cardiac
   (D) anterior cardiac
   (E) posterior vein of the left ventricle

23. Which of the following structures is located in the anterior interventricular sulcus?

   (A) sinoatrial nodal artery
   (B) atrioventricular nodal artery
   (C) middle cardiac vein
   (D) small cardiac vein
   (E) great cardiac vein

24. All the following statements concerning the right ventricle are correct EXCEPT

   (A) it is longer and more conical in shape than the left
   (B) it is triangular in the frontal plane
   (C) the muscular wall of the right ventricle is only one-third as thick as that of the left ventricle
   (D) it contains a supraventricular crest
   (E) it contains a septomarginal trabecula

25. The fibrous skeleton of the heart serves all the following functions EXCEPT

   (A) it provides attachment for the myocardium
   (B) it provides attachment for the cusps of the aortic semilunar valve

   (C) it provides circular form and rigidity to the atrioventricular apertures
   (D) it serves as an electrical insulator between the atria and ventricles
   (E) it joins the septum membranaceum with the anterior papillary muscle

26. The lunula is located on the

   (A) cephalic end of the crista terminalis
   (B) septomarginal trabecula
   (C) free margin of the semilunar valves
   (D) septal papillary muscle
   (E) distal end of the chordae tendineae

27. The atrioventricular node is located in which of the following areas?

   (A) at the right atrial septal wall immediately above the openings of the coronary sinus
   (B) at the cephalic end of the sulcus terminalis
   (C) in the right fibrous trigone
   (D) in the septum membranaceum
   (E) in the septomarginal trabeculae

28. Which of the following nerves contribute primarily to the superficial cardiac plexus?

   (A) inferior cervical cardiac branch of the left vagus and superior cervical cardiac branch of the left sympathetic trunk
   (B) greater splanchnic
   (C) phrenic
   (D) upper thoracic (T1–T4) intercostal nerves
   (E) lower thoracic (T6–T11) intercostal nerves

29. The trachea is separated from the bodies of the upper four thoracic vertebrae by the

   (A) aorta
   (B) esophagus
   (C) azygos vein
   (D) thoracic duct
   (E) heart

30. The trachea divides into the right and left bronchi at the level of which of the following structures?

   (A) jugular notch
   (B) sternal angle
   (C) xiphosternal junction
   (D) sternoclavicular joint
   (E) head of the 1st rib

31. The esophagus passes onto the front of the aorta at the level of the

 (A) sternal angle
 (B) jugular notch
 (C) 8th thoracic vertebra
 (D) 6th cervical vertebra
 (E) 2nd lumbar vertebra

32. All the following arteries are branches of the thoracic aorta EXCEPT the

 (A) pericardiacophrenic
 (B) bronchial
 (C) superior phrenic
 (D) mediastinal
 (E) posterior intercostal

33. The azygos vein arches anteriorly over the root of the right lung to end in the superior vena cava at the level of the

 (A) xiphosternal junction
 (B) 12th thoracic vertebra
 (C) 4th thoracic vertebra
 (D) sternal angle
 (E) 2nd cervical vertebra

34. The hemiazygos vein ascends on the left side of the vertebral bodies behind the thoracic aorta as far as which of the following vertebral levels?

 (A) 5th thoracic
 (B) 2nd thoracic
 (C) 2nd lumbar
 (D) 9th thoracic
 (E) 1st thoracic

35. The thoracic duct passes through which of the following structures?

 (A) right crus of the diaphragm
 (B) vertebrocostal trigone
 (C) esophageal hiatus   + vagus
 (D) aortic hiatus
 (E) caval foramen

36. All the following statements concerning the greater thoracic splanchnic nerves are correct EXCEPT

 (A) they are direct visceral branches to thoracic organs from the upper 4 or 5 thoracic ganglia
 (B) they arise from the 5th to the 9th (or 10th) thoracic ganglia
 (C) they perforate the crus of the diaphragm

 (D) they end in the abdomen in the lateral aspect of the celiac ganglion
 (E) they are preganglionic fibers

37. The mediastinum contains all the following structures EXCEPT the

 (A) heart
 (B) lungs
 (C) pulmonary arteries
 (D) trachea
 (E) esophagus

38. Anatomically, components of the thoracic wall proper include the

 (A) pectoral muscles
 (B) serratus anterior
 (C) trapezius
 (D) intercostal muscles
 (E) latissimus dorsi

39. The superior thoracic aperture can be described correctly by which of these statements?

 (A) it is large and irregular
 (B) it is bounded by the 3rd thoracic vertebra
 (C) its plane slopes downward and forward
 (D) it includes the costal arch   1st rib
 (E) it involves costal cartilages of the 10th rib

40. The sternal angle is found at which of these locations?

 (A) jugular notch
 (B) xiphoid process
 (C) level with the 4th costal cartilage   Thoraco vertebral
 (D) level with the lower border of the 6th thoracic vertebra
 (E) manubriosternal joint

41. Ossification of the parts of the body of the sternum usually is complete by age (in years)

 (A) 1
 (B) 3
 (C) 6
 (D) 15
 (E) 21

42. Which of the following defines true ribs?

 (A) upper 7 pairs
 (B) all 12 pairs
 (C) lower 5 pairs
 (D) 10th and 11th pairs
 (E) 12th pair

43. The vertical length of the rib cage is increased by which of the following?

    (A) movement of ribs at the costovertebral joints
    (B) movement of the diaphragm
    (C) movement of ribs at the costotransverse joint
    (D) pump-handle movement of ribs
    (E) bucket-handle movement of ribs

44. Which of these statements correctly describes intercostal muscles?

    (A) external intercostals begin anteriorly
    (B) external intercostal membrane is posterior
    (C) fibers of external intercostals slant upward and backward
    (D) fibers of internal intercostals run upward and forward
    (E) innermost intercostals are the best developed of the intercostals

45. Innervation of the thoracic wall can be described correctly by all the following statements EXCEPT

    (A) it receives a nerve supply from spinal nerves T1–T12
    (B) it receives no nerve supply from cervical nerves
    (C) cutaneous innervation of skin over paravertebral regions of the thorax is provided by dorsal rami of spinal nerves
    (D) ventral rami of T1–T11 are called intercostal nerves
    (E) the ventral ramus of T12 is the subcostal nerve

46. Which of these statements is correct in relation to intercostal nerves?

    (A) in the intercostal space, they run between the internal and external intercostal muscles
    (B) they are located in the costal groove above the artery and vein
    (C) they are all confined to the thorax
    (D) they are entirely cutaneous to the thoracic wall
    (E) the upper six nerves terminate as anterior cutaneous branches

47. Which of the following statements is correct regarding the blood vessels of the thoracic wall?

    (A) in the intercostal space, the vessels run just below the respective intercostal nerve
    (B) branches of the vessels vary widely from those of the intercostal nerves
    (C) superficial structures of the thorax are served by intercostal vessels

    (D) posterior intercostal arteries are branches of the internal thoracic artery
    (E) branches of the descending thoracic aorta become anterior intercostal arteries

48. All the following are correct statements concerning the internal thoracic artery EXCEPT

    (A) it is a branch of the arch of the aorta
    (B) it descends behind the subclavian vein
    (C) it divides into two terminal branches
    (D) it gives branches to the mediastinum
    (E) the musculophrenic artery is one of its terminal branches

49. Two-thirds of the increase in thoracic capacity in respiratory movements is the result of

    (A) pump-handle movement of ribs
    (B) bucket-handle movement of ribs
    (C) diaphragmatic movement
    (D) accessory respiratory muscle contraction
    (E) elastic recoil of lungs and rib cage

50. All the following statements concerning the lungs are correct EXCEPT

    (A) squamous epithelium forms alveoli
    (B) alveoli account for the greatest volume of the lung
    (C) alveoli lose all their air during expiration
    (D) lungs filled with air sound hollow to percussion
    (E) bronchial circulation supplies connective tissue of the lung

51. Which of the following statements is correct in relation to internal anatomy of the lung?

    (A) bronchopulmonary segments are the anatomic units
    (B) arteries and veins provide the major lung framework
    (C) bronchi branch symmetrically
    (D) bronchi are hollow tubes without particular wall support
    (E) pulmonary vessels show no particular relationship to bronchial branching

52. Which of these items is true regarding external anatomy of the lung?

    (A) the upper tapered end of the lung is its base
    (B) the root of the lung is located at its base
    (C) visceral pleura covers all lung surfaces
    (D) lobes are comparable to bronchopulmonary segments
    (E) each lung has three lobes

53. Which of these statements is correct regarding pulmonary circulation of the lung?

    (A) it is the main blood supply to the bronchi
    (B) it is the main blood supply to the connective tissue of the lung
    (C) the pulmonary trunk goes directly to the left lung
    (D) pulmonary veins enter the right atrium of the heart
    (E) the pulmonary trunk arises from the right ventricle

54. The ligamentum arteriosum is located between the

    (A) left pulmonary artery and the aortic arch
    (B) pulmonary trunk and the right pulmonary artery
    (C) left pulmonary vein and the aorta
    (D) right pulmonary vein and the pulmonary trunk
    (E) left bronchial artery and the aortic arch

55. All the following statements are correct concerning pulmonary veins EXCEPT

    (A) two veins pass from the hilum of each lung
    (B) usually they enter the right atrium of the heart
    (C) they show more variation than do the pulmonary arteries
    (D) they are formed by confluence of capillaries in the lung
    (E) their primary tributaries are related to particular bronchopulmonary segments

56. The bronchial arteries may arise from all the following EXCEPT the

    (A) descending aorta
    (B) right intercostal artery
    (C) arch of the aorta
    (D) subclavian artery
    (E) internal thoracic artery

57. All the following statements concerning the pericardial sac are correct EXCEPT

    (A) the outer layer is fibrous
    (B) epicardium completely invests the heart
    (C) the pericardial sac and its content comprise the middle mediastinum
    (D) the fibrous pericardium lubricates the moving surfaces of the heart
    (E) the pericardial sac is fused to the central tendon of the diaphragm

58. Which of these statements correctly describes the heart?

    (A) all the great veins enter its apex
    (B) its base is made largely of the left atrium and a portion of the right atrium
    (C) the apex points forward and toward the right
    (D) the diaphragmatic surface is formed largely by the right ventricle and atrium
    (E) the coronary sinus occupies the posterior interventricular sulcus

59. The right atrium includes all these structures EXCEPT the

    (A) tricuspid valve
    (B) crista terminalis
    (C) musculi pectinati
    (D) fossa ovalis
    (E) trabeculae carneae

60. Which of these statements correctly describes the azygos venous system?

    (A) primarily, it drains blood from the body wall
    (B) normally, it drains into the inferior vena cava
    (C) it is located entirely on the right side of the vertebral column
    (D) it receives no blood from thoracic viscera
    (E) it has a number of valves

61. All these items correctly describe the thoracic duct EXCEPT

    (A) it returns lymph from the greater part of the body to the venous system
    (B) it is the upward continuation of the cisterna chyli
    (C) it ends at the confluence of the right subclavian and brachiocephalic veins
    (D) in most of its course, it lies behind the esophagus
    (E) it contains valves

62. Characteristics of thoracic vertebrae include all the following EXCEPT

    (A) long vertical spinous processes of T5, T6, T7, and T8
    (B) a transverse foramen in each vertebra
    (C) a small circular vertebral foramen
    (D) progressively shorter transverse processes from T10–T12
    (E) thoracic articular processes set on an arc to permit rotation

63. Correct description of structure of the sternum includes which of the following statements?

   (A) the jugular notch is located at the lower border of the manubrium
   (B) the upper border of the body is located at the level of the costal cartilage of the 2nd rib
   (C) the sternal angle is located at the articulation of the body and the xiphoid process
   (D) the body consists of five fused sternebrae
   (E) the xiphoid process consists of bone thicker than that of the body

64. Ribs may be described correctly by all the following EXCEPT

   (A) every rib articulates with the vertebral column
   (B) the upper 7 pairs of ribs are called vertebrosternal
   (C) ribs 8, 9, and 10 are called vertebrochondral ribs
   (D) floating ribs are the last 2 pairs
   (E) ribs 1 through 12 are called true ribs

65. All the following statements concerning ribs are correct EXCEPT

   (A) the typical rib takes an upward slope
   (B) the sternal end of each arch lies at a lower level than the vertebral end
   (C) ribs and cartilages increase in length progressively from 1st to 7th rib
   (D) the transverse diameter of the thorax increases progressively from 1st to 8th rib
   (E) the 9th is the most obliquely placed rib

66. All the following statements concerning intercostal arteries are correct EXCEPT

   (A) the upper 2 posterior intercostal arteries arise from the supreme intercostal artery
   (B) the lower 9 posterior intercostal arteries arise from the aorta
   (C) the superior epigastric artery supplies anterior intercostal arteries
   (D) intercostal arteries run under the shelter of a costal groove
   (E) intercostal arteries accompany each intercostal nerve

67. Which of the following structures is NOT located in the mediastinum?

   (A) heart and pericardium
   (B) trachea
   (C) vessels proceeding to and from the heart
   (D) lungs
   (E) vagus nerves

68. All the following are parts of the parietal pleura EXCEPT

   (A) costal
   (B) mediastinal
   (C) diaphragmatic
   (D) pulmonary
   (E) cervical

69. If the root of the left lung was completely severed, which of these structures would be spared?

   (A) pulmonary ligament
   (B) pulmonary veins
   (C) vagus nerve
   (D) pulmonary artery
   (E) bronchus

70. Each segmental bronchus together with the portion of lung it supplies is called

   (A) primary segment
   (B) bronchopulmonary segment
   (C) lobar segment
   (D) epiarterial segment
   (E) alveolar segment

71. Correct information about bronchial arteries includes all the following statements EXCEPT

   (A) they arise by a stem from the aorta
   (B) they supply the pulmonary pleura
   (C) they supply the bronchi
   (D) the pressure within them is low
   (E) they run through the interlobar structures

72. The tracheal bifurcation can be seen at which of these levels?

   (A) T4–T5 in the supine living subject
   (B) T8 in the erect subject
   (C) T6 during inspiration
   (D) T12 during expiration
   (E) T2–T3 in the supine cadaver

73. The brachiocephalic veins are formed from the union of the
    (A) external jugular and inferior vena cava
    (B) ductus arteriosum and superior vena cava
    (C) azygos vein and axillary vein
    (D) internal jugular and subclavian
    (E) pulmonary vein and inferior vena cava

74. All the following structures empty into the right atrium of the heart EXCEPT the
    (A) coronary sinus
    (B) inferior vena cava
    (C) superior vena cava
    (D) anterior cardiac veins
    (E) pulmonary veins

75. Which of the following statements is an exception to the typical arrangement of costovertebral joints?
    (A) costovertebral articulations consist of synovial joints
    (B) the head of the rib articulates with its own vertebral body
    (C) an articular capsule surrounds each joint
    (D) the tubercle of a rib articulates with the tip of a transverse process
    (E) the head of the rib articulates with an intervertebral disk

76. In an adult, all of the following structures are prominent in the anterior mediastinum EXCEPT
    (A) loose areolar tissue
    (B) lymph vessels and nodes
    (C) fat
    (D) thymus gland
    (E) sternopericardial ligaments

77. Which of these statements correctly describes the position of the esophagus?
    (A) it passes anterior to the left principal bronchus
    (B) it begins at the level of the cricoid cartilage
    (C) it descends on the left of the aortic arch
    (D) it runs in the anterior mediastinum
    (E) it passes through the hiatus formed by the median arcuate ligament of the diaphragm

78. Which of the following statements is true of the trachea?
    (A) it descends behind the esophagus
    (B) its posterior surface is convex
    (C) it ends at the level of the sternal angle

    (D) during inspiration, its bifurcation ascends
    (E) it contains O-shaped bars of cartilage

79. The superior vena cava returns blood from all of these structures EXCEPT the
    (A) head
    (B) neck
    (C) upper limb
    (D) lungs
    (E) thoracic wall

80. All the following statements correctly describe the brachiocephalic veins EXCEPT
    (A) each is formed by the union of the internal jugular and the subclavian veins
    (B) they contain valves to prevent backflow of blood
    (C) they unite to form the superior vena cava
    (D) each vein receives the internal thoracic vein
    (E) they arise posterior to the medial ends of the clavicle

81. All these structures occupy the superior mediastinum EXCEPT the
    (A) heart and pericardium
    (B) thymus
    (C) aortic arch
    (D) trachea
    (E) esophagus

82. Which of the following statements is correct regarding the coronary arteries?
    (A) sharp lines of demarcation exist between their distribution to right and left ventricles
    (B) most of the blood in these arteries returns to the left atrium
    (C) they arise from the right and left aortic sinuses
    (D) variations of these arteries are uncommon
    (E) they are infrequent sites of arteriosclerosis

83. Initiation of the impulse for contraction of the heart is accomplished by the
    (A) atrioventricular node (AV node)
    (B) atrioventricular bundle (AV bundle)
    (C) sinoatrial node (SA node)
    (D) sympathetics
    (E) bundle of His

84. All the following statements concerning the left ventricle are correct EXCEPT

(A) its wall is much thicker than that of the right ventricle
(B) its interior is covered by trabeculae carneae
(C) the chordae tendineae of papillary muscles are distributed to cusps of the atrioventricular valve
(D) it forms the base of the heart
(E) the aorta arises from its anterior uppermost part

85. Characteristics of the left atrium consist of all the following EXCEPT

(A) it forms most of the base of the heart
(B) it contains a few musculi pectinati
(C) it receives the pulmonary arteries
(D) much of this atrium lies posterior to the right atrium
(E) the auricle overlaps the root of the pulmonary trunk

86. Which of the following is characteristic of the right ventricle?

(A) it gives origin to the pulmonary trunk
(B) usually it has only two papillary muscles
(C) it receives blood through the mitral valve
(D) it has internal muscular ridges, the musculi pectinati
(E) it contains the fossa ovalis

87. Which of the following statements correctly describes chambers of the heart?

(A) the coronary sulcus separates the two ventricles
(B) the right ventricle forms the right border of the heart
(C) the valve of the superior vena cava directs blood downward
(D) the superior vena cava opens into the right atrium
(E) the interventricular septum contains the fossa ovalis

88. The heart may correctly be described by all the following EXCEPT

(A) an apex formed by the tip of the left ventricle
(B) a diaphragmatic surface formed by both ventricles
(C) a base formed by the atria

(D) a location in the middle mediastinum
(E) an anterior surface formed mainly by the left atrium

89. The epicardium receives its arterial blood supply from which of the following arteries?

(A) pericardiophrenic
(B) coronary arteries
(C) musculophrenic
(D) superior phrenic
(E) bronchial

90. Which of these statements is true of the fibrous pericardium?

(A) it has no close relationship with the central tendon of the diaphragm
(B) it extends upward to the level of the sternal angle
(C) it moves freely within the thoracic cavity
(D) its base is pierced by the aorta
(E) it has no attachment to the sternum

91. Which of the following structures is not located in the mediastinum?

(A) heart
(B) thymus
(C) vertebral bodies
(D) great vessels
(E) vagus nerve

92. Which of these statements correctly describes lymphatic drainage of the lungs?

(A) usually both bronchomediastinal lymph trunks terminate in the thoracic duct
(B) only one lymphatic plexus is involved in this drainage
(C) little transfer of lymph drainage from side to side occurs
(D) no lymph vessels are located in the walls of the pulmonary alveoli
(E) rarely is this lymph drainage responsible for transfer of cancer cells to other organs

93. In what way does the root of the right lung differ from that of the left lung?

(A) in numbers of pulmonary arteries
(B) in numbers of pulmonary veins
(C) in numbers of primary bronchi
(D) in the presence of a pulmonary plexus of nerves
(E) in numbers of bronchial veins

94. Characteristics of the left lung include

  (A) it is heavier than the right lung
  (B) it is composed of three lobes
  (C) the azygos vein arches over its root
  (D) it has a horizontal fissure
  (E) the cardiac notch is found on its superior lobe

95. The central part of the parietal diaphragmatic pleura is supplied by which of these nerves?

  (A) intercostals
  (B) vagus
  (C) phrenic
  (D) sympathetics
  (E) parasympathetics

96. Which of the following items correctly describes the visceral pleura?

  (A) it receives its arterial supply from pulmonary arteries
  (B) its lymphatic vessels drain directly into the thoracic duct
  (C) its nerves accompany the pulmonary veins
  (D) it receives its nerve supply from autonomic nerves to the lung
  (E) it is intensely sensitive to pain (Somatic)

97. Which of the following statements correctly describes the pleural cavities?

  (A) they contain much lubricating fluid
  (B) each pleural cavity is a closed potential space
  (C) visceral and parietal pleura never become continuous
  (D) costal pleura covers the apex of the lung
  (E) at no point does the pleura extend below the costal margin

98. All of these statements describe dermatomes correctly EXCEPT

  (A) there is practically no overlapping of contiguous dermatomes
  (B) dermatomes are areas of skin supplied by the sensory root of a spinal nerve
  (C) areas of touch are more extensive than those for temperature
  (D) T10 nerve supplies the area of the umbilicus
  (E) the lower six intercostal nerves supply both thoracic and abdominal walls

DIRECTIONS (Questions 99 through 117): Each group of items in this section consists of lettered headings followed by a set of numbered words or phrases. For each numbered word or phrase, select the ONE lettered heading that is most closely associated with it. Each lettered heading may be selected once, more than once, or not at all.

Questions 99 through 102

  (A) cervical vertebrae
  (B) thoracic vertebrae
  (C) coccyx
  (D) sacrum
  (E) lumbar vertebrae

99. Costal facets

100. Wedge-shaped structure

101. Foramen transversarium

102. Large, kidney-shaped bodies

Questions 103 through 106

  (A) head of the rib
  (B) neck of the rib
  (C) body of the rib
  (D) tubercle of the rib
  (E) scalene tubercle

103. Costal groove

104. Two articular facets

105. Located between head and tubercle

106. Angle

Questions 107 through 110

  (A) sternum
  (B) costal margin
  (C) vertebral articulation with rib
  (D) jugular notch
  (E) cervical rib

107. Synovial joint

108. Upper 7 costal cartilages

109. Neurovascular symptoms

110. 7th through 10th costal cartilages

Questions 111 through 114

    (A) increase in vertical diameter of the thorax
    (B) increase in transverse diameter of the thorax
    (C) increase in anteroposterior diameter of the thorax
    (D) increase in pulmonary compression
    (E) expiration

111. Elastic recoil

112. Diaphragm

113. Pump-handle movement

114. Bucket-handle movement

Questions 115 through 118

    (A) fixes the arm in respiration
    (B) inspiratory muscles
    (C) keeps intercostal spaces rigid
    (D) depresses ribs
    (E) stabilizes scapula

115. Intercostal muscles

116. Pectoralis minor

117. Serratus posterior muscles

118. Subcostal muscles

ANSWERS AND EXPLANATIONS

1. (E) The inferior thoracic aperture (thoracic outlet) is large and irregular in outline. It is bounded by the 12th thoracic vertebra and the 12th ribs behind it, the cartilages of ribs 12 to 7 at the sides, and the xiphosternal junction in front. The aperture is closed by the diaphragm. The superior thoracic aperture (thoracic inlet) is small and kidney-shaped. *(Woodburne, p 347)*

2. (E) The xiphosternal junction marks the lower limit of the thoracic cavity in front. It is a landmark in the median line for the upper surface of the liver, the diaphragm, and the lower border of the heart. The xiphoid process usually bears a demifacet for the articulation of the 7th costal cartilage. The xiphosternal junction is located at the level of the 9th thoracic vertebra. *(Woodburne, pp 100, 349)*

3. (E) The 1st rib has a single facet for articulation with the 1st thoracic vertebra. The subclavian grooves are separated at the inner border of the rib by the scalene tubercle for the insertion of the anterior scalene muscle. The 2nd rib is marked by a marked tuberosity for the second digitation of the serratus anterior muscle. *(Woodburne, p 350)*

4. (B) The costal cartilages are bars of hyaline cartilage which prolong the ribs anteriorly and contribute materially to the elasticity of the walls of the chest. The upper 7 cartilages join the sternum. The cartilage of the 1st rib joins the manubrium. Costal cartilages 2 to 7 join the body of the sternum. *(Woodburne, p 351)*

5. (D) The transversus thoracis muscle lies on the inner surface of the sternochondral portion of the chest. It arises from the lower half of the body of the sternum and the xiphoid process. Directed upward and lateralward, its fibers insert into the 2nd to the 6th costal cartilage. *(Woodburne, p 354)*

6. (B) The thoracic wall is covered internally by a parietal thoracic (endothoracic) fascia. It is continuous with the prevertebral layer of cervical fascia and with the scalene fascia along the inner border of the 1st rib and, behind the sternum, with the fascia of the infrahyoid muscles. Inferiorly, the parietal thoracic fascia has continuity through the openings of the diaphragm with the parietal abdominopelvic (transversalis) fascia. *(Woodburne, p 354)*

7. (B) The thoracoabdominal intercostal nerves are the ventral rami of the thoracic spinal nerves 7 to 11 inclusive. At the anterior ends of the intercostal spaces, these nerves pass behind the costal cartilages and proceed forward into the abdominal wall between the transversus abdominis and internal abdominal oblique muscles. *(Woodburne, p 356)*

8. (B) The intercostal veins accompany the intercostal arteries and nerves, lying highest in the costal groove. There are 11 posterior intercostal veins and one subcostal vein on each side. They contain valves which direct the flow of blood posteriorly, and they anastomose with anterior intercostal veins which are tributary to the internal thoracic vein. *(Woodburne, p 357)*

9. (A) The pericardiacophrenic artery accompanies the phrenic nerve to the diaphragm. It gives branches to the pleura and the pericardium and supplies the upper surface of the diaphragm. The branches of the internal thoracic artery are the pericardiacophrenic, the anterior mediastinal, the pericardial, the sternal, the anterior intercostal, the anterior perforating, the musculophrenic, and the superior epigastric. *(Woodburne, p 358)*

10. (E) The superior mediastinum contains the great vessels related to the heart and pericardium—the arch of the aorta, the beginnings of the brachiocephalic trunk, the left common carotid and sub-clavian arteries, the brachiocephalic veins, and the upper portion of the superior vena cava. The thymus, thoracic parts of the trachea, and the esophagus are also included with the superior mediastinum. The vagus and phrenic nerves, the left recurrent laryngeal nerve, and the thoracic duct are also included. The arch of the azygos is located in the middle mediastinum. *(Woodburne, p 360)*

11. **(D)**   The posterior mediastinum contains the thoracic portion of the descending aorta, the azygos and hemiazygos veins, the esophagus, the vagus and thoracic splanchnic nerves, the thoracic duct, and the posterior mediastinal lymph nodes. The bronchi are located in the middle mediastinum. *(Woodburne, pp 360–361)*

12. **(A)**   The cervical dome of the pleura (cupula) projects slightly through the superior aperture but does not rise above the level of the neck of the first rib. The lungs and their covering membranes, the pleurae, occupy the lateral portions of the thoracic cavity. All other structures contained in the chest are crowded into a thick partition of tissue at and on either side of the median plane known as the mediastinum. The cervical dome of the pleura is parietal pleura, not visceral pleura. *(Woodburne, pp 360–362)*

13. **(E)**   The cervical pleura is maintained in position by a dome-like fascial expansion known as Sibson's fascia. This is an offshoot of the prevertebral layer of cervical fascia on the deep side of the scalene muscles, which is attached in front to the inner border of the first rib. *(Woodburne, p 362)*

14. **(C)**   The upper portion of the pericardium is separated from the sternum by the anterior portions of the pleurae and the lungs. Below, it is in direct relation with the left half of the lower portion of the body of the sternum and with the medial ends of the sixth and seventh costal cartilages and the left transversus thoracis muscle. *(Woodburne, p 365)*

15. **(B)**   The space between the arterial and venous mesocardia is the transverse sinus of the pericardium. It is situated deep to the great arterial channels and superior to the pulmonary veins. The oblique sinus of the pericardium is a box-like diverticulum of the pericardial cavity within the irregularities of the venous mesocardium between the right and left pulmonary veins. *(Woodburne, p 365)*

16. **(D)**   The posterior interventricular sulcus lodges the posterior interventricular branch of the right coronary artery and the middle cardiac vein. *(Woodburne, p 369)*

17. **(B)**   The aortic arch is the continuation of the ascending aorta and emerges from the pericardium behind the right half of the sternum at the level of the sternal angle. The arch terminates at the level of the disk between the 4th and 5th thoracic vertebrae by becoming continuous with the thoracic aorta. The underside of the arch is at the level of the sternal angle. *(Woodburne, p 370)*

18. **(E)**   The right pulmonary artery runs horizontally to the right under the arch of the aorta, behind the ascending aorta and the superior vena cava, and in front of the right bronchus. The left pulmonary artery is connected to the underside of the aortic arch by the ligamentum arteriosum. *(Woodburne, p 374)*

19. **(E)**   The right vagus nerve enters the chest on the right side between the brachiocephalic arterial trunk and the brachiocephalic vein. It passes dorsalward to the root of the right lung, where it forms the posterior pulmonary plexus. The left vagus crosses the aortic arch and passes the ligamentum arteriosum. *(Woodburne, p 374)*

20. **(D)**   The phrenic nerves are branches of the cervical plexus. At the base of the neck, the phrenic nerves overlie the anterior scalene muscles under the prevertebral layer of cervical fascia. They enter the chest by passing superficial to the subclavian arteries and deep to the subclavian veins, crossing the origin of the internal thoracic artery and joined by the pericardiacophrenic artery and vein. The nerves descend in front of the roots of the lungs between the parietal layers of the pericardium and the pleurae. *(Woodburne, p 374)*

21. **(B)**   The right coronary artery arises from the right aortic sinus and, passing forward, reaches the coronary sulcus between the pulmonary trunk and the right auricle. The terminal part of the right coronary is known as the posterior interventricular branch. It supplies both ventricles and anastomoses, near the apex, with the anterior interventricular branch of the left coronary artery. *(Woodburne, p 376)*

22. **(D)**   The tributaries of the coronary sinus are the great, middle, and small cardiac veins; the posterior vein of the left ventricle; and the oblique vein of the left atrium. The anterior cardiac veins and the smallest cardiac veins do not empty into the coronary sinus but empty directly into the right atrium. *(Woodburne, pp 377–378)*

23. **(E)**   The great cardiac vein begins at the apex of the heart and ascends in the anterior interventricular sulcus. The sinoatrial artery usually arises from the right coronary artery and circles the base of the superior vena cava, anteriorly or posteriorly,

to end in the sinoatrial node at the cephalic end of the sulcus terminalis. The atrioventricular nodal artery arises from the right coronary artery and penetrates the atrioventricular node at the base of the interatrial septum. The middle cardiac vein is located in the posterior interventricular sulcus and the small cardiac vein in the coronary sulcus. *(Woodburne, pp 376–378)*

24. **(A)** The right ventricle is triangular in the frontal plane. The muscular wall of the right ventricle is only one-third as thick as that of the left ventricle. A muscular ridge, the supraventricular crest, arches toward and over the anterior cusp of the tricuspid valve and separates the muscular ventricle from the pulmonary conus. The septomarginal trabecula extends from the septum to the anterior papillary muscle. The left ventricle is longer and more conical in shape than the right, and its walls are three times as thick. *(Woodburne, p 381)*

25. **(E)** The fibrous connective tissue of the heart which serves as the "skeleton" provides circular form and rigidity to the atrioventricular apertures and to the roots of the aorta and pulmonary trunk. Besides providing attachment for the myocardium and valves, the fibrous skeleton serves as an electrical insulator between atria and ventricles. *(Woodburne, p 383)*

26. **(C)** The convex margins of the semilunar valves are attached to the wall of the artery, and their free borders are directed upward into the lumen of the vessel. The free margin of each valve exhibits a centrally placed nodule of dense connective tissue and, on either side of it, a crescentic thinned-out area, the lunula. *(Woodburne, p 384)*

27. **(A)** The atrioventricular node is a nodule of specialized myocardium that is situated in the septal wall of the right atrium immediately above the opening of the coronary sinus. The atrioventricular bundle is a stand of specialized myocardium which passes through the right fibrous trigone into the musculature of the ventricular septum. It courses along the lower margin of the septum membranaceum. The SA node is located at the cephalic end of the sulcus terminalis. *(Woodburne, pp 386–387)*

28. **(A)** The superficial cardiac plexus lies in the concavity of the aortic arch to the right of the ligamentum arteriosum. The plexus receives the inferior cervical cardiac branch of the left vagus nerve and the superior cervical cardiac branch of the left sympathetic trunk. *(Woodburne, pp 387–388)*

29. **(B)** The thoracic part of the trachea lies posteriorly in the superior mediastinum, where it is separated from the bodies of the upper 4 thoracic vertebrae by the esophagus. In quiet respiration, the trachea ends at the level of the sternal angle slightly to the right of the median line, being diverted to that side by the arch of the aorta. *(Woodburne, p 389)*

30. **(B)** The trachea averages 1.7 cm in diameter. It ends at the level of the sternal angle by dividing into the right and left bronchi. *(Woodburne, p 389)*

31. **(C)** Passing behind and to the right of the arch of the aorta, the esophagus descends into the posterior mediastinum along the right side of the thoracic aorta. As the esophagus continues toward the left and as the thoracic aorta attains more nearly the median line over the vertebral bodies, the esophagus passes onto the front of the aorta at about the 8th thoracic vertebral level. *(Woodburne, p 399)*

32. **(A)** The pericardiacophrenic artery is a branch of the internal thoracic artery. The branches of the thoracic aorta, all small, include the pericardial, bronchial, esophageal, mediastinal, posterior intercostal, subcostal, and the superior phrenic. *(Woodburne, pp 358,400)*

33. **(C)** At the level of the 4th thoracic vertebra, the azygos vein arches anteriorly over the root of the right lung to end in the superior vena cava just before that vessel pierces the pericardium. *(Woodburne, p 401)*

34. **(D)** The hemiazygos vein ascends on the left side of the vertebral bodies behind the thoracic aorta as far as the 9th thoracic vertebra. At this level, the hemiazygos vein passes to the right across the vertebral column behind the aorta, the esophagus, and the thoracic duct, and ends in the azygos vein. *(Woodburne, p 402)*

35. **(D)** The thoracic duct passes through the aortic hiatus of the diaphragm, lying between the aorta and the azygos vein, and ascends in this relationship through the posterior mediastinum. *(Woodburne, p 402)*

36. **(A)** Direct visceral branches to thoracic organs arise from the trunk and ganglia of the upper 4 or 5 thoracic segments. The greater thoracic splanchnic nerves arise from the 5th to the 9th (or 10th) thoracic ganglia. They perforate the crus of the diaphragm and end in the abdomen in the lateral aspect of the celiac ganglion. They are preganglionic fibers which pass through the diaphragm, synapse in collateral ganglia in the abdomen, and provide the sympathetic innervation for most of the abdominal visceral. *(Woodburne, p 402)*

37. **(B)** The mediastinum is a broad median septum that partitions the thoracic cavity and separates the two hollow spaces filled by the right and left lungs. The bulk of the mediastinum is made up of the heart, enclosed in the pericardial sac, and of the major pulmonary and systemic arteries and veins. The trachea and esophagus enter the mediastinum from the neck through the superior thoracic aperture. *(Hollinshead, p 465)*

38. **(D)** The walls of the thoracic cavity are made up of layers of muscle and fascia supported by the thoracic skeleton. The thoracic cage supports the bones and muscles of the pectoral girdle. Much of the thoracic skeleton is covered by muscles that belong to the upper limb or vertebral column (eg, pectoral muscles, serratus anterior, trapezius, and latissimus dorsi). These muscles, supplied by nerves other than those serving the true body wall, anatomically are not considered as components of the thoracic wall. Intercostal muscles are layers of the thoracic wall proper. *(Hollinshead, pp 466–467)*

39. **(C)** The superior thoracic aperture slopes downward and forward. This aperture is small, and its boundaries are the first thoracic vertebra, the first pair of ribs with their cartilages, and the superior margin of the manubrium of the sternum. The costal arch, made up of costal cartilages 7 through 10, forms part of the inferior thoracic aperture, not the superior aperture. *(Hollinshead, p 468)*

40. **(E)** The joint between the manubrium and body of the sternum is palpable as the sternal angle; this is a smooth ridge produced by the angulation of the bones and their slightly everted articular edges. The sternal angle lies at the level of the 2nd costal cartilage and the lower border of the 4th thoracic vertebra. This angle serves as a reference point for counting the ribs, as it identifies the 2nd rib. *(Hollinshead, pp 469,472)*

41. **(E)** The sternum ossifies from a number of centers that form independently of the ribs. Usually there is a single center for the manubrium and a single one for the uppermost part of the body. Each of the remaining three segments that contribute to the body may have a single or paired center of ossification. Fusion of the parts of the body begins below and extends upward, being completed at the 21st year. *(Hollinshead, p 469)*

42. **(A)** There are 12 pairs of ribs, of which the upper 7 are called true ribs because they form complete arches between the vertebrae and the sternum. The lower 5 ribs, which fail to reach the sternum, are regarded as false ribs. Ten of the 12 pairs of ribs form arches between respective vertebrae and the sternum, whereas the last 2 pairs of ribs float freely anteriorly (floating ribs). *(Hollinshead, pp 467–469,471)*

43. **(B)** Vertical increase in the diameter of the thoracic cavity is the result of movement of the diaphragm. The anteroposterior and lateral increase depends on movement of the ribs. All of the choices listed, except B, relate to thoracic cage increased measurement caused by movement of the ribs. *(Hollinshead, pp 472–474)*

44. **(D)** The fibers of internal intercostal muscles run upward and forward from one rib to the one above. The external intercostals begin posteriorly just lateral to the tubercle of the rib; anteriorly, the muscle is represented in the upper intercostal spaces by the external intercostal membrane. Fibers of external intercostal muscles slant downward and forward from one rib to the next one below. Innermost intercostal muscles are less well developed than the other two intercostal muscles. *(Hollinshead, pp 474–475)*

45. **(B)** All choices are correct, except B, which states that the thoracic wall receives no innervation from cervical nerves. Anteriorly, as far down as the sternal angle, the skin is innervated by supraclavicular nerves, ventral rami of C4 and C5. Ventral rami of spinal nerves T1–T12 supply the thoracic wall, those of T1–T11 being called intercostal nerves and that of T12, the subcostal nerve. Over the paravertebral area of the back, the skin is supplied by dorsal rami of corresponding spinal nerves, which also innervate the erector spinae muscles. *(Hollinshead, p 476)*

46. **(E)** Intercostal nerves are examples of typical spinal nerves; the 2nd through the 6th intercostals are confined to the thorax. The 7th to 11th intercostals and subcostal nerve continue into the abdominal wall. The upper 6 intercostal nerves follow the curve of the ribs and costal cartilages toward the sternum and terminate as anterior cutaneous branches. The nerves run in the costal groove of the intercostal space between the internal and innermost intercostal muscles. *(Hollinshead, pp 477–478)*

47. **(C)** The thoracic wall is supplied chiefly by intercostal arteries and is drained by intercostal veins. These vessels are found in each intercostal space running in the costal groove just above the respective intercostal nerve. Their course and branches conform closely to those of the nerve. Superficial structures of the thorax are served by intercostal vessels and also by branches of the axillary and subclavian arteries and veins. Most anterior intercostal arteries are branches of the internal thoracic artery. Posterior intercostal arteries of all but the first two intercostal spaces are branches of

the descending thoracic aorta. (*Hollinshead, pp 478–479*)

48. **(A)**   The internal thoracic artery is given off by the subclavian artery at the base of the neck. This artery, like the intercostal vessels, runs in the neuromuscular plane of the thorax, that is, anterior to the transversus thoracis muscle and on the internal surface of the costal cartilage and the internal intercostal muscles. The other items listed are correct. (*Hollinshead, p 479*)

49. **(C)**   Ribs increase the anteroposterior and transverse diameters of the thorax by their pump-handle- and bucket-handle-type movements. It has been stated that two-thirds of the increase in thoracic capacity is due to diaphragmatic movements. This is true even in those in whom costal breathing is quite prominent. In normal breathing, expiration is largely passive, due to elastic recoil of the lungs and rib cage and the relaxation of the diaphragm. (*Hollinshead, p 487*)

50. **(C)**   Choice C is incorrect because the alveoli are connected to the exterior by a branching system of tubes (the bronchial tree) and remain filled with air even during expiration. They account for the greatest volume of lung, by far. The lung has two circulations—the pulmonary and the bronchial. The latter is part of the systemic circulation and carries blood for nutrition of the bronchi and connective tissue of the lung. (*Hollinshead, pp 489,497*)

51. **(A)**   The internal anatomy of the lungs conforms to a segmental pattern laid down during development by the budding of bronchi. The bronchopulmonary segments are the anatomic units of the lung. Clinical evaluation, as well as surgical resection, of diseased portions of the lungs, relies on the anatomy of bronchopulmonary segmentation. A bronchopulmonary segment is a pyramidal-shaped unit of the lung aerated by a segmental bronchus. Each segment is served principally by a segmental branch of the pulmonary artery and a segmental vein. The bronchopulmonary segments can be conceived of as the anatomic bronchovascular units of the lungs. (*Hollinshead, pp 490,493–494,506*)

52. **(C)**   Each lung presents a tapered upper end (the apex) and a broad base. All lung surfaces are covered completely by visceral pleura that unites with mediastinal parietal pleura around the root of the lung. The root of the lung is a narrow pedicle that suspends the lung from the mediastinum in the pleural cavity and enters the lung at the pulmonary hilum. Although the right lung has three lobes and the left only two, the bronchopulmonary segments in right and left lungs correspond. (*Hollinshead, pp 490–492*)

53. **(E)**   The lung has two circulations—the pulmonary and the bronchial. The pulmonary trunk arises from the right ventricle of the heart and divides into right and left pulmonary arteries. These arteries end in the capillary networks around the alveolar sacs of the lung. Venules arise from these capillaries and form the pulmonary veins, which enter the left atrium of the heart. The bronchial circulation, which is a part of the systemic circulation, carries blood to the bronchi and connective tissue of the lungs. (*Hollinshead, pp 497–499*)

54. **(A)**   The left pulmonary artery is connected to the aortic arch by the ligamentum arteriosum, the fibrous remains of the ductus arteriosum. In the fetus this structure serves as a shunt between the two vessels. Following birth, the ductus closes and becomes the ligamentum arteriosum. (*Hollinshead, p 499*)

55. **(B)**   The two pulmonary veins running from each lung enter the left, not the right, atrium of the heart. Their pattern shows more variation than that of the pulmonary arteries. Anomalous pulmonary veins may drain into systemic veins and prevent oxygenated blood from being delivered to the left side of the heart for circulation to the body. Such a condition also overloads the right side of the heart and, if widespread enough, may be incompatible with life. (*Hollinshead, p 500*)

56. **(E)**   Descriptions of the internal thoracic artery do not state that any bronchial arteries arise from it. All the other listed sources of bronchial arteries are correct. Both the descending portion and arch of the aorta, along with the subclavian artery, provide sources of blood for the bronchi. (*Hollinshead, pp 479,500–501*)

57. **(D)**   All the choices listed are correct except D. The function of the fibrous pericardium is to retain the heart in position within the thoracic cavity and to limit distention of the heart. The function of the serous sac is to lubricate the moving surfaces of the heart. (*Hollinshead, pp 518–519*)

58. **(B)**   The base of the heart largely is made up of the left atrium and a portion of the right atrium. All of the great veins enter the base of the heart and fix it posteriorly to the pericardial wall. The diaphragmatic surface is formed largely by the left ventricle and a narrower portion of the right ventricle. The coronary sulcus separates the right atrium from the right ventricle, and a large vein, the coronary sinus, is lodged in the sulcus. (*Hollinshead, pp 522–523*)

59. **(E)**   All the structures listed are found in the right atrium except trabeculae carneae. These

structures are fleshy ridges found in the right ventricles, not the atria. *(Hollinshead, pp 527–528)*

60. **(A)** The azygos venous system drains blood from the body wall into the superior vena cava. It does, however, receive venous blood from some of the thoracic viscera. The azygos system consists of two longitudinal venous channels, one on each side of the vertebral column. The channel on the right is called the azygos vein; on the left, it usually consists of two veins—the hemiazygos and the accessory hemiazygos veins. The two left veins are interconnected with each other, and both empty independently into the azygos vein through connecting transverse veins. *(Hollinshead, pp 570–571)*

61. **(C)** The incorrect statement is related to the ending of the thoracic duct. In the base of the neck, the duct ends at the confluence of the left subclavian and the left internal jugular veins. The thoracic duct is the upward continuation of the cisterna chyli. It lies behind the esophagus in most of its course, and its beaded appearance is due to the presence of valves. *(Hollinshead, pp 90,572–573)*

62. **(B)** All the other choices listed correctly describe thoracic vertebrae. The structural characteristic that thoracic vertebrae do not have is a transverse foramen. This foramen is characteristic of cervical vertebrae and functions to transmit the vertebral artery and vein. *(Basmajian, pp 69–70,482–483)*

63. **(B)** The sternum consists of the manubrium, the body, and the xiphoid process. The upper border of the body of the bone articulates with the lower border of the manubrium, forming the sternal angle. This location is at the level of the costal cartilage of the second rib. *(Basmajian, pp 70–71)*

64. **(E)** The true ribs are the upper 7 pairs of ribs that articulate directly with the sternum. They are otherwise known as the vertebrosternal ribs. The remaining 5 pairs are false ribs. The cartilages of ribs 8, 9, and 10 articulate with the cartilages immediately above them and are called vertebrochondral ribs. The last 2 pairs of ribs form floating or vertebral ribs. *(Basmajian, p 72)*

65. **(A)** The typical rib takes a downward, not an upward slope. The 1st arch slopes downward throughout. The ribs increase in obliquity progressively from the 1st to the 9th; the 9th rib is the most obliquely placed. Choices B, C, and D are correct statements. *(Basmajian, pp 72–73)*

66. **(C)** The internal thoracic artery supplies most of the branches that are anterior intercostal arteries. The superior epigastric artery is one of the two terminal branches of the internal thoracic artery; it descends behind the 7th costal cartilage and rec-

tus abdominis muscle to anastomose with the inferior epigastric branch of the external iliac artery, thereby bringing the great vessels of the upper and lower limbs into communication. The other choices are correct. *(Basmajian, p 76)*

67. **(D)** The mediastinum lies between the right and left pleural cavities. These are closed potential spaces within thin-walled sacs of serous membrane. The lung, in development, invaginates the pleural cavity. The other structures listed are contents of the mediastinum. *(Basmajian, pp 77–84)*

68. **(D)** The parietal layer of pleura lines each pleural cavity. This cavity possesses two walls (costal and mediastinal), a base, and an apex. Therefore, its parts are (1) the costal pleura lining the rib cage, (2) the mediastinal pleura applied to the mediastinum, (3) the diaphragmatic pleura, and (4) the cupola, or cervical, pleura that rises into the neck. The pulmonary, or visceral, pleura coats the lung. *(Basmajian, p 77)*

69. **(C)** The root or connecting portion of the mediastinal and pulmonary pleura is a tube or sleeve of pleura in whose upper half lie all the structures that pass to and from the lung. Its lower half is collapsed and is known as the pulmonary ligament. If the root was sectioned, it would sever this ligament, as well as all structures listed except the vagus nerve. The left vagus nerve passes in the mediastinum behind, not through, the root of the lung; it, therefore, would not be severed. *(Basmajian, pp 77,81–83)*

70. **(B)** The trachea bifurcates into a right and left primary bronchus for supply of the respective lungs. Primary bronchi give off secondary bronchi (lobar), three on the right side and two on the left, for the corresponding lobes of the lung. The secondary bronchi divide into tertiary segmental bronchi. Each segmental bronchus, together with the portion of the lung it supplies, is called a bronchopulmonary segment. *(Basmajian, pp 88–89)*

71. **(D)** All the statements about bronchial arteries are correct except that the pressure in them is low. The pressure in these vessels is high; in the pulmonary arteries, it is low. Nevertheless, anastomoses between bronchial and pulmonary vessels occur at capillaries of the respiratory bronchioles and even earlier. *(Basmajian, p 90)*

72. **(A)** The tracheal bifurcation both in the cadaver and supine living subject lies at about the level of T4–T5. When the subject is erect, it usually lies at T6 or lower. It descends during inspiration. The domes of the diaphragm fall 2 to 3 cm when the erect posture is assumed. *(Basmajian, p 92)*

73. **(D)** On each side the internal jugular and the subclavian veins unite to form the brachiocephalic vein. This occurs behind the sternal end of the clavicle. The left brachiocephalic vein passes obliquely behind the upper half of the manubrium and joins the right brachiocephalic vein to form the superior vena cava. *(Basmajian, p 96)*

74. **(E)** The four pulmonary veins carrying oxygenated blood from the lungs, enter the left, not the right, atrium. The other vessels listed enter the right atrium. In addition to the tributaries of the coronary sinus, there are several small anterior cardiac veins that arise on the surface of the right ventricle and pass across the coronary sulcus to penetrate directly the anterior wall of the right atrium. *(Basmajian, p 104; Hollinshead, pp 536–537)*

75. **(B)** In the typical arrangement of costovertebral joints, the head of each rib articulates with the demifacets of two adjacent vertebrae and the intervertebral disk between them. There are some exceptions to this general arrangement. The heads of the first and the last three ribs articulate only with the bodies of their own vertebra. The other choices listed are correct. *(Moore, p 39)*

76. **(D)** In infants and children, the anterior mediastinum may contain the lower part of the thymus gland. During childhood, the thymus begins to diminish in relative size (undergoes involution). By adulthood, it is often scarcely recognizable. *(Moore, pp 79–80)*

77. **(B)** The esophagus extends from the lower end of the pharynx, at the level of the cricoid cartilage, to the stomach. The esophagus enters the superior mediastinum between the trachea and the vertebral column and passes posterior, not anterior, to the left principal bronchus. It descends behind and to the right, not the left, of the aortic arch. It occupies the posterior, not the anterior, mediastinum. It passes through the esophageal hiatus, not the hiatus formed by the median arcuate ligament of the diaphragm (aortic hiatus). *(Moore, p 114)*

78. **(C)** The trachea begins in the neck as a continuation of the lower end of the larynx. It ends at the level of the sternal angle by dividing into right and left principal bronchi. During inspiration, the tracheal bifurcation descends. The trachea is kept open by a series of C-shaped bars of cartilage. It descends in front of the esophagus, and its posterior side is flat where it is applied to the esophagus. *(Moore, p 114)*

79. **(D)** The superior vena cava enters the right atrium vertically from above. It returns blood from everything above the diaphragm (parts listed) except the lungs. The blood from the lungs enters the left atrium via the pulmonary veins. *(Moore, p 109)*

80. **(B)** The brachiocephalic veins have no valves. Each is formed by union of the internal jugular and subclavian veins. Each receives the internal thoracic, vertebral, inferior thyroid, and highest intercostal veins. The brachiocephalic veins unite to form the superior vena cava. *(Moore, p 107)*

81. **(A)** All the structures listed are found in the superior mediastinum except the heart and pericardium. The middle mediastinum contains the heart and pericardium, with the adjacent phrenic nerves and the roots of the great vessels passing to and from the heart. *(Moore, p 107)*

82. **(C)** The coronary arteries arise from the right and left aortic sinuses, respectively, at the root of the aorta just after it leaves the heart. They are the first vessels given off by the aorta. Most of the blood in these vessels returns to the chambers of the heart via the coronary sinus. Some small venous channels, however, empty directly into its chambers. The coronary sinus drains all the venous blood from the heart except that carried by the anterior cardiac veins and the venae cordis minimae, which open directly into the right atrium. *(Moore, pp 99–109)*

83. **(C)** The SA node initiates the impulse for contraction, which is conducted rapidly to the cardiac muscle cells of the atria, causing them to contract. The impulse enters the AV node and is transmitted through the AV bundle and its branches to the papillary muscles and then throughout the walls of the ventricles. The bundle of His is the old name for the AV bundle. *(Moore, pp 104–105)*

84. **(D)** The point of the left ventricle forms the apex, not the base, of the heart. All the other choices are correct. *(Moore, p 89)*

85. **(C)** All the choices are correct except C. The left atrium receives the four pulmonary veins, not the pulmonary arteries. The pulmonary veins carry oxygenated blood returning from the lungs. *(Moore, pp 94–95)*

86. **(A)** The right ventricle gives origin to the pulmonary trunk. This vessel leaves the right ventricle and divides into the right and left pulmonary arteries that take blood to the lungs. There are three papillary muscles in the right ventricle. Their chordae tendineae are inserted into the free edges and ventricular surfaces of the right atrioventricular (tricuspid) valve. *(Moore, pp 93–94)*

87. **(D)** The coronary sulcus separates both atria from both ventricles. The right atrium, not the

right ventricle, forms the right border of the heart. The superior vena cava opening into the right atrium does not have a valve. The fossa ovalis is a prominent feature of the interatrial, not the interventricular, septum. *(Moore, pp 91–94)*

88. (E) The heart is described correctly by all the choices except E. The anterior (sternocostal) surface of the heart is formed mainly by the right ventricle and the right atrium, not by the left atrium, as stated in E. The left ventricle and left atrium lie more posteriorly and form only a small strip on the sternocostal surface. *(Moore, p 89)*

89. (B) The epicardium of the heart is supplied by the coronary arteries. The blood supply to the pericardium is derived from the internal thoracic artery via its branches and from pericardial branches of the bronchial, esophageal, and superior phrenic arteries. The veins of the pericardium are tributaries of the azygos system. *(Moore, p 82)*

90. (B) The ascending aorta carries the pericardium upward beyond the heart to the level of the sternal angle. The base of the fibrous pericardium is fused to the central tendon of the diaphragm. Owing to its many connections, the pericardium is anchored firmly, not freely, within the thoracic cavity. Its truncated apex, not its base, is pierced by the aorta. In the anterior median line, the pericardium is attached to the posterior surface of the sternum by the superior and inferior sternopericardial ligaments. *(Moore, p 80)*

91. (C) The median region between the two pleural sacs is called the mediastinum. It extends from the sternum and costal cartilages in front to the anterior surfaces of the 12 thoracic vertebrae behind. The vertebral bodies, however, are not in the mediastinum. All the other structures listed are contents of the mediastinum. *(Moore, p 79)*

92. (D) No lymph vessels are located in the walls of the pulmonary alveoli. The bronchomediastinal lymph trunks usually terminate on each side at the junction of the subclavian and internal jugular veins; the left trunk may terminate in the thoracic duct. There are two lymphatic plexuses—a superficial and a deep plexus. Cancer cells may spread to the opposite side through the lymphatics because some lymph from the left lung also drains into nodes on the right. Lymph from the lungs drains into the venous system; hence, lymph from the lungs may carry cancer cells into the blood. Common sites of spread of cancer cells via the blood from a bronchogenic carcinoma are the brain, bones, and adrenal glands. *(Moore, p 77)*

93. (A) The roots of the left and right lungs are similar, except that there is only one pulmonary artery in the root of the left lung and two pulmonary arteries on the right. Each side has two pulmonary veins, a bronchus, a pulmonary plexus of nerves, lymph vessels, and lymph nodes enclosed in connective tissue. *(Moore, pp 73–74)*

94. (E) The left lung is divided into inferior and superior lobes by a long, deep, oblique fissure. The superior lobe has a wide cardiac notch on its anterior border where the lung is deficient, owing to the bulge of the heart. The right lung is larger and heavier than the left lung. The azygos vein arches over the root of the right, not the left, lung. A horizontal fissure is found in the right, not the left, lung. *(Moore, pp 66–67)*

95. (C) The central part of the parietal diaphragmatic pleura is supplied by the phrenic nerve; it also supplies the mediastinal pleurae. The costal pleura and the pleura on the peripheral part of the diaphragm are supplied by the intercostal nerves. *(Moore, p 60)*

96. (D) The visceral pleura receives nerve supply from autonomic nerves to the lung. It receives its arterial supply from the bronchial arteries. Its numerous lymphatics drain into nodes at the hila of the lungs. The visceral pleura is insensitive to pain; the parietal pleura is very sensitive to pain. *(Moore, p 60)*

97. (B) The only correct choice is B, which states that each pleural cavity is a closed potential space. Normally the pleural cavity contains only a capillary layer of serous lubricating fluid. This substance lubricates the surface and reduces friction between parietal and visceral layers of pleura. Visceral and parietal pleura become continuous at the root of the lung. The apex of the lung is covered by cervical pleura (cupola of the pleura). The pleurae descend below the costal margin in three regions, where an abdominal incision might enter a pleural sac. These regions are (1) the right xiphisternal angle, (2) the right costovertebral angle, and (3) the left costovertebral angle. *(Moore, p 60)*

98. (A) A dermatome is an area of skin supplied by a dorsal (sensory) root of a spinal nerve. There is considerable overlapping of contiguous dermatomes. The area around the umbilicus is a helpful landmark for identification of innervation level because it is supplied by T10. *(Moore, p 58)*

99–102. (99-B, 100-D, 101-A, 102-E) The thoracic vertebrae are characterized by having articular facets for articulation with ribs. There is one facet or more on each side of the vertebral body for articulation with the head of a rib and one on each transverse process of the upper ten vertebrae for the tubercle of a rib. The sacrum is a large, triangular, wedge-shaped bone that usually is composed of five fused sacral vertebrae in the adult. On the pelvic and dorsal surfaces of the sacrum, there are typically four pairs of foramina for exit of the anterior and posterior primary divisions of the sacral nerves. The cervical vertebrae form the bony axis of the neck. Their distinctive feature is the large, oval-shaped foramen transversarium (transverse foramen) in each transverse process. The vertebral arteries pass through these foramina, except in C7, which transmit only small accessory veins. Lumbar vertebrae may be distinguished by their relatively large bodies, as compared with thoracic and cervical vertebrae and by the absence of costal facets; their vertebral bodies, seen from above, are kidney-shaped, and their vertebral foramina are oval to triangular. *(Moore, pp 615–618)*

103–106.   (103-C, 104-A, 105-B, 106-C)   The body of a rib is thin, flat, long, and curved. The sharp inferior border of the rib projects downward and is located external to the costal groove on the internal surface of the body, near its inferior border. The point of greatest change in curvature is called the angle of the rib. The head of the rib is wedge-shaped and presents two articular facets for articulation with the numerically corresponding vertebra and the vertebra superior to it. These facets are separated by the crest of the head, which is joined to the intervertebral disk by an intra-articular ligament. The neck of the rib is the stout, flattened part located between the head and the tubercle; the neck lies anterior to the transverse process of the corresponding vertebra. Its upper border, called the neck, is sharp, and its lower border is rounded. *(Moore, pp 34–35)*

107–110.   (107-C, 108-A, 109-E, 110-B)   Synovial joints connect the rib with the facets of the vertebral bodies and transverse processes of the vertebrae. They are the plane type of synovial joint that allows gliding movement. The head of each typical rib articulates with the demifacets of two adjacent vertebrae and the intervertebral disk between them. The first 7 pairs of ribs are called true ribs or vertebrosternal ribs because they articulate with the sternum through their costal cartilages. The true ribs increase in length from above downward. The 7th through the 10th costal cartilages meet on each side, and their inferior edges form the costal margin. The diverging costal margins form an infrasternal (subcostal) angle below the xiphisternal joint. Cervical ribs are in about 0.5% to 1% of people and articulate with the 7th cervical vertebra. Usually these ribs produce no symptoms, but in some cases the subclavian artery and the lower trunk of the brachial plexus are kinked where they pass over the cervical rib. Compression of these structures between the extra rib and the anterior scalene muscle produces symptoms of nerve and arterial compression, called the neurovascular compression syndrome. *(Moore, pp 39–40)*

111–114.   (111-E, 112-A, 113-C, 114-B)   During normal expiration, the elastic recoil of the lungs produces a subatmospheric pressure in the pleural cavities. This and the weight of the thoracic walls cause the lateral and anteroposterior diameters of the thorax to return to normal following inspiration. Movements of the thorax primarily are concerned with increasing and decreasing the intrathoracic volume. The resulting changes in pressure result in air being alternately drawn into and expelled from the lungs. The vertical diameter of the thorax is increased primarily when the diaphragm contracts, lowering it. The transverse diameter of the thorax is increased by the ribs swinging outward during the so-called "bucket-handle" movement; this elevates ribs 2 through 10, approximately, and everts their lower borders. This pulls the lateral portions of the ribs away from the midline, thereby increasing the transverse diameter of the thorax. The anteroposterior diameter of the thorax also is increased by raising the ribs. Movement of the costovertebral joints through the long axes of the necks of the ribs results in raising and lowering their sternal ends— the "pump-handle" movement. *(Moore, pp 48–49)*

115–118.   (115-C, 116-E, 117-B, 118-D)   The exact role of the intercostal muscles in the widening of intercostal spaces on inspiration is controversial. It is known that all three layers of intercostal muscles act together in keeping the intercostal spaces rigid. This action prevents the spaces from bulging out during expiration and from being drawn in during inspiration. The serratus posterior superior and serratus posterior inferior muscles run from the vertebrae to the ribs. Both of these muscles are concerned with inspiration. The pectoralis minor muscle arises from the 3rd, 4th, and 5th ribs and inserts on the coracoid of the scapula. It stabilizes the scapula by drawing it forward and downward and elevates the ribs from which it arises; thus, it is an accessory respiratory muscle. The subcostal muscles are thin, muscular slips, variable in size and shape. They extend from the inside of the angle of one rib to the internal surface of the rib below, crossing one or two intercostal spaces. They run in the same direction as the internal intercostal muscles and lie internal to them. These muscles probably depress the ribs. *(Moore, p 50)*

Clinical Thoracic Questions

1. A cervical rib is due to

    (A) proliferation of the nucleus pulposus
    (B) hyperplasia of the annulus fibrosus
    (C) elongation of the transverse process of the 7th cervical vertebra
    (D) fusion of the transverse processes of the 6th and 7th cervical vertebra
    (E) an accessory cervical vertebra

2. In coarctation of the aorta, blood is fed into the distal thoracic aorta through which of the following arteries?

    (A) renal
    (B) internal thoracic
    (C) inferior epigastric
    (D) intercostal
    (E) superficial circumflex iliac

3. Which of the following structures is the more vulnerable to aneurysms?

    (A) ascending aorta
    (B) arch of the aorta
    (C) thoracic aorta
    (D) abdominal aorta
    (E) carotid arteries

    (A) interatrial septal defect
    (B) interventricular septal defect
    (C) coarctation of the aorta
    (D) stenosis
    (E) valvular incompetence

4. Narrowing of the passageways

5. Failure of complete closure of the valve

6. Abnormal narrowing that deprives much of the body of a normal circulation

7. Inadequate development of the septum secundum

8. Excessive resorption of the septum primum

9. Usually involves the membranous portion of the septum

10. The "tetralogy of Fallot" involves all the following EXCEPT

    (A) pulmonary stenosis
    (B) interventricular septal defect
    (C) right ventricular enlargement
    (D) the aorta sitting over the interventricular septal defect
    (E) an interatrial septal defect

11. All the following are correct statements about rib fractures EXCEPT

(A) most frequently they occur as a result of compression forces on the thorax
(B) most often they occur just anterior to the costal angle
(C) splinting the chest wall is essential treatment
(D) broken rib ends tend to spring outward
(E) fractured bone ends may injure the lungs

12. Which of these statements is true about inflammation of the pleura?

(A) usually lung infections do not involve the pleura
(B) formation of pleural exudate may minimize mechanical irritation
(C) inflammation affects motor nerves to the pleura
(D) pleural pain is caused by irritation of autonomic nerves
(E) usually pleural inflammation does not result in formation of pleural adhesions

13. If the phrenic nerve was cut close to its origin, which of these effects could be seen?

(A) loss of bronchoconstriction
(B) loss of sensation in the middle diaphragm
(C) loss of power in intercostal muscles
(D) difficulty in expiration
(E) loss of the respiratory reflex arc

14. Which of these statements correctly describes sensation of the heart?

(A) referred pain from the heart rarely occurs
(B) heart ischemia rarely results in generation of painful stimuli
(C) afferent pain fibers from the heart run in the vagus nerve
(D) pain from the heart is usually felt only in the left chest
(E) the heart is insensitive to cold, heat, and touch

15. Results of an abnormal aortic valve may include all the following EXCEPT

(A) hypertrophy of the right ventricle
(B) production of a heart murmur
(C) aortic regurgitation
(D) collapsing pulse
(E) valvular incompetence

16. The heart valve most frequently diseased is the

(A) aortic
(B) mitral
(C) pulmonary
(D) tricuspid
(E) coronary sinus valve

ANSWERS AND EXPLANATIONS

1. **(C)** A cervical rib is due to elongation of the transverse process of the 7th cervical vertebra. The elongated process is most commonly continued by a fibrous strand that attaches to the first thoracic rib. These structures elevate the great vessels and the brachial plexus cords as they cross the upper rib cage and may produce symptoms referable to the tension thereby imposed on them. *(Woodburne, p 351)*

2. **(D)** In coarctation of the aorta, blood is fed into the distal thoracic aorta through the intercostal arteries, and these may become so large as to erode the adjacent surfaces of the ribs. This circumstance is clearly seen in x-rays of the chest, giving evidence of the condition and a striking example of collateral circulation. *(Woodburne, p 357)*

3. **(A)** The ascending aorta is more subject to aneurysm than the succeeding parts. It receives the strongest thrust of blood from the ventricle, and its wall is not reinforced by the apposition of the fibrous pericardium. *(Woodburne, p 370)*

4. **(D)** Stenosis, or narrowing of the passageways, may develop either congenitally or as a result of disease. *(Woodburne, p 385)*

5. **(E)** Valvular incompetence reflects failure of complete closure of the valve. *(Woodburne, p 385)*

6. **(C)** An abnormal narrowing that deprives much of the body of a normal circulation, coarctation of the aorta, takes place occasionally at the site of the aortic isthmus. *(Woodburne, p 372)*

7. **(A)** An interatrial septal defect larger than a probe, patent foramen ovale, can result from inadequate development of the interatrial septum secundum. *(Woodburne, p 384)*

8. **(A)** An interatrial septal defect may develop because of an excessive resorption of the interatrial septum primum. *(Woodburne, p 384)*

9. **(B)** Interventricular septal defects also occur and usually involve the membranous portion of the septum. *(Woodburne, p 384)*

10. **(E)** The "tetralogy of Fallot" combines pulmonary stenosis and an interventricular septal defect with a shift of the ostium of the aorta over the septal defect and enlargement of the right ventricle. *(Woodburne, p 385)*

11. **(C)** Although ribs may fracture at any point under direct violence, the most frequent fractures are due to compression forces on the thorax. These forces occur most frequently just anterior to the costal angle, the weakest part of the rib. Usually rib fractures heal without any splinting. The broken rib ends tend to spring outward; however, a direct force may drive them inward, causing hemorrhage or injury to the lung. *(Hollinshead, p 471)*

12. **(B)** Inflammation resulting from infection, irritation, emboli, or neoplasms in segments of the lung causes hyperemia of the overlying pleura, which leads to exudate formation. Respiratory movements become painful primarily when the parietal pleura is involved because somatic pain afferents are excited. Sufficient exudate sooner or later separates the pleural layers and minimizes the mechanical irritation. Resolution of the inflammation often leaves adhesions between parietal and visceral pleura; usually these are painless. *(Hollinshead, p 485)*

13. **(B)** If the phrenic nerve was cut at its origin, the only result listed would be B. This is because the phrenic nerve not only is motor to its own half of the diaphragm but also is sensory to the central part of the diaphragmatic pleura. *(Basmajian, pp 91–92)*

14. **(E)** The heart is insensitive to touch, cutting, cold, and heat, but ischemia and the resulting accumulation of metabolic products stimulate pain endings in the myocardium. The pain of angina pectoris and of myocardial infarction commonly radiates to the left shoulder and the medial aspect of the arm (referred pain). The afferent pain fibers run centrally in the middle and inferior cervical branches and the thoracic cardiac branches of the sympathetic trunk. *(Moore, pp 81–82)*

15. **(A)** In aortic valve stenosis, the edges of the valve are usually fused together. The valvular stenosis causes extra work for the left, not the right, ventricle, resulting in left ventricular hypertrophy. A heart murmur is also produced. If the aortic valve is damaged by disease, the valvular incompetence results in aortic regurgitation that produces a heart murmur and a collapsing pulse. *(Moore, p 96)*

16. **(B)** The mitral valve is the most frequently diseased of the heart valves. Rheumatic fever was formerly a common cause of this type of heart disease. Nodules on the valve cusps roughen them, resulting in irregular blood flow and a heart murmur. Later, the diseased cusps undergo scarring and shortening, resulting in a condition called valvular incompetence. With this, blood in the left ventricle regurgitates into the left atrium, producing a murmur when the ventricles contract. *(Moore, p 96)*

Developmental Thoracic Questions

DIRECTIONS (Questions 1 through 3): Each of the numbered items or incomplete statements in this section is followed by answers or by completions of the statement. Select the ONE lettered answer or completion that is BEST in each case.

1. The surface of the developing lung is covered by a layer of mesothelium designated as the

    (A) parietal pleura
    (B) visceral pleura
    (C) diaphragmatic pleura
    (D) costal pleura
    (E) mediastinal pleura

2. Establishment of internal gross anatomy of the lung takes place during which of these developmental periods?

    (A) primitive
    (B) canalicular
    (C) pseudoglandular
    (D) neonatal
    (E) terminal sac

3. The segment of the primitive heart tube giving rise to the aortic sac is the

    (A) bulbis cordis
    (B) primitive ventricle
    (C) truncus arteriosus
    (D) primitive atrium
    (E) sinus venosus

ANSWERS AND EXPLANATIONS

1. **(B)** The developing lungs are covered by a layer of mesothelium designated as the visceral, or pulmonary, pleura. As the lungs grow more and more into the pleural cavity, their pulmonary mesothelial surface contacts the parietal pleura, the outer wall of the sac that is draped over the thoracic wall and the fibrous pericardium. The costal pleura is the parietal pleura lining the thoracic wall. The mediastinal pleura is continuous anteriorly and posteriorly with the costal pleura. The diaphragmatic pleura is an inferior reflection of the costal pleura over the diaphragm, thus forming the floor of the pleural and thoracic cavities. *(Hollinshead, pp 480–482)*

2. **(C)** The development of the lung is divided into five periods: the embryonic, pseudoglandular, canalicular, terminal sac, and neonatal periods. Establishment of the internal gross anatomy of the lung takes place during the first two periods. The pseudoglandular period (8th to 16th week) is the principal growth time of the bronchi and of the future respiratory bronchioles and alveolar ducts. The first period, the embryonic period (4th to 7th weeks) is the period of budding. *(Hollinshead, p 512)*

3. **(C)** In development of the primitive heart tube, differential growth defines five segments of the tube, which receive the names listed as choices A through E in this question. Of these segments, at the rostral end is the truncus arteriosus, and the aortic sac appears as a dilatation of the truncus. Six pairs of aortic arches that arise from this sac skirt around the foregut and link the truncus to the bilateral dorsal aorta. *(Hollinshead, pp 516–517)*

Nervous Thoracic
Questions

DIRECTIONS (Questions 1 through 8): Each of the numbered items or incomplete statements in this section is followed by answers or by completions of the statement. Select the ONE lettered answer or completion that is BEST in each case.

1. Innervation of pleura can be described correctly by all of these statements EXCEPT

   (A) costal pleura is supplied by intercostal nerves
   (B) the central portion of diaphragmatic pleura is supplied by the phrenic nerve
   (C) peripheral diaphragmatic pleura is supplied by intercostal nerves
   (D) the pain of pleurisy is mediated by autonomic nerves
   (E) mediastinal pleura is supplied by the phrenic nerve

2. Which of the following statements describes the nerve supply of the lungs correctly?

   (A) sympathetic fibers in the pulmonary plexus are preganglionic fibers
   (B) vagal fibers in the pulmonary plexus are post-ganglionic fibers
   (C) visceral afferents from the lung have been demonstrated only in the vagus nerve
   (D) the vagus innervates the smooth muscle in walls of pulmonary vessels
   (E) sympathetic fibers control constriction of the bronchi

3. Which of the following statements is correct in relation to the thoracic splanchnic nerves?

   (A) their fibers synapse in the sympathetic chain ganglion
   (B) they are part of the cardiac plexus
   (C) usually they are five in number
   (D) they consist of parasympathetic nerve fibers
   (E) they are composed predominantly of preganglionic fibers

4. Which of the following statements concerning the recurrent laryngeal nerves is correct?

   (A) they are branches of the phrenic nerve
   (B) they branch from the sympathetic trunk
   (C) their neuronal cell bodies are in the cervical spinal cord
   (D) the left nerve recurs around the ligamentum arteriosum
   (E) the right nerve recurs around the superior vena cava

5. All the following statements correctly describe the sympathetic trunk EXCEPT

   (A) ganglia are limited to those for the 12 thoracic nerves
   (B) the trunk lies a little wide of the mediastinum
   (C) intercostal arteries and veins cross the trunk posteriorly
   (D) inferior cervical and first thoracic ganglia form the stellate ganglion
   (E) postganglionic fibers pass from the upper 5 thoracic ganglia to the cardiac plexus

6. Regarding nerves of the lungs and pleura, all the following statements are true EXCEPT

   (A) branches of the vagus contribute to the pulmonary plexus
   (B) branches of the thoracic sympathetic ganglia 1 through 5 help to form the pulmonary plexus
   (C) sensory vagal fibers constitute the afferent limb of the respiratory reflex arc
   (D) efferent vagal fibers are secretomotor
   (E) visceral pleura has many afferent nerves sensitive to mechanical stimulation

7. All the following statements correctly describe the left vagus nerve EXCEPT

   (A) it gives off the left recurrent laryngeal nerve
   (B) posterior to the left bronchus, it breaks up into the left pulmonary plexus
   (C) it supplies the left side of the diaphragm
   (D) it forms part of the esophageal plexus
   (E) it descends from the neck posterior to the left common carotid artery

8. All the following correctly describe innervation of the heart EXCEPT

   (A) sympathetics increase rate of heartbeat
   (B) parasympathetics reduce rate and force of heartbeat
   (C) the impulse-conducting system of the heart is controlled by the autonomic nervous system
   (D) the parasympathetic cardiac nerves supply three branches to each side
   (E) vagal stimulation dilates coronary arteries

ANSWERS AND EXPLANATIONS

1. **(D)** All the choices are correct except D. The pain of pleurisy (pleural inflammation or irritation) is mediated along somatic afferent pathways of these nerves. By contrast, visceral pleura, being supplied by autonomic nerves of the lung, is insensitive to pain stimuli. *(Hollinshead, pp 484–485)*

2. **(C)** Each lung is supplied by visceral afferent and visceral efferent nerve fibers through the pulmonary plexus. Visceral efferents are contributed to the plexus by the vagus and thoracic sympathetic ganglia. The sympathetic fibers in the plexus are postganglionic, and the vagal fibers are preganglionic. Visceral afferents from the lung have been demonstrated only in the vagus. Apparently, the vagus does not innervate smooth muscle in the walls of pulmonary vessels. The vagus, not the sympathetics, is responsible for constriction of the bronchi. *(Hollinshead, pp 501–503)*

3. **(E)** Preganglionic fibers leave the thoracic sympathetic trunks as thoracic splanchnic nerves destined for the innervation of abdominal or pelvic viscera. These nerves relay in collateral ganglia of the abdomen (celiac, superior, and inferior mesenteric ganglia). They also contain afferent fibers (pain sensation) from abdominal and pelvic viscera. These nerves usually are three in number, called the greater, lesser, and lowest splanchnic nerves. *(Hollinshead, pp 573–575)*

4. **(D)** The left recurrent laryngeal nerve springs from the vagus, where the latter crosses the aortic arch. Embryologically, the left recurrent laryngeal nerve recurs around the ligamentum arteriosum rather than the aorta, as the ligamentum arteriosum is the obliterated half of the primitive VI left aortic arch. The right recurrent nerve recurs around the right subclavian artery. None of the other choices is correct. *(Basmajian, pp 83,116)*

5. **(A)** The sympathetic trunks are paired, each consisting of a series of ganglia connected by intervening fibers. Each trunk extends from the level of the first cervical vertebra to the tip of the coccyx, where the two trunks may meet. Choice A thus is erroneous in stating that ganglia are limited to the thoracic segments. *(Basmajian, pp 84–85; Hollinshead, p 60)*

6. **(E)** Branches of the vagus and of the thoracic sympathetic ganglia form pulmonary plexuses, and these supply the lungs. Vagal fibers form the afferent limb of the respiratory reflex arc. Efferent vagal fibers are secretomotor. The visceral pleura is insensitive to mechanical stimulation. *(Basmajian, pp 91–92)*

7. **(C)** All the statements about the left vagus nerve are correct except that it supplies the left diaphragm. The phrenic nerves are the sole motor supply to the diaphragm. They arise from ventral rami of the 3rd, 4th, and 5th cervical nerves. *(Moore, p 114)*

8. **(E)** All the statements regarding innervation of the heart are true except that vagal stimulation dilates the coronary arteries. The vagus—the parasympathetic cardiac nerve—constricts the coronary arteries. It also slows the rate and reduces the force of the heartbeat. The intrinsic impulse-conducting system of the heart is under control of the cardiac nerves of the autonomic nervous system; this enables the heart to respond to changing physiological needs of the body. *(Moore, p 106)*

Illustrations
Questions

THE INFERIOR SURFACE OF THE DIAPHRAGM
(Questions 1 through 18)

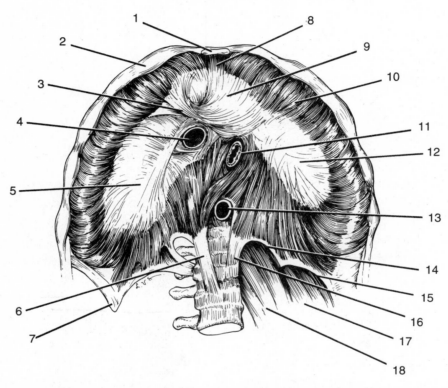

Figure 1–1. The inferior surface of the diaphragm. (Modified and reproduced, with permission, from Way LW [editor]: *Current Surgical Diagnosis & Treatment,* 10th ed. Appleton & Lange, 1994.)

DIRECTIONS: With reference to the diagram, match the numbered structures with their corresponding lettered items.

(A) xiphoid process

(B) middle leaflet

(C) central tendon

(D) left leaflet

(E) 12th rib

(F) costochondral fibers

(G) esophageal hiatus

(H) costal cartilage

(I) vena cava foramen

(J) right leaflet

(K) aortic hiatus

(L) sternal fibers

(M) right crus

(N) psoas major muscles

(O) medial lumbocostal arch

(P) left crus

(Q) quadratus lumborum muscle

(R) lateral lumbocostal arch

TRACHEA AND BRONCHI
(ANTERIOR VIEW)
(Questions 19 through 32)

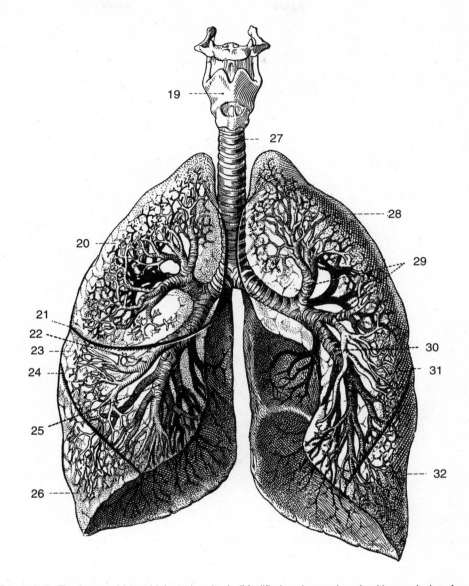

Figure 1–2. Trachea and bronchi (anterior view). (Modified and reproduced, with permission, from Montgomery RL: *Basic Anatomy,* Urban & Schwarzenberg, p. 374, 1980.)

Directions: With reference to the diagram, match the numbered structures with their corresponding lettered items.

(A) oblique fissure

(B) inferior lobe bronchus

(C) superior lobe bronchus

(D) middle lobe right lung

(E) larynx

(F) inferior lobe left lung

(G) middle lobe bronchus

(H) superior lobe right bronchus

(I) trachea

(J) inferior lobe right lung

(K) horizontal fissure

(L) superior lobe right lung

(M) superior lobe left lung

DIAGRAM OF THE HEART
(Questions 33 through 41)

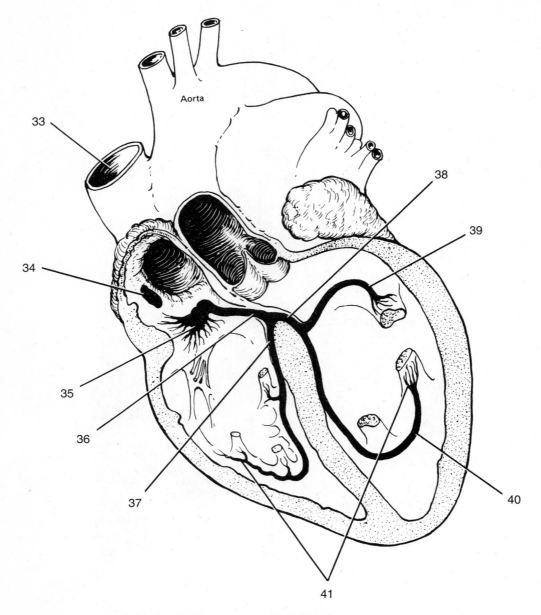

Figure 1–3. Diagram of the heart showing the impulse-generating and impulse-conducting systems. (Modified and reproduced, with permission, from Junqueira LC, Carneiro J, Kelley RO: *Basic Histology,* 7th ed. Appleton & Lange, 1992.)

Directions: With reference to the diagram, match the numbered structures with their corresponding lettered items.

(A) anterior fascicle

(B) sinoatrial node

(C) atrioventricular node

(D) left bundle branch

(E) superior vena cava

(F) atrioventricular bundle (His)

(G) posterior fascicle

(H) right bundle branch

(I) Purkinje system

AZYGOS AND HEMIAZYGOS VEINS
(Questions 42 through 55)

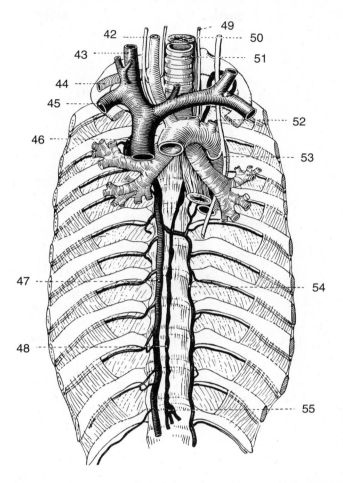

Figure 1–4. Azygos and hemiazygos vein. (Modified and reproduced, with permission, from Montgomery RL: *Basic Anatomy,* Urban & Schwarzenberg, p. 332, 1980.)

Directions: With reference to the diagram, match the numbered structures with their corresponding lettered items.

(A) internal jugular vein

(B) trachea

(C) subclavian artery

(D) common carotid artery

(E) thoracic duct

(F) vagus nerve

(G) hemiazygos vein

(H) arch of the azygos vein

(I) cisterna chyli

(J) azygos vein

(K) inferior laryngeal nerve

(L) esophagus

(M) thoracic duct

(N) subclavian vein

VIEW OF THE LEFT HEART WITH THE LEFT VENTRICULAR WALL TURNED BACK
TO SHOW THE MITRAL VALVE
(Questions 56 through 67)

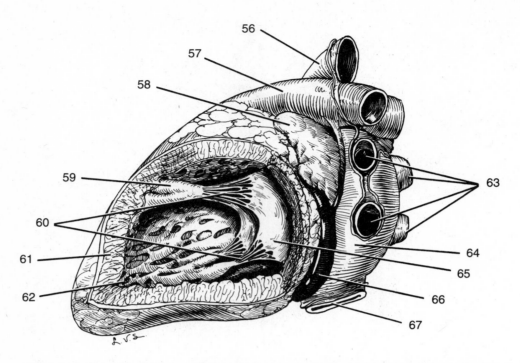

Figure 1–5. View of the left heart with the left ventricular wall turned back to show the mitral valve. (Modified and reproduced, with permission, from Cheitlin MD, Sokolow M, McIllroy MB [editors]: *Clinical Cardiology,* 4th ed. Appleton & Lange, 1993.)

Directions: With reference to the diagram, match the numbered structures with their corresponding lettered items.

(A) pulmonary veins

(B) anterior papillary muscles

(C) posterior papillary muscles

(D) mitral valve

(E) aorta

(F) left atrial appendage

(G) inferior vena cava

(H) chordae tendineae

(I) coronary sinus

(J) left atrium

(K) pulmonary trunk

(L) left ventricle

ANTERIOR VIEW OF THE HEART WITH THE ANTERIOR WALL REMOVED TO SHOW THE RIGHT VENTRICULAR CAVITY
(Questions 68 through 80)

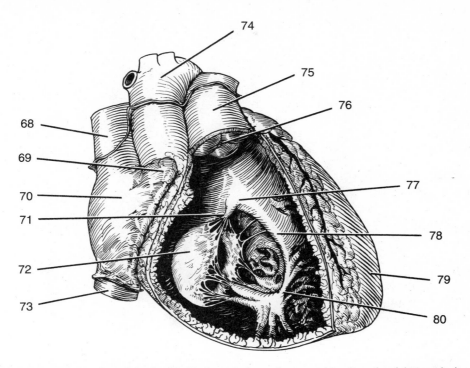

Figure 1–6. Anterior view of the heart with the anterior wall removed to show the right ventricular cavity. (Modified and reproduced, with permission, from Cheitlin MD, Sokolow M, McIllroy MB [editors]: *Clinical Cardiology,* 4th ed. Appleton & Lange, 1993.)

Directions: With reference to the diagram, match the numbered structures with their corresponding lettered items.

(A) pulmonary trunk

(B) moderator band

(C) inferior vena cava

(D) superior vena cava

(E) parietal band

(F) crista supraventricularis

(G) aorta

(H) right atrial appendage

(I) septal band

(J) right atrium

(K) pulmonary valve

(L) tricuspid valve

(M) left ventricle

VIEW OF THE RIGHT HEART WITH THE RIGHT WALL REFLECTED TO SHOW
THE RIGHT ATRIUM
(Questions 81 through 91)

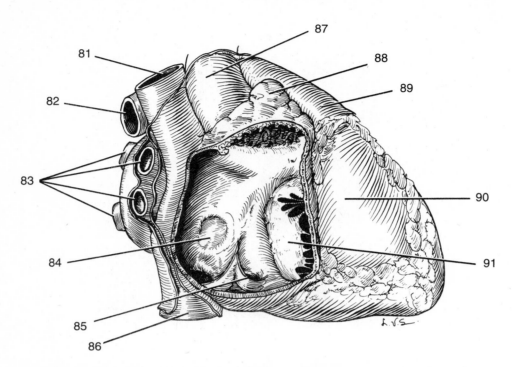

Figure 1–7. View of the right heart with the right wall reflected to show the right atrium. (Modified and reproduced, with permission, from Cheitlin MD, Sokolow M, McIllroy MB [editors]: *Clinical Cardiology,* 4th ed. Appleton & Lange, 1993.)

Directions: With reference to the diagram, match the numbered structures with their corresponding lettered items.

(A) pulmonary trunk

(B) aorta

(C) tricuspid valve

(D) fossa ovalis

(E) right atrial appendage

(F) right ventricle

(G) pulmonary veins

(H) superior vena cava

(I) right pulmonary artery

(J) orifice of coronary sinus

(K) inferior vena cava

EARLY (TOP) AND LATE (BOTTOM) STAGES OF ATRIAL AND VENTRICULAR SEPTATION
(Questions 92 through 117)

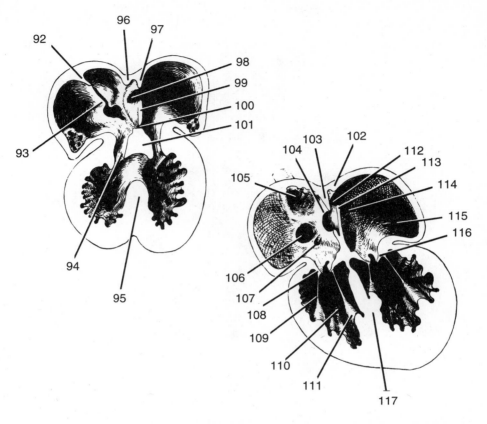

Figure 1–8. Early (*top*) and late (*bottom*) stages of atrial and ventricular septation. (Modified and reproduced, with permission, from Cheitlin MD, Sokolow M, McIllroy MB [editors]: *Clinical Cardiology,* 4th ed. Appleton & Lange, 1993.)

Directions: With reference to the diagram, match the numbered structures with their corresponding lettered items.

(A) septum II
(B) tendinous cord
(C) interatrial foramen II
(D) interatrial foramen I (almost closed)
(E) septum spurium
(F) right atrium
(G) right atrioventricular canal
(H) mitral valve
(I) papillary muscle
(J) interventricular septum

(K) septum I
(L) inferior vena cava
(M) coronary sinus
(N) left atrium
(O) superior vena cava
(P) pulmonary veins
(Q) tricuspid valve
(R) right ventricle
(S) atrioventricular canal endocardial cushion
(T) foramen ovale

HEART CHAMBERS
(Questions 118 through 134)

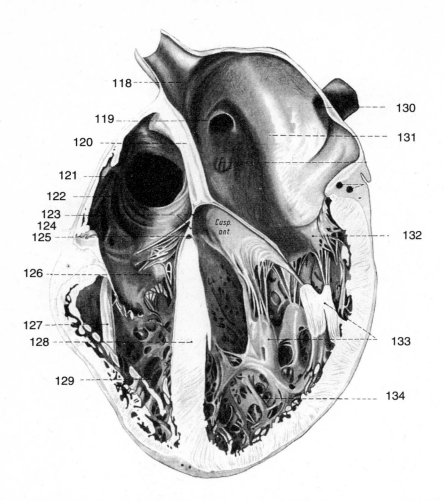

Figure 1–9. Heart chambers. (Modified and reproduced, with permission, from Montgomery RL: *Basic Anatomy,* Urban & Schwarzenberg, p. 284, 1980.)

Directions: With reference to the diagram, match the numbered structures with their corresponding lettered items.

(A) interventricular septum

(B) left ventricle

(C) atrioventricular bundle

(D) opening for pulmonary vein

(E) pars membranacea

(F) right atrioventricular valve

(G) left atrium

(H) left atrioventricular valve

(I) interatrial septum

(J) atrioventricular bundle

(K) papillary muscle

(L) opening of inferior vena cava

(M) right ventricle

(N) pectinate muscle

PATH OF BLOOD FLOW
(Questions 135 through 142)

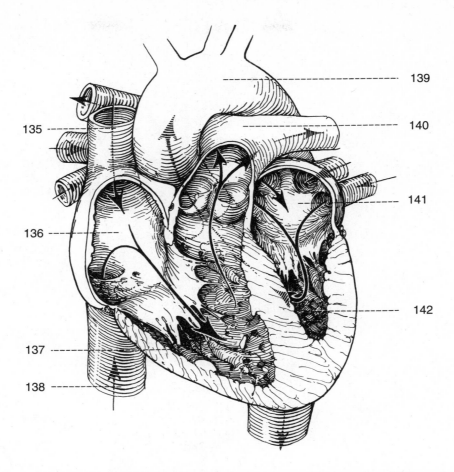

Figure 1–10. Path of blood flow. (Modified and reproduced, with permission, from Montgomery RL: *Basic Anatomy,* Urban & Schwarzenberg, p. 285, 1980.)

Directions: With reference to the diagram, match the numbered structures with their corresponding lettered items.

(A) pulmonary trunk
(B) aorta
(C) left ventricle
(D) right atrium

(E) left atrium
(F) inferior vena cava
(G) right ventricle
(H) superior vena cava

Answers

THE INFERIOR SURFACE OF THE DIAPHRAGM

1.	(A)	10.	(F)
2.	(H)	11.	(G)
3.	(C)	12.	(D)
4.	(I)	13.	(K)
5.	(J)	14.	(O)
6.	(M)	15.	(R)
7.	(E)	16.	(P)
8.	(L)	17.	(Q)
9.	(B)	18.	(N)

TRACHEA AND BRONCHI (ANTERIOR VIEW)

19.	(E)	26.	(J)
20.	(L)	27.	(I)
21.	(K)	28.	(M)
22.	(G)	29.	(C)
23.	(D)	30.	(B)
24.	(A)	31.	(A)
25.	(B)	32.	(F)

DIAGRAM OF THE HEART

33.	(E)	38.	(D)
34.	(B)	39.	(A)
35.	(C)	40.	(G)
36.	(F)	41.	(I)
37.	(H)		

AZYGOS AND HEMIAZYGOS VEINS

42.	(D)	49.	(K)
43.	(A)	50.	(L)
44.	(C)	51.	(B)
45.	(N)	52.	(C)
46.	(H)	53.	(F)
47.	(J)	54.	(G)
48.	(E)	55.	(I)

VIEW OF THE LEFT HEART WITH THE LEFT VENTRICULAR WALL TURNED BACK TO SHOW THE MITRAL VALVE

56.	(E)	62.	(C)
57.	(K)	63.	(A)
58.	(F)	64.	(J)
59.	(B)	65.	(D)
60.	(H)	66.	(I)
61.	(L)	67.	(G)

ANTERIOR VIEW OF THE HEART WITH THE ANTERIOR WALL REMOVED TO SHOW THE RIGHT VENTRICULAR CAVITY

68.	(D)	75.	(A)
69.	(H)	76.	(K)
70.	(J)	77.	(F)
71.	(E)	78.	(I)
72.	(L)	79.	(M)
73.	(C)	80.	(B)
74.	(G)		

VIEW OF THE RIGHT HEART WITH THE RIGHT WALL REFLECTED TO SHOW THE RIGHT ATRIUM

81.	(H)	87.	(B)
82.	(I)	88.	(E)
83.	(G)	89.	(A)
84.	(D)	90.	(F)
85.	(J)	91.	(C)
86.	(K)		

EARLY (TOP) AND LATE (BOTTOM) STAGES OF ATRIAL AND VENTRICULAR SEPTATION

92.	(E)	105.	(O)
93.	(F)	106.	(L)
94.	(G)	107.	(M)
95.	(J)	108.	(Q)
96.	(A)	109.	(B)
97.	(K)	110.	(R)
98.	(C)	111.	(I)
99.	(K)	112.	(C)
100.	(D)	113.	(K)
101.	(S)	114.	(P)
102.	(K)	115.	(N)
103.	(A)	116.	(H)
104.	(T)	117.	(J)

HEART CHAMBERS

118.	(D)	127.	(K)
119.	(D)	128.	(A)
120.	(I)	129.	(M)
121.	(L)	130.	(D)
122.	(N)	131.	(G)
123.	(A)	132.	(H)
124.	(E)	133.	(K)
125.	(J)	134.	(B)
126.	(F)		

PATH OF BLOOD FLOW

135.	(H)	139.	(B)
136.	(D)	140.	(A)
137.	(G)	141.	(E)
138.	(F)	142.	(C)

CHAPTER 2

Head and Neck
Questions

DIRECTIONS (Questions 1 through 92): Each of the numbered items or incomplete statements in this section is followed by answers or by completions of the statement. Select the ONE lettered answer or completion that is BEST in each case.

1. Which of the following arteries provide the blood supply for the hypophysis?

   (A) common carotid
   (B) internal carotid
   (C) external carotid
   (D) vertebral
   (E) subclavian

2. Which of the following nerves is a continuation of the internal carotid nerve?

   (A) lesser petrosal
   (B) greater petrosal
   (C) pterygoid plexus
   (D) caroticotympanic nerve
   (E) cervical plexus

3. All the following structures pass through the superior orbital fissure EXCEPT the

   (A) ophthalmic vein
   (B) oculomotor nerve
   (C) abducens nerve
   (D) optic nerve
   (E) trochlear nerve

4. Which of the following structures pass through the foramen ovale?

   (A) mandibular division of the trigeminal nerve
   (B) middle meningeal artery
   (C) ophthalmic artery
   (D) abducens nerve
   (E) greater petrosal nerve

5. All the following structures are part of the ethmoid bone EXCEPT the

   (A) crista galli
   (B) superior nasal concha
   (C) medial pterygoid plate
   (D) middle nasal concha
   (E) cribriform plate

6. The spine of the sphenoid bone gives attachment to the

   (A) tensor veli palatini muscle
   (B) medial pterygoid muscle
   (C) temporomandibular ligament
   (D) stylomandibular ligament
   (E) zygomaticus major muscle

7. The posterior nasal spine is located on which of the following bones?

   (A) maxilla
   (B) palatine
   (C) vomer
   (D) occipital
   (E) ethmoid

8. Which of the following muscles is associated with the spine of the sphenoid, the scaphoid fossa, and the pterygoid hamulus?

   (A) medial pterygoid
   (B) lateral pterygoid
   (C) tensor veli palatini
   (D) tensor tympani
   (E) levator veli palatini

9. Which of the following structures is located between the superciliary ridges?

   (A) anterior lacrimal crest
   (B) supraorbital notch
   (C) superior orbital fissure
   (D) glabella
   (E) anterior nasal spine

10. The infratemporal fossa accommodates all the following structures EXCEPT

    (A) principal muscles of mastication
    (B) maxillary artery
    (C) pterygoid plexus
    (D) mandibular division of the trigeminal
    (E) pterygopalatine ganglion

11. The body of the mandible has a sharp inferior margin that ends posteriorly in the

    (A) mental protuberance
    (B) mental tubercle
    (C) angle of the mandible
    (D) mandibular condyle
    (E) mandibular notch

12. Which of the following muscles is considered the principal muscular landmark of the neck?

    (A) mylohyoid
    (B) sternocleidomastoid
    (C) sternohyoid
    (D) stylohyoid
    (E) anterior scalene

13. The digastric muscle is a two-bellied muscle that attaches by an intermediate tendon to the

    (A) mandibular condyle
    (B) thyroid cartilage
    (C) cricoid cartilage
    (D) styloid process
    (E) hyoid bone

14. The omohyoid, the sternocleidomastoid, and the posterior belly of the digastric muscle form the boundary for which of the following triangles?

    (A) occipital
    (B) submandibular
    (C) submental
    (D) carotid
    (E) omoclavicular

15. As a rule, the isthmus of the thyroid gland crosses the

    (A) hyoid bone
    (B) 2nd to 4th tracheal rings
    (C) cricoid cartilage
    (D) thyroid cartilage
    (E) inferior belly of the omohyoid muscle

16. The prevertebral layer of cervical fascia forms the floor for which of the following triangles?

    (A) submental
    (B) posterior cervical
    (C) submandibular
    (D) carotid
    (E) muscular

17. Which of the following muscles aids in depressing the corner of the mouth downward and widens the aperture, as in expressions of sadness or fright?

    (A) orbicularis oris
    (B) buccinator
    (C) mylohyoid
    (D) mentalis
    (E) platysma

18. The cervical branch of the facial nerve innervates which of the following muscles?

    (A) sternocleidomastoid
    (B) geniohyoid
    (C) sternothyroid
    (D) platysma
    (E) masseter

19. Which of the following veins unites with the retromandibular to form the external jugular vein?

    (A) posterior auricular
    (B) superficial temporal
    (C) transverse facial
    (D) internal jugular
    (E) facial

20. Which of the following veins crosses perpendicularly to the superficial surface of the sternocleidomastoid beneath the platysma muscle?

    (A) internal jugular
    (B) anterior jugular
    (C) posterior jugular
    (D) external jugular
    (E) retromandibular

21. Which of the following nerves is a dorsal ramus of the second cervical nerve?

    (A) great auricular
    (B) greater occipital
    (C) lesser occipital
    (D) transverse cervical
    (E) supraclavicular

22. Which of the following nerves is formed by contributions from the ventral rami of cervical nerves 3 and 4?

    (A) supraclavicular
    (B) greater occipital
    (C) great auricular
    (D) transverse cervical
    (E) occipitalis tertius

23. The superficial layer of cervical fascia splits into two sheets to enclose which of the following muscles?

    (A) sternothyroid
    (B) anterior scalene
    (C) trapezius
    (D) mylohyoid
    (E) semispinalis capitis

24. Which of the following ligaments is formed from a thickening of the deep parotid fascia?

    (A) temporomandibular
    (B) stylohyoid
    (C) stylomandibular
    (D) sphenomandibular
    (E) nuchal

25. Which of the following fascial layers gives rise to the axillary sheath?

    (A) superficial layer of cervical fascia
    (B) prevertebral
    (C) carotid sheath
    (D) buccopharyngeal
    (E) pretracheal

26. The sheath of the thyroid gland is formed from which of the following fascial layers?

    (A) carotid sheath
    (B) prevertebral
    (C) superficial layer of the cervical fascia
    (D) pretracheal
    (E) alar

27. Which of the following structures is located within the cervical visceral fasciae?

    (A) cervical sympathetic trunk
    (B) pharynx
    (C) external jugular vein
    (D) common carotid artery
    (E) hypoglossal nerve

28. The largest and most important interfascial interval in the neck is which of the following spaces?

    (A) suprasternal
    (B) retropharyngeal
    (C) submandibular
    (D) lateral pharyngeal
    (E) parotid

29. The sternohyoid muscle is innervated by which of the following nerves?

    (A) hypoglossal
    (B) ansa cervicalis
    (C) transverse cervical
    (D) supraclavicular
    (E) vagus

30. The superior thyroid artery is usually the first branch of which of the following arteries?

    (A) common carotid
    (B) external carotid
    (C) internal carotid
    (D) subclavian artery
    (E) maxillary artery

31. The inferior thyroid artery is a branch of which of the following arteries?

    (A) dorsal scapular
    (B) costocervical
    (C) external carotid
    (D) thyrocervical
    (E) vertebral

32. The middle thyroid vein empties into which of the following veins?

    (A) external jugular
    (B) anterior jugular
    (C) posterior jugular
    (D) internal jugular
    (E) vertebral

33. Which of the following structures is embedded in the anterior sheath of the carotid sheath?

    (A) sympathetic trunk
    (B) thyrocervical trunk
    (C) vertebral artery
    (D) prevertebral fascia
    (E) superior ramus of the ansa cervicalis

34. The common carotid artery usually bifurcates into the external and internal carotids at the level of the

    (A) jugular notch
    (B) cricoid cartilage
    (C) upper border of the thyroid cartilage
    (D) neck of the mandible
    (E) sternoclavicular joint

35. Which of the following arteries enters the cranium to become the principal artery of the brain?

    (A) external carotid
    (B) internal carotid
    (C) maxillary
    (D) vertebral
    (E) common carotid

36. Which of the following arteries passes obliquely upward deep to the posterior belly of the digastric and the stylohyoid muscles running deep to the submandibular gland?

    (A) lingual
    (B) facial
    (C) maxillary
    (D) superior thyroid
    (E) occipital

37. Which of the following arteries arises from the posterior aspect of the external carotid at the level of the upper border of the posterior belly of the digastric?

    (A) facial
    (B) occipital
    (C) lingual
    (D) posterior auricular
    (E) ascending pharyngeal

38. The vagus nerve leaves the skull through which of the following foramina?

    (A) jugular
    (B) internal acoustic
    (C) foramen spinosum
    (D) foramen ovale
    (E) foramen lacerum

39. The cell bodies of the superior ganglion of the vagus nerve are concerned primarily with which of the following components of the nerve?

    (A) general visceral efferent
    (B) general somatic afferent
    (C) general somatic efferent
    (D) general visceral afferent
    (E) special visceral afferent

40. Which of the following nerves innervate the cricothyroid and the inferior constrictor muscle of the pharynx?

    (A) inferior cervical cardiac
    (B) external branch of the superior laryngeal
    (C) inferior laryngeal
    (D) recurrent laryngeal
    (E) superior cervical cardiac

41. The superior deep cervical lymph nodes occupy which of the following cervical triangles?

    (A) carotid
    (B) omoclavicular
    (C) submandibular
    (D) occipital
    (E) submental

42. Which of the following ganglia is commonly located at the level of the 2nd cervical vertebra?

    (A) stellate ganglion
    (B) inferior cervical ganglion
    (C) vertebral ganglion
    (D) middle cervical ganglion
    (E) superior cervical ganglion

43. Which of the following ganglia is commonly located at the level of the cricoid cartilage?

    (A) superior ganglion of the vagus
    (B) inferior ganglion of the glossopharyngeal
    (C) otic
    (D) middle cervical sympathetic
    (E) submandibular

44. Which of the following ganglia is commonly located at the base of the transverse process of the 7th cervical vertebrae?

    (A) pterygopalatine
    (B) submandibular
    (C) cervicothoracic
    (D) vertebral
    (E) geniculate

45. The posterior belly of the digastric muscle is innervated by which of the following nerves?

    (A) trigeminal
    (B) facial
    (C) vagus
    (D) ansa subclavia
    (E) hypoglossal

46. Which of the following arteries passes through the brachial plexus either above or below the middle trunk?

    (A) costocervical
    (B) suprascapular
    (C) transverse scapular
    (D) dorsal scapular
    (E) vertebral

47. The subclavian vein joins the internal jugular vein to form the brachiocephalic vein at which of the following structures?

    (A) the outer border of the first rib
    (B) behind the acromioclavicular joint
    (C) behind the coracoclavicular joint
    (D) in front of the coracohumeral ligament
    (E) behind the sternal end of the clavicle

48. The costocervical trunk usually gives rise to which of the following arteries?

    (A) highest intercostal
    (B) inferior thyroid
    (C) suprascapular
    (D) transverse cervical
    (E) ascending cervical

49. Which of the following muscles is an essential muscular landmark of the neck?

    (A) longus colli
    (B) longus capitis
    (C) rectus capitis
    (D) scalenus anterior
    (E) scalenus posterior

50. Which of the following laryngeal cartilages has a triangular base with vocal and muscular processes?

    (A) cricoid
    (B) corniculate
    (C) arytenoid
    (D) cuneiform
    (E) epiglottis

51. Which of the following structures contributes to the formation of the vocal ligaments?

    (A) thyrohyoid membrane
    (B) cricotracheal ligament
    (C) quadrangular membrane
    (D) conus elasticus
    (E) hypoepiglottic ligament

52. Which of the following structures constitutes the vestibular ligament of the false vocal fold?

    (A) quadrangular membrane
    (B) median cricothyroid ligament
    (C) thyrohyoid membrane
    (D) thyroepiglottic ligament
    (E) cricotracheal ligament

53. The space between the apposed vocal folds and arytenoid cartilages is known as the

    (A) glottis
    (B) rima glottidis
    (C) vestibule
    (D) rima vestibuli
    (E) piriform recess

54. Which of the following muscles of the larynx is an abductor of the vocal ligament?

    (A) posterior cricoarytenoid
    (B) lateral cricoarytenoid
    (C) transverse arytenoid
    (D) thyroarytenoid
    (E) cricothyroid

55. Which of the following muscles of the larynx increases tension on the vocal folds?

    (A) cricothyroid
    (B) lateral cricoarytenoid
    (C) posterior cricoarytenoid
    (D) thyroarytenoid
    (E) transverse arytenoid

56. The vocalis muscles are composed of those internal fibers of which of the following muscles?

    (A) lateral cricoarytenoid
    (B) cricothyroid
    (C) thyroarytenoid
    (D) posterior cricoarytenoid
    (E) oblique arytenoid

57. The principal sensory nerve of the larynx is the

    (A) recurrent laryngeal
    (B) inferior laryngeal
    (C) superior laryngeal
    (D) glossopharyngeal
    (E) cervical sympathetic trunk

58. Which of the muscles of the larynx is innervated by the external branch of the superior laryngeal nerve?

    (A) lateral cricoarytenoid
    (B) posterior cricoarytenoid
    (C) thyroarytenoid
    (D) transverse arytenoid
    (E) cricothyroid

59. The superior laryngeal artery is a branch of which of the following arteries?

    (A) lingual
    (B) superior thyroid
    (C) costocervical trunk
    (D) thyrocervical trunk
    (E) transverse cervical

60. The trachea begins at the level of the

    (A) hyoid bone
    (B) thyroid cartilage
    (C) 4th cervical vertebra
    (D) cricoid cartilage
    (E) 2nd cervical vertebra

61. The carina is part of the

    (A) hyoid bone
    (B) epiglottis
    (C) trachea
    (D) larynx
    (E) pharynx

62. The pharynx terminates at the level of the

    (A) hyoid bone
    (B) 2nd cervical vertebra
    (C) thyroid cartilage
    (D) cricoid cartilage
    (E) jugular notch

63. The pharyngobasilar fascia contributes to which of the following layers of the pharyngeal wall?

    (A) mucous membrane
    (B) submucosa

    (C) longitudinal muscle layer
    (D) circular muscle layer
    (E) buccopharyngeal fascia

64. The middle pharyngeal constrictor arises from the

    (A) pterygomandibular raphe
    (B) cricoid cartilage
    (C) thyroid cartilage
    (D) torus tubarius
    (E) hyoid bone

65. Which of the following muscles enters the pharyngeal wall in the gap between the origins of the middle and superior pharyngeal constrictor muscles?

    (A) stylopharyngeus
    (B) palatopharyngeus
    (C) salpingopharyngeus
    (D) thyrohyoid
    (E) sternohyoid

66. Which of the following muscles of the pharynx is innervated by the glossopharyngeal nerve?

    (A) superior pharyngeal constrictor
    (B) salpingopharyngeus
    (C) stylopharyngeus
    (D) palatopharyngeus
    (E) middle pharyngeal constrictor

67. Which of the following ganglia is a peripheral ganglion in the course of the parasympathetic innervation of the parotid gland?

    (A) ciliary
    (B) pterygopalatine
    (C) submandibular
    (D) otic
    (E) geniculate

68. Which of the following nerves supplies parasympathetic fibers through the otic ganglion to the parotid gland?

    (A) vagus
    (B) glossopharyngeal
    (C) facial
    (D) hypoglossal
    (E) accessory

69. Which of the following nerves innervates the genioglossus muscle?

   (A) hypoglossal
   (B) ansa cervicalis
   (C) glossopharyngeal
   (D) vagus
   (E) trigeminal

70. The esophagus begins at the level of the

   (A) hyoid bone
   (B) thyroid cartilage
   (C) 4th cervical vertebra
   (D) cricoid cartilage
   (E) jugular notch

71. Which of the following nerves is a cutaneous branch of the maxillary division of the trigeminal nerve?

   (A) lacrimal
   (B) infratrochlear
   (C) auriculotemporal
   (D) buccal
   (E) superior labial

72. The levator anguli oris muscle is innervated by which of the following nerves?

   (A) auriculotemporal
   (B) facial
   (C) ansa cervicalis
   (D) inferior alveolar
   (E) inferior palpebral nerve

73. The pterygomandibular raphe is a ligamentous band that stretches between the pterygoid hamulus and the

   (A) spine of the sphenoid
   (B) hyoid bone
   (C) mental protuberance
   (D) posterior end of the mylohyoid line
   (E) posterior nasal spine

74. The angular artery is the terminal part of which of the following arteries?

   (A) superficial temporal
   (B) posterior auricular
   (C) maxillary
   (D) facial
   (E) occipital

75. The infraorbital artery is one of the terminal branches of which of the following arteries?

   (A) facial
   (B) transverse facial
   (C) superficial temporal
   (D) lingual
   (E) maxillary

76. The mental artery is a terminal branch of which of the following arteries?

   (A) superficial temporal
   (B) transverse facial
   (C) inferior alveolar
   (D) facial
   (E) lingual

77. The retromandibular vein is formed by the confluence of the superficial temporal and which of the following veins?

   (A) transverse facial
   (B) maxillary
   (C) facial
   (D) lingual
   (E) submental

78. The parotid duct penetrates which of the following muscles?

   (A) masseter
   (B) medial pterygoid
   (C) buccinator
   (D) superior pharyngeal constrictor
   (E) levator anguli oris

79. The deep portion of the parotid fascia forms the

   (A) stylomandibular ligament
   (B) sphenomandibular ligament
   (C) pterygomandibular raphe
   (D) carotid sheath
   (E) buccopharyngeal fascia

80. The facial nerve enters the temporal bone by way of which of the following openings?

   (A) carotid canal
   (B) foramen lacerum
   (C) stylomastoid foramen
   (D) internal acoustic meatus
   (E) jugular foramen

81. Which of the following nerves is usually the first extracranial branch of the facial nerve?

    (A) cervical branch
    (B) marginal mandibular branch
    (C) buccal branch
    (D) zygomatic branch
    (E) posterior auricular

82. The 4th layer of the scalp is represented by which of the following?

    (A) an aponeurotic
    (B) a muscular
    (C) a dense connective
    (D) a periosteal
    (E) a loose connective

83. The blood vessels of the scalp are located primarily in the

    (A) skin
    (B) dense subcutaneous layer
    (C) aponeurotic layer
    (D) loose connective tissue layer
    (E) periosteal layer

84. The supraorbital artery is a branch of which of the following arteries?

    (A) superficial temporal
    (B) transverse facial
    (C) maxillary
    (D) facial
    (E) ophthalmic

85. The muscles of the scalp are innervated by which of the following nerves?

    (A) supraorbital
    (B) auriculotemporal
    (C) temporal and auricular branches of the facial
    (D) greater occipital
    (E) lesser occipital

86. The masseteric fascia is formed from which of the following?

    (A) superficial layer of cervical fascia
    (B) carotid sheath
    (C) prevertebral fascia
    (D) buccopharyngeal
    (E) pretracheal fascia

87. The sphenomandibular ligament is a thickening of the

    (A) carotid sheath
    (B) pterygoid fascia
    (C) prevertebral fascia
    (D) pretracheal fascia
    (E) buccopharyngeal

88. The innervation of the masseter muscle is provided by which of the following nerves?

    (A) buccal branch of the facial
    (B) buccal branch of the trigeminal
    (C) maxillary division of the trigeminal
    (D) inferior alveolar
    (E) mandibular division of the trigeminal

89. The sphenomeniscus inserts into the

    (A) mandibular condyle
    (B) articular tubercle
    (C) postglenoid tubercle
    (D) articular disk
    (E) lingula

90. The jaws are opened by forward traction on the neck of the mandible by which of the following muscles?

    (A) masseter
    (B) temporalis
    (C) lower portion of the lateral pterygoid
    (D) upper fibers of the medial pterygoid
    (E) sphenomeniscus

91. Which of the following muscles positions or stabilizes the condyle and disk against the articular eminence during closing movements of the mandible?

    (A) temporalis
    (B) masseter
    (C) medial pterygoid
    (D) anterior belly of the digastric
    (E) sphenomeniscus portion of the lateral pterygoid

92. The medial pterygoid muscle assists which of the following muscles in protrusion of the mandible?

    (A) mylohyoid
    (B) lateral pterygoid
    (C) geniohyoid
    (D) temporalis
    (E) sphenomeniscus

DIRECTIONS (Questions 93 through 112): Each group of items in this section consists of lettered headings followed by a set of numbered words or phrases. For each numbered word or phrase, select the ONE lettered heading that is most closely associated with it. Each lettered heading may be selected once, more than once, or not at all.

Questions 93 through 96

For each insertion below, select the muscle with which it is associated.

    (A) temporalis
    (B) sphenomeniscus
    (C) masseter
    (D) medial pterygoid
    (E) inferior belly of the lateral pterygoid

93. Articular disk

94. Pterygoid fovea

95. Lateral surfaces of the coronoid process, ramus, and angle of the mandible

96. Anterior border and medial surface of the coronoid process

Questions 97 through 100

For each muscle listed below, select the nerve that provides branches for its innervation.

    (A) masseteric
    (B) medial pterygoid
    (C) meningeal
    (D) inferior alveolar
    (E) auriculotemporal

97. Tensor veli palatine

98. Mylohyoid

99. Tensor tympani

100. Anterior belly of the digastric

Questions 101 through 104

For each artery listed below, select the structure associated with it.

    (A) mandibular foramen
    (B) mandibular notch
    (C) foramen spinosum
    (D) infraorbital canal
    (E) sphenopalatine foramen

101. Middle meningeal

102. Inferior alveolar

103. Masseteric

104. Anterior superior alveolar

Questions 105 through 108

For each function associated with the tongue, select the nerve that carries those fibers.

    (A) trigeminal
    (B) facial
    (C) hypoglossal
    (D) glossopharyngeal
    (E) vagus

105. Taste to the anterior two-thirds of the tongue

106. Motor fibers to the styloglossus

107. General sensation to the posterior one-third of the tongue

108. General sensation to the anterior two-thirds of the tongue

Questions 109 through 112

For each muscle listed below, select the nerve that provides the innervation for it.

    (A) vagus
    (B) glossopharyngeal
    (C) trigeminal
    (D) facial
    (E) hypoglossal

109. Levator veli palatini

110. Tensor veli palatini

111. Palatoglossus

112. Palatopharyngeus

DIRECTIONS (Questions 113 through 133): Each of the numbered items or incomplete statements in this section is followed by answers or by completions of the statement. Select the ONE lettered answer or completion that is BEST in each case.

113. All the following statements apply to the fibrous outer layer of the eye EXCEPT

    (A) the sclera constitutes the posterior five-sixths of the outer layer of the eye
    (B) it is continuous in front with the cornea
    (C) transparent cornea constitutes the anterior one-sixth of the outer layer
    (D) it is perforated by vorticose veins
    (E) it gives rise to the optic disk

114. All the following statements apply to the choroid layer of the eye EXCEPT

    (A) it is brown in color
    (B) it consists of a dense capillary plexus
    (C) the ciliary body is part of the choroid layer
    (D) the iris is part of the choroid layer
    (E) it is the innermost layer of the eye

115. All the following statements correctly apply to the lens EXCEPT

    (A) the lens is a transparent biconvex body
    (B) the shape of the lens is modified by the ciliary muscle
    (C) the lens is held in place by the suspensory ligament
    (D) the lens is the principal refractive structure of the eye
    (E) the lens is flatter on its posterior surface and more curved anteriorly

116. The middle ear includes the

    (A) tragus
    (B) anthelix
    (C) cochlea
    (D) auditory ossicles
    (E) membranous labyrinth

117. All the following statements correctly apply to the tympanic membrane EXCEPT

    (A) it is set obliquely into the external acoustic meatus
    (B) it is composed of 3 layers
    (C) it forms the lateral wall of the middle ear
    (D) the umbo is at the most indrawn part of the membrane
    (E) the lower limit of the membrane is called membrane flaccida

118. Which of the following arteries provide branches to the middle ear?

    (A) maxillary
    (B) posterior auricular
    (C) ascending pharyngeal
    (D) middle meningeal
    (E) superficial temporal

119. The internal ear consists of all the following structures EXCEPT

    (A) cochlea
    (B) semicircular canals
    (C) utricle
    (D) saccule
    (E) epitympanic recess

120. All the following statements correctly apply to the cochlear duct EXCEPT

    (A) it is the membranous part of the bony cochlea
    (B) it is rectangular in cross-section
    (C) it is bounded below by a fibrous extension of the osseous spiral lamina—the basilar membrane
    (D) it is bounded above by the more delicate vestibular membrane
    (E) it is continuous with the remainder of the membranous tubules through the ductus reuniens connecting it to the sacculus

121. All the following structures traverse the internal acoustic meatus EXCEPT the

    (A) facial nerve
    (B) vestibulocochlear nerve
    (C) labyrinthine artery
    (D) labyrinthine vein
    (E) deep auricular artery

122. Which of the following statements correctly apply to the geniculate ganglion?

    (A) it is the sensory ganglion of the trigeminal nerve
    (B) it contains motor neurons
    (C) it is located in the pterygoid canal
    (D) it is located at the junction of the internal acoustic meatus and the facial canal
    (E) it is located in the stylomastoid foramen

123. All the following statements correctly apply to the chorda tympani nerve EXCEPT

    (A) it arises from the facial nerve
    (B) it passes through the tympanic cavity
    (C) it passes forward over the medial surface of the tympanic membrane
    (D) it passes through the petrotympanic fissure
    (E) it passes through the foramen ovale

124. The peripheral processes of the cochlear nerve are located in the

    (A) saccule
    (B) utricle
    (C) ampulla of the posterior semicircular duct
    (D) organ of Corti
    (E) vestibule

125. Which of the following foramina open into the infratemporal fossa?

    (A) foramen rotundum
    (B) jugular foramen
    (C) stylomastoid
    (D) foramen ovale
    (E) foramen lacerum

126. Which of the following muscles is associated with the medial pterygoid plate?

    (A) stapedius
    (B) tensor tympani
    (C) palatopharyngeus
    (D) tensor veli palatini
    (E) palatoglossus

127. The jugular foramen transmits all the following structures EXCEPT

    (A) internal jugular vein
    (B) glossopharyngeal nerve
    (C) vagus nerve
    (D) accessory nerve
    (E) hypoglossal nerve

128. All the following statements correctly apply to the cavernous sinuses EXCEPT

    (A) it has nerves in its outer wall
    (B) it has a nerve and a major artery coursing through it
    (C) it lies on either side of the body of the sphenoid
    (D) it is formed between the meningeal and periosteal layers of the dura
    (E) the mandibular nerve passes through the sinus

129. The meningeal arteries arise from all the following arteries EXCEPT the

    (A) maxillary
    (B) anterior ethmoidal
    (C) ascending pharyngeal
    (D) occipital
    (E) superficial temporal

130. Which of the following vessels supply approximately four-fifths of the dura mater?

    (A) occipital artery
    (B) posterior meningeal
    (C) anterior meningeal
    (D) middle meningeal
    (E) middle cerebral

131. All the following statements correctly apply to the contracting ciliary muscle EXCEPT

    (A) the ciliary processes and ring are drawn toward the corneoscleral junction
    (B) it reduces tension on the fibers of the suspensory ligament
    (C) the lens increases its curvatures
    (D) it creates greater refractive power for vision of close object
    (E) it is innervated by the trigeminal nerve

132. Which of the following structures is characterized by nervous elements?

    (A) pars ciliaris retinae
    (B) pars iridica retinae
    (C) ora serrata
    (D) pars optica retinae
    (E) lens

133. All the following statements correctly apply to the maxillary division of the trigeminal EXCEPT

    (A) it is entirely sensory
    (B) it supplies the skin of the cheek
    (C) it supplies the lower eyelid
    (D) it supplies the upper lip
    (E) it traverses the infratemporal fossa

ANSWERS AND EXPLANATIONS

1. **(B)** The blood supply of the hypophysis is provided by two inferior hypophyseal branches of the internal carotid arteries, and by one or two superior hypophyseal arteries which spring from the internal carotid artery just as it leaves the cavernous sinus. (Woodburne, p 322)

2. **(D)** The internal carotid nerve, the postganglionic cranial continuation of the superior cervical sympathetic ganglion, accompanies the internal carotid artery into the cranium. The internal carotid plexus surrounds the lateral aspect of the artery and gives off the caroticotympanic nerves and the deep petrosal nerve. *(Woodburne, p 320)*

3. **(D)** The optic nerve passes through the optic canals: the ophthalmic vein, ophthalmic division of the trigeminal nerve, oculomotor, abducens, and trochlear nerves pass through the superior orbital fissure. *(Woodburne, p 312)*

4. **(A)** The mandibular division of the trigeminal nerve transverses the foramen ovale along with the accessory meningeal artery. *(Woodburne, p 312)*

5. **(C)** The medial pterygoid is part of the sphenoid bone. The crista galli, cribriform plate, superior nasal concha, middle nasal concha, and perpendicular plate are parts of the ethmoid. *(Woodburne, p 310)*

6. **(A)** Behind the foramen spinosum is the spine of the sphenoid bone which gives attachment to the sphenomandibular ligament and the tensor veli palatini muscle. *(Woodburne, p 308)*

7. **(B)** Behind the hard palate is the posterior nasal apertures, which are separated by the vomer. Also in the median line at the posterior margin of the palatine bone is the posterior nasal spine. *(Woodburne, p 307)*

8. **(C)** The spine of the sphenoid gives attachment of the sphenomandibular ligament and the tensor veli palatini muscle. The tensor veli palatini takes origin from the scaphoid fossa and its tendon turns around the hamulus. *(Woodburne, p 308)*

9. **(D)** The smooth depressed area between the two superciliary arches is the glabella. It may show an inferior remnant of the metopic suture. *(Woodburne, p 305)*

10. **(E)** The infratemporal fossa accommodates the principal muscles of mastication, the maxillary artery, the pterygoid plexus of veins, and the mandibular division of the trigeminal nerve. The pterygopalatine ganglion is located in the pterygopalatine fossa. *(Woodburne, p 304)*

11. **(C)** The prominence of the chin is the mental protuberance. The body of the mandible has a sharp inferior margin that ends posteriorly in the angle of the mandible. The ramus continues upward toward the ear and ends in the mandibular condyle. *(Woodburne, p 253)*

12. **(B)** The principal muscular landmark of the neck is the sternocleidomastoid. The infrahyoid and suprahyoid muscles are located within the anterior cervical triangle, in which the sternocleidomastoid forms one boundary. *(Woodburne, p 179)*

13. **(E)** The digastric muscle is a two-bellied muscle that attaches by an intermediate tendon to the hyoid bone. The digastric muscle completes the boundaries of the submandibular triangle with the base formed by the mandible. *(Woodburne, p 179)*

14. **(D)** The omohyoid muscle passes downward and laterally from the hyoid bone to disappear behind the sternocleidomastoid muscle and thus subdivides this area of the anterior triangle into two triangles. The upper triangle, bordered by the omohyoid, the sternocleidomastoid, and the posterior belly of the digastric muscle, is known as the carotid triangle. *(Woodburne, p 179)*

15. **(B)** Usually, the isthmus of the thyroid gland crosses the 2nd, 3rd, and 4th tracheal rings. *(Woodburne, p 179)*

16. **(B)** The posterior cervical triangle has as its floor the prevertebral layer of cervical fascia covering the splenius, levator scapulae, scalenus medius, and scalenus posterior muscles. *(Woodburne, p 179)*

17. **(E)** The platysma muscle draws the corner of the mouth downward and widens the aperture, as in expressions of sadness or fright. *(Woodburne, p 180)*

18. **(D)** The platysma muscle is innervated by the cervical branch of the fascial nerve. *(Woodburne, p 180)*

19. **(A)** The external jugular vein is formed a little below and behind the angle of the mandible by the union of the retromandibular vein and the posterior auricular vein. *(Woodburne, pp 180–181)*

20. **(D)** The external jugular crosses perpendicularly to the superficial surface of the sternocleidomastoid muscle directly under the platysma muscle. *(Woodburne, p 180)*

21. **(B)** The greater occipital nerve is a dorsal ramus of the 2nd cervical nerve. The lesser occipital, great auricular, transverse cervical, and supraclavicular nerves are cutaneous branches of the ventral rami of the cervical plexus. *(Woodburne, p 181)*

22. **(A)** The supraclavicular nerves are branches of a large trunk formed by contributions from the ventral rami of cervical nerves 3 and 4. *(Woodburne, p 183)*

23. **(C)** The superficial layer of cervical fascia splits into two sheets to enclose the sternocleidomastoid and trapezius muscles. *(Woodburne, p 183)*

24. **(C)** The stylomandibular ligament is a thickening of the deep parotid fascia extending from the tip of the styloid process to the angle of the mandible. *(Woodburne, p 242)*

25. **(B)** As the lower cervical spinal nerves emerge between the anterior and middle scalene muscles and are extended laterally over the first rib as the brachial plexus, they carry with them a prolongation of the prevertebral fascia known as the axillary sheath. *(Woodburne, p 186)*

26. **(D)** The sheath of the thyroid gland is a well-differentiated portion of the pretracheal fascia and encloses the gland on all sides. *(Woodburne, p 186)*

27. **(B)** In the central part of the neck lie the cervical viscera—pharynx, esophagus, larynx, trachea, thyroid, and parathyroid glands—enclosed within a cylindrical cervical visceral fasciae. *(Woodburne, p 186)*

28. **(B)** The largest and most important interfascial interval in the neck is the retropharyngeal space. This is an areolar interval between the buccopharyngeal fascia anteriorly and the prevertebral fascia posteriorly. *(Woodburne, p 187)*

29. **(B)** The sternohyoid muscle is innervated by one or more branches of the superior ramus of the ansa cervicalis, which enter its lateral margin. *(Woodburne, p 189)*

30. **(B)** The superior thyroid artery is usually the first branch of the external carotid artery. *(Woodburne, p 194)*

31. **(D)** The inferior thyroid artery is the largest branch of the thyrocervical trunk, which is a branch of the subclavian artery. *(Woodburne, p 214)*

32. **(D)** The middle thyroid vein crosses the common carotid artery and empties into the lower end of the internal jugular vein. *(Woodburne, p 192)*

33. **(E)** The superior ramus of the ansa cervicalis nerve, conducting motor impulses to the infrahyoid muscles from the upper cervical nerves, lies on the anterior sheath of the carotid sheath. *(Woodburne, p 211)*

34. **(C)** The external carotid artery extends from the upper border of the thyroid cartilage to the neck of the mandible, where it divides into the superficial temporal and maxillary arteries. *(Woodburne, pp 194–195)*

35. **(B)** The internal carotid has no branches in the neck but continues within the carotid sheath to the base of the skull, where it enters the cranium to become the principal artery of the brain. *(Woodburne, p 194)*

36. **(B)** The facial artery arises immediately above the lingual. It passes obliquely upward, deep to the posterior belly of the digastric and the stylohyoid muscles, over which it arches to lie in a groove on the deep surface of the submandibular gland. *(Woodburne, pp 194–195)*

37. **(D)** The posterior auricular artery arises from the posterior aspect of the external carotid at the level of the upper border of the posterior belly of the digastric muscle. It ascends through the parotid fossa to the notch between the external acoustic meatus and the mastoid process. *(Woodburne, p 195)*

38. **(A)** The vagus nerve leaves the skull through the jugular foramen, contained in the same dural sheath with the accessory nerve. *(Woodburne, p 197)*

39. **(B)** The cell bodies of the superior ganglion of the vagus are concerned primarily with the general somatic afferent (cutaneous) component of the nerve. *(Woodburne, p 197)*

40. **(B)** The external branch of the superior laryngeal nerve descends on the inferior constrictor of the pharynx to the lower border of the thyroid cartilage, where it terminates in the cricothyroid muscle. It also supplies the inferior constrictor muscle of the pharynx. *(Woodburne, p 198)*

41. **(A)** The deep cervical lymph nodes, as is generally true elsewhere in the body, are arranged along the blood vessels, arteries, or veins. The superior deep cervical nodes thus occupy the carotid triangle of the neck. *(Woodburne, pp 200–201)*

42. **(E)** The superior cervical ganglion is the largest of the three cervical ganglia. It is usually broad, flattened, and tapered at the ends and lies in front on the transverse process of the 2nd cervical vertebra. *(Woodburne, p 203)*

43. **(D)** The middle cervical sympathetic ganglion commonly lies at the level of the cricoid cartilage in the bend of the inferior thyroid artery. *(Woodburne, pp 203–204)*

44. **(C)** The cervicothoracic ganglion represents a combination of the inferior cervical and the first, or the first several, thoracic ganglia. It lies anterior to the base of the transverse process of the 7th cervical vertebra and is usually posteromedial to the origin of the vertebral artery. *(Woodburne, p 204)*

45. **(B)** The anterior belly receives its innervation at its lateral border from the nerve to the mylohyoid, a branch of the mandibular division of the trigeminal nerve. The posterior belly is supplied by a branch of the facial nerve. *(Woodburne, p 205)*

46. **(D)** The dorsal scapular artery has an intimate relation to the brachial plexus, passing posteriorly through it, most frequently either above or below the middle trunk. *(Woodburne, p 215)*

47. **(E)** The subclavian vein is the continuation of the axillary vein at the outer border of the 1st rib. The subclavian vein joins the internal jugular vein to form the brachiocephalic vein behind the sternal end of the clavicle. *(Woodburne, p 215)*

48. **(A)** The costocervical trunk arises from the posterior aspect of the subclavian artery behind the anterior scalene muscle. It passes backward over the cervical pleura and the apex of the lung to the neck of the 1st rib, where it divides into the highest intercostal and the deep cervical. *(Woodburne, p 215)*

49. **(D)** The anterior scalene is one of the essential muscular landmarks of the neck. The phrenic nerve is formed at its lateral margin, descends on the muscle under the prevertebral fascia, and enters the thorax by passing its medial border. The roots of the brachial plexus and the subclavian artery emerge between the anterior and middle scalene muscles, and the subclavian vein passes anterior to the insertion of the anterior scalene. *(Woodburne, p 216)*

50. **(C)** The base of the arytenoid cartilage is triangular. Of the three borders of the pyramid, one forms the sharp, anteriorly directed vocal process to which the vocal ligament is attached. The laterally directed angle ends in the muscular process on which insert the posterior and lateral cricoarytenoid muscles. *(Woodburne, p 219)*

51. **(D)** The median part of the conus elasticus is the median cricothyroid ligament. The lateral parts of the conus end above in parallel thickenings, known as vocal ligaments, uniting the thyroid and the arytenoid cartilages. *(Woodburne, p 220)*

52. **(A)** The quadrangular membrane is a submucosal sheet of connective tissue ending in the aryepiglottic fold posterosuperiorly and inferiorly in a free margin that constitutes the vestibular ligament of the false vocal (vestibular) fold. *(Woodburne, p 220)*

53. **(B)** The vocal folds and the space between them are designated as the glottis and are the part of the larynx most directly concerned in the production of sounds. The rima glottidis—the space between the apposed vocal folds and arytenoid cartilages—is the narrowest part of the laryngeal cavity. *(Woodburne, p 221)*

54. **(A)** The posterior cricoarytenoid muscles are the abductors of the vocal folds; drawing the muscular processes backwards turns the vocal processes in a lateral direction. *(Woodburne, p 222)*

55. **(A)** The cricothyroid muscle draws the thyroid cartilage downward and forward toward the cricoid, which increases the distance between the thyroid and the arytenoid cartilages (mounted on the cricoid). Thus, the anterior and posterior attachments of the vocal ligaments are carried further apart, and the tension of the vocal folds is made greater. *(Woodburne, p 222)*

56. **(C)** The vocalis muscles are composed of those internal fibers of the thyroarytenoid muscles most closely related to the vocal ligament. Such fibers are considered to be chiefly responsible for the control of pitch through their ability to regulate the vibrating part of the vocal ligaments. *(Woodburne, p 223)*

57. **(C)** The superior laryngeal nerve is the principal sensory nerve of the larynx and sends branches to the surfaces of the epiglottis and to the aryepiglottic fold. *(Woodburne, p 224)*

58. **(E)** The long, slender external branch of the superior laryngeal nerve descends along the oblique line of the thyroid cartilage to the cricothyroid muscle, which it supplies. All the other intrinsic muscles of the larynx are innervated by the inferior laryngeal nerve. *(Woodburne, p 224)*

59. **(B)** The arteries of the larynx are the superior laryngeal, the inferior laryngeal, and the cricothyroid. The superior laryngeal artery is a branch of the superior thyroid artery, which pierces the thyrohyoid membrane in company with the internal branch of the superior laryngeal nerve. *(Woodburne, p 224)*

60. **(D)** The trachea begins at the lower border of the cricoid cartilage at the level of the 6th cervical vertebra and terminates at the sternal angle (upper border of the 5th thoracic vertebra). *(Woodburne, p 225)*

61. **(C)** The last tracheal cartilage is thick and broad in the middle, and its lower border is prolonged downward and backward in a hooked process. This is the carina, which forms a keel-like projection between the origins of the right and left bronchi. *(Woodburne, p 225)*

62. **(D)**   The pharynx is approximately 12 cm long. It begins at the base of the skull and terminates below at the level of the lower border of the cricoid cartilage. *(Woodburne, pp 225–226)*

63. **(B)**   The submucosa is a strong, fibrous sheet, known as the pharyngobasilar fascia, which is uncovered by the muscular layer of the pharynx in its uppermost part and is especially strong there. *(Woodburne, p 226)*

64. **(E)**   The middle pharyngeal constrictor muscle arises from the upper border of the greater horn of the hyoid bone, from the lesser horn, and from the stylohyoid ligament. *(Woodburne, p 228)*

65. **(A)**   The stylopharyngeus muscle enters the pharyngeal wall in the gap between the origins of the middle and superior pharyngeal constrictors. *(Woodburne, p 228)*

66. **(C)**   The pharyngeal plexus provides the innervation of the muscles of the pharynx, with the exception of the stylopharyngeus. The pharyngeal plexus is formed by the pharyngeal and vagal nerves and of the superior cervical sympathetic ganglion. *(Woodburne, p 229)*

67. **(D)**   The otic ganglion is a peripheral ganglion in the course of the parasympathetic innervation of the parotid gland; the postganglionic neurons arising in the ganglion distribute by way of the auriculotemporal branch of the trigeminal nerve to the gland. *(Woodburne, pp 230–231)*

68. **(B)**   The tympanic nerve, a branch of the glossopharyngeal, supplies parasympathetic fibers through the otic ganglion, to the parotid gland and sensory fibers, to the mucous membrane of the middle ear. *(Woodburne, p 230)*

69. **(A)**   The terminal branches of the hypoglossal nerve distribute to the styloglossus, hyoglossus, genioglossus, and the intrinsic muscles of the tongue. *(Woodburne, p 231)*

70. **(D)**   The esophagus begins at the level of the lower border of the cricoid cartilage and ends below the diaphragm opposite the 11th thoracic vertebra. *(Woodburne, pp 231–232)*

71. **(E)**   The superior labial branches, three or four in number, descend to the skin and mucous membrane of the upper lip and gingiva and to the labial glands. The lacrimal and infratrochlear nerves are cutaneous branches of the ophthalmic division of the trigeminal. Both the buccal and the auriculotemporal are cutaneous branches of the mandibular division of the trigeminal nerve. *(Woodburne, p 234)*

72. **(B)**   The levator anguli oris muscle elevates the angle of the mouth, at the same time drawing it in a medial direction, and is innervated by a buccal branch of the facial nerve. *(Woodburne, p 236)*

73. **(D)**   The pterygomandibular raphe is a ligamentous band that, stretched between the pterygoid hamulus superiorly and the posterior end of the mylohyoid line of the mandible inferiorly, separates the fibers of the buccinator from those of the superior pharyngeal constrictor muscle. *(Woodburne, p 237)*

74. **(D)**   The angular artery is the terminal part of the facial artery. Ascending to the medial angle of the orbit, it supplies orbicularis oculi and the lacrimal sac. *(Woodburne, p 239)*

75. **(E)**   The infraorbital artery is one of the terminal branches of the maxillary artery and reaches the face by traversing the infraorbital groove and canal in company with the infraorbital vein and nerve. *(Woodburne, p 240)*

76. **(C)**   The mental artery is a terminal branch of the inferior alveolar artery that, as a branch of the first part of the maxillary artery, passes through a canal in the mandible to supply the lower teeth. *(Woodburne, p 240)*

77. **(B)**   The retromandibular vein is formed in the upper portion of the parotid gland, deep to the neck of the mandible, by the confluence of the superficial temporal vein and the maxillary vein. *(Woodburne, pp 240–241)*

78. **(C)**   Crossing the masseter muscle and the buccal fat pad, the parotid duct turns deeply at the anterior border of the buccal pad of fat and penetrates the buccinator muscle, opening in the interior of the mouth opposite the second upper molar tooth. *(Woodburne, p 241)*

79. **(A)**   The parotid fascia is an extension into the face of the superficial layer of the cervical fascia. The deep portion of the parotid fascia also forms a thickening, the stylomandibular ligament, which passes downward and lateralward from the styloid process to the angle of the mandible. *(Woodburne, p 242)*

80. **(D)**   The facial nerve enters the temporal bone by way of the internal acoustic meatus and leaves it through the stylomastoid foramen. *(Woodburne, p 243)*

81. **(E)**   The posterior auricular is the first extracranial branch of the facial nerve. It ascends between the external acoustic meatus and the mastoid process. *(Woodburne, p 243)*

82. **(E)** The 3rd layer of the scalp is musculoaponeurotic. The 2nd layer is a dense connective layer. The 4th layer is both loose and scanty, which permits a wide spread of fluid accumulations in this layer. *(Woodburne, p 245)*

83. **(B)** The blood vessels of the scalp are firmly held by the strong fibers of the subcutaneous connective tissue and are prevented thereby from retracting or contracting their lumina when severed. *(Woodburne, p 245)*

84. **(E)** The supraorbital artery is a branch of the ophthalmic artery, which is a branch of the internal carotid. *(Woodburne, p 247)*

85. **(C)** The occipital portion of the muscle is innervated by the posterior auricular branch of the facial nerve. The temporal branch of the facial nerve supplies the frontal portion of the muscle. The posterior auricular branch of the facial nerve supplies the posterior muscle; the anterior and superior auricular muscles are innervated by the temporal branch of the facial. *(Woodburne, pp 248–249)*

86. **(A)** The superficial layer of cervical fascia, after attachment to the inferior border of the mandible, continues into the face as both the parotid and masseteric fascia. *(Woodburne, p 250)*

87. **(B)** The sphenomandibular ligament is a thickening of the pterygoid fascia, which extends between the spine of the sphenoid bone and the lingula of the mandible. *(Woodburne, p 250)*

88. **(E)** The nerve to the masseter muscle is a branch of the mandibular division of the trigeminal nerve, which reaches it by passing through the mandibular notch and penetrating its deep surface. *(Woodburne, p 250)*

89. **(D)** The upper head of the lateral pterygoid is designated as the sphenomeniscus and inserts into the articular disk of the temporomandibular joint and into the upper part of the neck of the condyle. *(Woodburne, pp 251–252)*

90. **(C)** The jaws are opened by forward traction on the neck of the mandible by the lower portion of the lateral pterygoid muscles, assisted by the digastric, mylohyoid, and geniohyoid muscles. *(Woodburne, p 253)*

91. **(E)** Electromyographic studies suggest that the sphenomeniscus portion of the lateral pterygoid muscle positions or stabilizes the condyle and disk against the articular eminence during closing movements of the mandible. *(Woodburne, p 253)*

92. **(B)** The medial pterygoid muscle assists the lateral pterygoid in protrusion of the mandible; the posterior fibers of the temporalis retract it, assisted by the suprahyoid group of muscles. *(Woodburne, p 218)*

93–96. **(93-B, 94-E, 95-C, 96-A)** The sphenomeniscus inserts into the articular disk of the temporomandibular joint. The inferior belly of the lateral pterygoid inserts into the pterygoid fovea. The masseter inserts into the lateral surfaces of the coronoid process, ramus, and angle of the mandible. The temporalis inserts into the anterior border and medial surface of the coronoid process of the mandible. *(Woodburne, pp 250–253)*

97–100. **(97-B, 98-D, 99-B, 100-D)** The medial pterygoid nerve provides the nerve to the tensor veli palatini muscle, which enters this muscle near its origin, and the nerve to the tensor tympani muscle. The mylohyoid nerve arises from the inferior alveolar nerve just before the latter enters the mandibular foramen and descends into the mylohyoid groove to provide the motor innervation of the mylohyoid muscle and the anterior belly of the digastric muscle. *(Woodburne, pp 257–258)*

101–104. **(101-C, 102-A, 103-B, 104-D)** The middle meningeal artery enters the middle cranial fossa by way of the foramen spinosum. The inferior alveolar artery enters the mandibular foramen with the inferior alveolar nerve. The masseteric artery passes through the mandibular notch with the masseteric nerve and supplies the masseter muscle. The anterior superior alveolar branches arise in the infraorbital canal and descend in the alveolar canals to the upper incisive and cuspid teeth. *(Woodburne, pp 258–260)*

105–108. **(105-B, 106-C, 107-D, 108-A)** Taste to the anterior two-thirds of the tongue is provided by the facial nerve. The hypoglossal nerve provides the motor innervation to all the extrinsic and intrinsic muscles of the tongue. The glossopharyngeal nerve provides general sensation to the posterior one-third of the tongue. The trigeminal nerve provides general sensation to the anterior two-thirds of the tongue. *(Woodburne, pp 266–267)*

109–112. **(109-A, 110-C, 111-A, 112-A)** The tensor veli palatini muscle is supplied by the mandibular division of the trigeminal nerve. All of the other palatal muscles are supplied by the contribution of the vagus nerve to the pharyngeal plexus. *(Woodburne, p 235)*

113. **(E)** The sclera is a firm, fibrous cup that constitutes the posterior five-sixths of the outer layer of the eye. It is continuous in front with the cornea at the corneoscleral junction. The sclera is perforated

by vorticose veins. The transparent cornea constitutes the anterior one-sixth of the fibrous tunic. The optic disk is not part of the sclera. (Woodburne, p 290)

114. **(E)** The choroid layer is brown in color due to the pigment cells of its outermost layer. It consists of a dense capillary plexus. The ciliary body is an elevated zone of the anterior portion of the choroid layer. The iris is a thin, contractile membrane having a central aperture, the pupil. It is the middle layer of the eye, not the innermost layer. (Woodburne, pp 290–291)

115. **(E)** The lens is a transparent biconvex body, flatter on its anterior surface and more curved posteriorly. The shape of the lens is modified by the ciliary muscle, as the eye focuses on objects at differing distances. The lens is held in place by a series of straight fibrils, constituting the suspensory ligament of the lens. The lens lies behind the cornea and is the principal refractive structure of the eye. The lens is flatter on its anterior surface and more curved posteriorly. (Woodburne, p 292)

116. **(D)** The middle ear is a narrow cavity in the temporal bone; here the energy of sound waves is converted into mechanical energy through a chain of ossicles. The tragus, anthelix, and cochlea are part of the external ear. The membranous labyrinth is part of the internal ear. (Woodburne, pp 293– 299)

117. **(E)** The upper limits of the tympanic membrane is designated as the membrana flaccida. The tympanic membrane is set obliquely into the external acoustic meatus and is composed of three layers: the modified skin of the external meatus on its outer surface, the mucous membrane of the cavity internally, and an intermediate fibrous stratum. The center point, the umbo, is at the most indrawn part of the membrane. (Woodburne, pp 295–296)

118. **(A)** The arteries of the middle ear are numerous. The two larger ones are the anterior tympanic branch of the maxillary artery to the tympanic membrane and the stylomastoid branch of the posterior auricular artery to the tympanic antrum and mastoid cells. Smaller arteries include the inferior tympanic branch of the ascending pharyngeal artery and the superficial petrosal branch of the middle meningeal artery. The superficial temporal does not send branches to the middle ear. (Woodburne, pp 297–298)

119. **(E)** The internal ear provides the essential organs of hearing and equilibrium. It consists of the cochlea, for the auditory sense, and a series of intercommunicating channels (the semicircular ducts, the utricle, and the saccule), for the sense of balance and position. The epitympanic recess is the space above the tympanic membrane. (Woodburne, p 261)

120. **(B)** The cochlear duct is the membranous part of the bony cochlea. The cochlear duct is triangular in cross-section, being bounded below by a fibrous extension of the osseous spiral lamina, the basilar membrane, and above by the more delicate vestibular membrane. It is continuous with the remainder of the membranous tubules through the ductus reuniens connecting it to the sacculus. (Woodburne, p 300)

121. **(E)** The facial nerve and the vestibulocochlear nerve traverse the internal acoustic meatus. Both the labyrinth artery and vein also traverse the internal acoustic meatus. (Woodburne, p 300)

122. **(D)** The geniculate ganglion is the sensory ganglion of the facial nerve. It is located at the abrupt bend taken by the nerve as it turns from the internal acoustic meatus into the posteriorly directed facial canal. It is not located in the stylomastoid foramen. (Woodburne, p 300)

123. **(E)** The chorda tympani arises from the facial nerve proximal to the stylomastoid foramen and enters the tympanic cavity. It passes forward over the medial surface of the tympanic membrane and arches across the handle of the malleus. It emerges from the skull through the petrotympanic fissure. It does not pass through the foramen ovale. (Woodburne, p 300)

124. **(D)** The peripheral processes of the cochlear nerve are located in the organ of Corti, their cell bodies forming the spiral ganglion of the cochlea, which is situated in the osseous spiral lamina. (Woodburne, p 301)

125. **(D)** The foramen ovale and foramen spinosum open into the roof of the infratemporal fossa. (Woodburne, p 301)

126. **(D)** At the base of the medial pterygoid plate, it is hollowed out in the oval scaphoid fossa for the origin of the tensor veli palatini muscle; at the inferior extremity of the plate, the tendon of the tensor turns around its recurved hamulus. (Woodburne, p 307)

127. **(E)** The jugular foramen transmits the jugular vein and the glossopharyngeal, vagus, and accessory nerves. It also transmits the inferior petrosal sinus. The hypoglossal foramen transmits the hypoglossal nerve. (Woodburne, p 308)

128. **(E)** The cavernous sinuses lie on either side of the body of the sphenoid. They are formed between the meningeal and periosteal layers of the dura.

This sinus has nerves in its outer wall and a nerve and a major artery coursing through it. The abducens nerve passes through the sinus. The mandibular nerve does not pass through the sinus. *(Woodburne, pp 315–316)*

129. (E) The middle meningeal artery is a branch of the maxillary artery. The anterior meningeal artery is a branch of the anterior ethmoidal artery. The posterior meningeal ethmoidal artery is a branch of the ascending pharyngeal, occipital, and vertebral arteries. None of the meningeal vessels arise from the superficial temporal artery. *(Woodburne, p 279)*

130. (D) The middle meningeal artery supplies four-fifths of the dura mater. *(Woodburne, p 316)*

131. (E) The ciliary muscle is the muscle of accommodation. By its contraction, the ciliary process and ring are drawn toward the corneoscleral junction, and the wedge-shaped ring is bulged toward its center. This reduces the tension on the fibers of the suspensory ligament, thereby allowing the natural elasticity of the lens to increase its curvatures, resulting in greater refractive power for vision of close objects. The muscle is innervated by parasympathetic fibers of the oculomotor nerve. *(Woodburne, p 291)*

132. (D) Three regions are differentiated in the retina. The pars optica retinae is that portion characterized by nervous elements. At the ora serrata the nervous elements of the retina cease. The lens is likewise not an area characterized by nervous elements. *(Woodburne, p 292)*

133. (E) The maxillary division of the trigeminal nerve is entirely sensory and supplies the skin of the cheek, the side of the nose, the lower eyelid, and the upper lip. It traverses the pterygopalatine fossa, not the infratemporal fossa. *(Woodburne, p 276)*

Clinical Head and Neck Questions

DIRECTIONS (Questions 1 through 10): Each of the numbered items or incomplete statements in this section is followed by answers or by completions of the statement. Select the ONE lettered answer or completion that is BEST in each case.

1. Bell's palsy is associated with which of the following nerves?

    (A) oculomotor
    (B) facial
    (C) optic
    (D) abducens
    (E) trigeminal

2. Tic douloureux is associated with which of the following nerves?

    (A) trochlear
    (B) facial
    (C) optic
    (D) vagus
    (E) trigeminal

3. The danger area of the scalp is recognized as which of the following layers?

    (A) loose areolar tissue
    (B) aponeurosis epicranialis
    (C) skin
    (D) connective tissue
    (E) pericranium

4. Pachymeningitis refers to inflammation of the

    (A) pia and arachnoid together
    (B) dura
    (C) pia
    (D) arachnoid
    (E) periosteum

5. A pulsating exophthalmos involves all the following EXCEPT the

    (A) cavernous sinus
    (B) internal carotid artery
    (C) ophthalmic veins
    (D) arteriovenous fistula
    (E) optic nerve

6. The condition known as hyperacusia is associated with a lesion of which of the following nerves?

    (A) oculomotor
    (B) facial
    (C) vestibulocochlear
    (D) trigeminal
    (E) trochlear

7. Congenital torticollis or wryneck is associated with injury to the

    (A) erector spinalis muscle
    (B) trapezius muscle
    (C) sternocleidomastoid muscle
    (D) 6th cervical vertebra
    (E) anterior scalene muscle

8. Which of the following cervical triangles is used surgically for approaches to the thyroid and parathyroid glands?

    (A) carotid
    (B) muscular
    (C) submandibular
    (D) occipital
    (E) supraclavicular

9. All the following are associated with Horner's syndrome EXCEPT

   (A) vasodilation
   (B) absence of sweating on the face and neck
   (C) exophthalmos
   (D) ptosis
   (E) pupillary constriction

10. Foreign bodies entering the pharynx may become lodged in which of the following areas?

    (A) pharyngeal recess
    (B) retropharyngeal space
    (C) supratonsilar fossa
    (D) piriform recess
    (E) lateral pharyngeal space

ANSWERS AND EXPLANATIONS

1. **(B)** Paralysis of the facial nerve for no obvious reason, known as Bell's palsy (paralysis), may occur after exposure to a cold draft. The most common cause of Bell's palsy is inflammation of the facial nerve near the stylomastoid foramen. This causes edema and swelling of the nerve and compression of its fibers in the facial canal or stylomastoid foramen. Patients with facial paralysis are unable to close their lips and eyelids on the affected side. *(Moore, p 661)*

2. **(E)** Trigeminal neuralgia (tic douloureux) is a condition characterized by sudden attacks of excruciating pain that are initiated by a mere touch in the area of distribution of one of the divisions of the trigeminal nerve, usually the maxillary division. The cause of the neuralgia is unknown. *(Moore, p 664)*

3. **(A)** The loose areolar connective tissue layer is the dangerous area of the scalp because pus or blood in it can spread easily. Infection in this layer can also be transmitted to the cranial cavity through emissary veins that pass from this layer through apertures in the cranial bones. *(Moore, p 673)*

4. **(B)** The dura mater is occasionally called the pachymenix; hence, you may hear the term pachymeningitis, which refers to inflammation of the dura mater. The pia and arachnoid together are referred to as the leptomeninges. *(Moore, p 681)*

5. **(E)** The fact that the cavernous sinus envelops the internal carotid artery and several cranial nerves is of clinical significance. In fractures of the base of the skull, the internal carotid artery may tear within the cavernous sinus, producing an arteriovenous fistula. In such cases, arterial blood rushes into the cavernous sinus, enlarging it and forcing blood into the connecting ophthalmic veins that normally drain the orbital cavity. The eye protrudes (exophthalmos) and conjunctiva becomes engorged in the side of the torn artery. The eye pulsates in synchrony with the radial pulse. *(Moore, p 692)*

6. **(B)** The tympanic muscles have a protective action in that they dampen large vibrations of the tympanic membrane resulting from loud noises. Thus, paralysis of the stapedius muscle, resulting from a lesion of the facial nerve is associated with excessive acuteness of hearing (a condition known as hyperacusia). This condition results from uninhibited movements of the stapes. *(Moore, p 773)*

7. **(C)** Occasionally, the sternocleidomastoid muscle is injured at birth, resulting in a condition known as congenital torticollis, or wryneck. There is fixed rotation and tilting of the head owing to contracture of this muscle. *(Moore, p 787)*

8. **(B)** The muscular triangle is used surgically for approaches to the thyroid and parathyroid glands and for exposure of the trachea, esophagus, and inferior levels of the carotid vascular system. *(Moore, p 803)*

9. **(C)** Severance of a sympathetic trunk in the neck interrupts the sympathetic nerve supply to the head and neck on that side. Patients have a severe sympathetic disturbance known as the Horner syndrome, consisting of pupillary constriction, ptosis, sinking of the eye, vasodilation, and absence of sweating on the face and neck. *(Moore, p 815)*

10. **(D)** Foreign bodies entering the pharynx may become lodged in the piriform recess. If sharp, they may pierce the mucous membrane and injure the internal laryngeal nerve. *(Moore, p 836)*

Developmental Head and Neck Questions

DIRECTIONS (Questions 1 through 10): Each group of items in this section consists of lettered headings followed by a set of numbered words or phrases. For each numbered word or phrase, select the ONE lettered heading that is most closely associated with it. Each lettered heading may be selected once, more than once, or not at all.

(A) 1st pharyngeal arch
(B) 2nd pharyngeal arch
(C) 3rd pharyngeal pouch
(D) 4th pharyngeal pouch
(E) 3rd pharyngeal arch
(F) 4th pharyngeal arch
(G) 1st pharyngeal pouch
(H) 2nd pharyngeal pouch

1. Mandibular process

2. Stylopharyngeus muscle

3. Auditory (eustachian) tube

4. Incus and malleus

5. Thyroid cartilage

6. Maxilla

7. Palatine tonsil

8. Inferior parathyroid

9. Mandible

10. Stapedius muscle

ANSWERS AND EXPLANATIONS

1. **(A)** The 1st pharyngeal arch consists of a dorsal portion, known as the maxillary process, extending forward beneath the region of the eye, and a ventral portion, the mandibular process, which contains Meckel's cartilage. *(Sadler, p 302)*

2. **(E)** The cartilage of this arch produces the lower part of the body and the greater horn of the hyoid bone. The musculature is limited to the stylopharyngeus muscle. *(Sadler, p 304)*

3. **(G)** The 1st pharyngeal pouch forms a stalk-like diverticulum, the tubotympanic recess, which comes in contact with the epithelial lining of the 1st pharyngeal cleft, the future external auditory meatus. The distal portion of the outpocketing widens into a sac-like structure, the primitive tympanic or middle ear cavity, whereas the proximal part remains narrow, forming the auditory (eustachian) tube. *(Sadler, p 305)*

4. **(A)** During further development, Meckel's cartilage located in the 1st pharyngeal arch retrogresses and disappears, except for two small portions at its dorsal end that persist and form the incus and malleus. *(Sadler, p 302)*

5. **(F)** The cartilaginous components of the 4th pharyngeal arch fuse with the 6th pharyngeal arch to form the thyroid, cricoid, arytenoid, corniculate, and cuneiform cartilages of the larynx. *(Sadler, p 305)*

6. **(A)** The mesenchyme of the maxillary process subsequently gives rise to the premaxilla, maxilla, zygomatic bone, and part of the temporal bone through membranous ossification. *(Sadler, p 302)*

7. **(H)** The epithelial lining of the 2nd pharyngeal pouch proliferates and forms buds which penetrate into the surrounding mesenchyme. The buds are

secondarily invaded by mesodermal tissue, thus forming the primordium of the palatine tonsil. *(Sadler, p 305)*

8. **(C)** The 3rd and 4th pouches are characterized at their distal extremity by a dorsal and a ventral wing. In the 5th week, the epithelium of the dorsal wing of the 3rd pouch differentiates into the inferior parathyroid gland, while that of the ventral part forms the thymus. *(Sadler, p 306)*

9. **(A)** The mandible is similarly formed by membranous ossification of the mesenchymal tissue surrounding Meckel's cartilage of the 1st pharyngeal arch. *(Sadler, p 302)*

10. **(B)** The muscles of the 2nd pharyngeal arch include the stapedius, the stylohyoid, the posterior belly of the digastric, the auricular, and the muscles of facial expression. *(Sadler, p 305)*

Nervous Head and Neck
Questions

(A) olfactory

(B) optic

(C) oculomotor

(D) trochlear

(E) trigeminal

(F) abducens

(G) facial

(H) vestibulocochlear

(I) glossopharyngeal

(J) vagus

(K) spinal accessory

(L) hypoglossal

1. Associated with the superior orbital fissure, supraorbital foramen, foramen rotundum, infraorbital foramen, foramen ovale, mandibular foramen, and mental foramen

2. Has axons that pass through the cribriform plate

3. Innervates the lateral rectus muscle

4. Innervates the genioglossus, hyoglossus, and styloglossus muscles

5. Passes through the foramen magnum and the jugular foramen

6. Innervates the buccinator muscle

7. Enters the internal acoustic meatus and exits the stylomastoid foramen

8. Innervates the stylopharyngeus muscle

9. Innervates the superior oblique muscle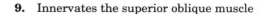

10. Innervates the muscles of mastication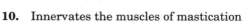

11. Innervates the medial rectus muscle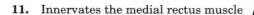

12. Supplied by the central artery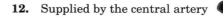

ANSWERS AND EXPLANATIONS

1. **(E)** The ophthalmic division of the trigeminal nerve passes through the superior orbital fissure and then passes through the supraorbital foramen. The maxillary division passes through the foramen rotundum, pterygopalatine fossa, inferior orbital fissure, infraorbital groove, infraorbital canal, and the infraorbital foramen. The mandibular division of the trigeminal nerve passes through the foramen ovale, infratemporal, fossa, mandibular foramen, mandibular canal, and mental foramen. *(Moore, p 680)*

2. **(A)** Axons of olfactory cells located in the olfactory epithelium pass through the cribriform plate to reach the olfactory bulbs. *(Moore, p 680)*

3. **(F)** All orbital muscles are supplied by the oculomotor except the superior oblique and the lateral rectus, which are supplied by the trochlear and abducens, respectively. *(Moore, p 716)*

4. **(L)** All muscles of the tongue except the palatoglossus are supplied by the hypoglossal nerve. *(Moore, p 747)*

5. **(K)** The accessory nerve is a motor nerve consisting of spinal and cranial roots. The spinal root is composed of fibers that arise from cervical segments of the spinal cord. They pass superiorly in the subarachnoid space to enter the posterior cranial fossa through the foramen magnum. Both roots leave the skull through the jugular foramen. *(Moore, p 791)*

6. **(G)** The buccinator muscle, as all muscles of facial expression, receives its motor innervation from the facial nerve. *(Moore, p 655)*

7. **(G)** The facial nerve enters the internal acoustic meatus and emerges from the skull through the stylomastoid foramen between the mastoid and styloid processes of the temporal bone. *(Moore, p 664)*

8. **(I)** The stylopharyngeus muscle is innervated by the glossopharyngeal nerve. *(Moore, p 828)*

9. **(D)** All orbital muscles are supplied by the oculomotor except the superior oblique and the lateral rectus, which are supplied by the trochlear and abducens, respectively. *(Moore, p 716)*

10. **(E)** The muscles of mastication are innervated by the mandibular division of the trigeminal nerve. *(Moore, p 716)*

11. **(C)** All orbital muscles are supplied by the oculomotor except the superior oblique and the lateral rectus, which are supplied by the trochlear and abducens, respectively. *(Moore, p 716)*

12. **(B)** The optic nerve is supplied by one of the smallest but most important branches of the ophthalmic artery. It pierces the optic nerve and runs within it to emerge through the optic disk. *(Moore, p 716)*

Illustrations
Questions

SUPERFICIAL VEINS OF THE NECK
(Questions 1 through 11)

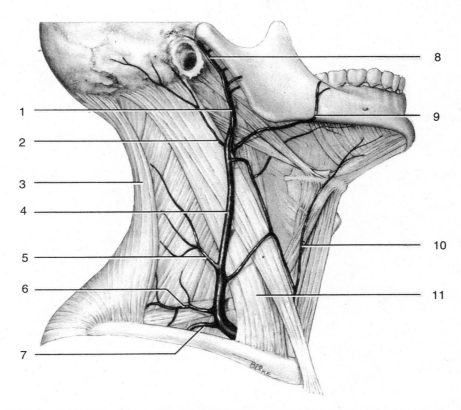

Figure 2–1. Superficial veins of the neck. (Modified and reproduced, with permission, from Montgomery RL: *Head and Neck,* McGraw-Hill, p. 27, 1980.)

Directions: With reference to the diagram, match the numbered structures with their corresponding lettered items.

(A) external jugular vein

(B) transverse cervical vein

(C) posterior auricular vein

(D) suprascapular vein

(E) trapezius muscle

(F) posterior external jugular vein

(G) superficial temporal vein

(H) retromandibular vein

(I) sternocleidomastoid muscle

(J) anterior jugular vein

(K) facial vein

TYPICAL CERVICAL VERTEBRAE
(Questions 12 through 23)

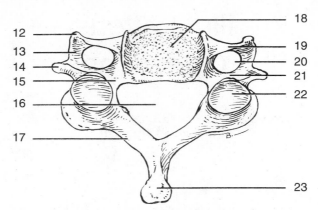

Figure 2–2. Typical cervical vertebrae. (Modified and reproduced, with permission, from Montgomery RL: *Head and Neck,* McGraw-Hill, p. 44, 1980.)

Directions: With reference to the diagram, match the numbered structures with their corresponding lettered items.

(A) pedicle

(B) superior articular surface

(C) spinous process

(D) vertebral foramen

(E) anterior tubercle

(F) lamina

(G) costal process

(H) costotransverse lamella

(I) transverse foramen

(J) body

(K) posterior tubercle

(L) lateral process

INFRAHYOID MUSCLES—LATERAL VIEW
(Questions 24 through 35)

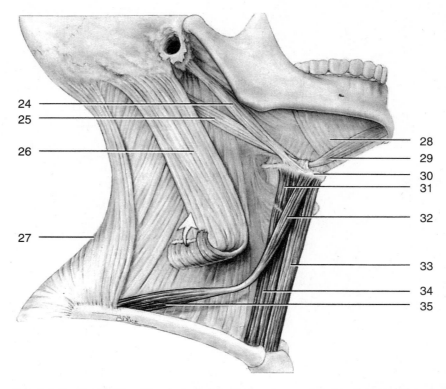

Figure 2–3. Infrahyoid muscles—lateral view. (Modified and reproduced, with permission, from Montgomery RL: *Head and Neck,* McGraw-Hill, p. 57, 1980.)

Directions: With reference to the diagram, match the numbered structures with their corresponding lettered items.

(A) trapezius

(B) omohyoid

(C) posterior belly of digastric

(D) sternohyoid

(E) mylohyoid

(F) stylohyoid

(G) sternocleidomastoid

(H) anterior belly of digastric

(I) sternothyroid

(J) hyoid

(K) thyrohyoid

INFRAHYOID MUSCLES—ANTERIOR VIEW
(Questions 36 through 50)

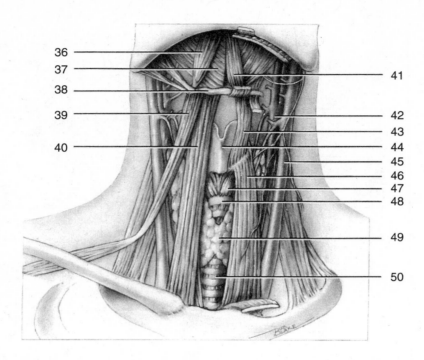

Figure 2–4. Infrahyoid muscles—anterior view. (Modified and reproduced, with permission, from Montgomery RL: *Head and Neck,* McGraw-Hill, p. 57, 1980.)

Directions: With reference to the diagram, match the numbered structures with their corresponding lettered items.

(A) thyroid gland
(B) common carotid
(C) thyroid cartilage
(D) anterior belly of digastric
(E) thyrohyoid
(F) cricoid cartilage
(G) mylohyoid
(H) sternothyroid

(I) trachea
(J) omohyoid
(K) internal jugular vein
(L) sternohyoid
(M) geniohyoid
(N) hyoid
(O) cricothyroid muscle

THE SUBMANDIBULAR TRIANGLE
(Questions 51 through 62)

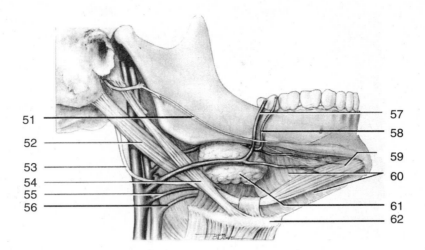

Figure 2–5. The submandibular triangle. (Modified and reproduced, with permission, from Montgomery RL: *Head and Neck,* McGraw-Hill, p. 88, 1980.)

Directions: With reference to the diagram, match the numbered structures with their corresponding lettered items.

(A) stylohyoid muscle

(B) facial vein

(C) mylohyoid muscle

(D) mandibular branch of facial nerve

(E) hyoid

(F) posterior belly of digastric

(G) lingual artery

(H) anterior belly of digastric muscle

(I) hypoglossal nerve

(J) submandibular gland

(K) facial artery

(L) lingual vein

THYROID GLAND
(Questions 63 through 75)

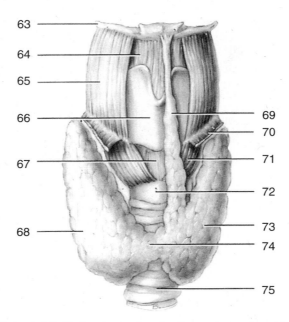

Figure 2–6. Thyroid gland. (Modified and reproduced, with permission, from Montgomery RL: *Head and Neck,* McGraw-Hill, p. 58, 1980.)

Directions: With reference to the diagram, match the numbered structures with their corresponding lettered items.

(A) thyrohyoid membrane

(B) thyroid cartilage

(C) sternothyroid

(D) hyoid

(E) cricothyroid

(F) thyrohyoid

(G) cricothyroid membrane

(H) cricoid cartilage

(I) left lobe of thyroid gland

(J) thyroid isthmus

(K) right lobe of thyroid gland

(L) pyramidal lobe

(M) trachea

THYROID GLAND, VENOUS DRAINAGE
(Questions 76 through 89)

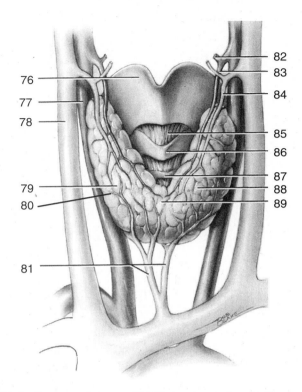

Figure 2–7. Thyroid gland, venous drainage. (Modified and reproduced, with permission, from Montgomery RL: *Head and Neck,* McGraw-Hill, p. 58, 1980.)

Directions: With reference to the diagram, match the numbered structures with their corresponding lettered items.

(A) right lobe of thyroid gland

(B) internal jugular vein

(C) inferior thyroid vein

(D) common carotid

(E) superior laryngeal artery

(F) thyroid cartilage

(G) middle thyroid vein

(H) superior thyroid artery

(I) cricothyroid membrane

(J) cricoid cartilage

(K) thyroid gland isthmus

(L) left lobe of thyroid gland

(M) superior thyroid vein

(N) trachea

PARATHYROID GLANDS
(Questions 90 through 101)

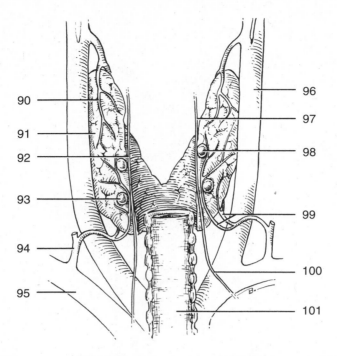

Figure 2–8. Parathyroid glands. (Modified and reproduced, with permission, from Montgomery RL: *Head and Neck,* McGraw-Hill, p. 61, 1980.)

Directions: With reference to the diagram, match the numbered structures with their corresponding lettered items.

(A) thyroid gland

(B) inferior parathyroid gland

(C) trachea

(D) common carotid

(E) superior thyroid artery

(F) left inferior laryngeal nerve

(G) inferior thyroid artery

(H) subclavian artery

(I) right recurrent laryngeal nerve

(J) right inferior laryngeal nerve

(K) superior parathyroid gland

(L) thyrocervical trunk

INTERNAL AND EXTERNAL CAROTID ARTERIES
(Questions 102 through 117)

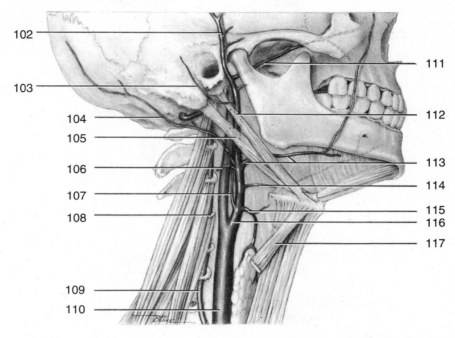

Figure 2–9. Internal and external carotid arteries. (Modified and reproduced, with permission, from Montgomery RL: *Head and Neck,* McGraw-Hill, p. 63, 1980.)

Directions: With reference to the diagram, match the numbered structures with their corresponding lettered items.

(A) posterior belly of the digastric
(B) internal carotid artery
(C) maxillary artery
(D) common carotid artery
(E) cervical portion of facial artery
(F) external carotid artery
(G) superficial temporal artery
(H) omohyoid muscle

(I) vertebral artery
(J) posterior auricular artery
(K) 4th cervical vertebra
(L) stylohyoid muscle
(M) ascending pharyngeal artery
(N) superior thyroid artery
(O) lingual artery
(P) occipital artery

CERVICAL SYMPATHETIC TRUNK
(Questions 118 through 129)

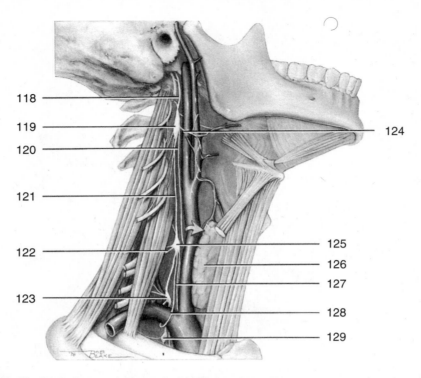

Figure 2–10. Cervical sympathetic trunk. (Modified and reproduced, with permission, from Montgomery RL: *Head and Neck,* McGraw-Hill, p. 80, 1980.)

Directions: With reference to the diagram, match the numbered structures with their corresponding lettered items.

(A) superior cervical cardiac nerve

(B) ansa subclavia

(C) 1st thoracic ganglion

(D) internal carotid nerve

(E) middle cervical cardiac nerve

(F) inferior cervical ganglion

(G) thyroid gland

(H) cervical sympathetic trunk

(I) external carotid nerve

(J) superior cervical ganglion

(K) middle cervical ganglion

(L) gray rami

DEEP MUSCULATURE OF THE NECK
(Questions 130 through 137)

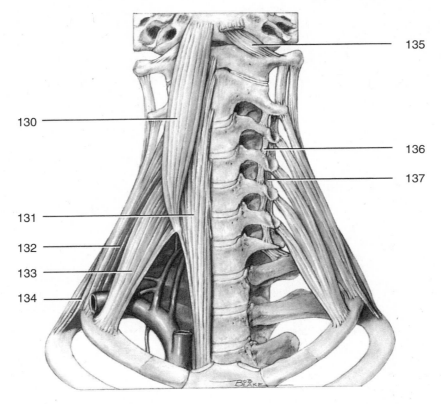

Figure 2–11. Deep musculature of the neck. (Modified and reproduced, with permission, from Montgomery RL: *Head and Neck,* McGraw-Hill, p. 107, 1980.)

Directions: With reference to the diagram, match the numbered structures with their corresponding lettered items.

(A) middle scalene muscle

(B) rectus capitis anterior

(C) longus colli muscle

(D) anterior intertransverse muscle

(E) longus capitis muscle

(F) posterior scalene muscle

(G) posterior intertransverse muscle

(H) anterior scalene muscle

ANTERIOR VIEW OF THE CARTILAGES OF THE LARYNX
(Questions 138 through 150)

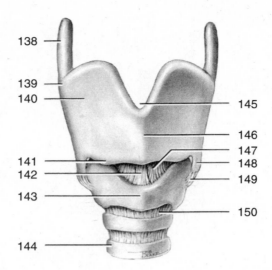

Figure 2–12. Anterior view of the cartilages of the larynx. (Modified and reproduced, with permission, from Montgomery RL: *Head and Neck,* McGraw-Hill, p. 112, 1980.)

Directions: With reference to the diagram, match the numbered structures with their corresponding lettered items.

(A) inferior thyroid tubercle

(B) arch of cricoid cartilage

(C) cricotracheal ligament

(D) elastic cone

(E) cricothyroid joint and capsule

(F) inferior horn of thyroid cartilage

(G) superior thyroid notch

(H) median cricothyroid ligament

(I) superior horn of thyroid cartilage

(J) tracheal cartilage

(K) lamina of thyroid cartilage

(L) superior thyroid tubercle

(M) laryngeal prominence

POSTERIOR VIEW OF THE CARTILAGES OF THE LARYNX
(Questions 151 through 162)

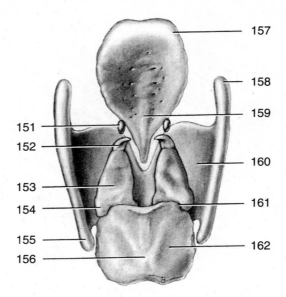

Figure 2–13. Posterior view of the cartilages of the larynx. (Modified and reproduced, with permission, from Montgomery RL: *Head and Neck,* McGraw-Hill, p. 112, 1980.)

Directions: With reference to the diagram, match the numbered structures with their corresponding lettered items.

(A) inferior horn of thyroid

(B) epiglottic cartilage

(C) epiglottic tubercle

(D) cuneiform cartilage

(E) cricoid cartilage

(F) arytenoid articular surface of cricoid cartilage

(G) corniculate cartilage

(H) lamina of thyroid cartilage

(I) arytenoid cartilage

(J) median crest of cricoid cartilage

(K) superior horn of thyroid cartilage

(L) muscular process

THE LARYNX
(Questions 163 through 173)

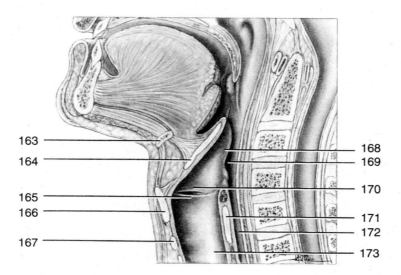

Figure 2–14. The larynx. (Modified and reproduced, with permission, from Montgomery RL: *Head and Neck,* McGraw-Hill, p. 111, 1980.)

Directions: With reference to the diagram, match the numbered structures with their corresponding lettered items.

(A) aryepiglottic fold

(B) trachea

(C) cricoid cartilage

(D) superior laryngeal aperture

(E) thyroid cartilage

(F) epiglottic cartilage

(G) esophagus

(H) hyoid bone

(I) vestibular fold

(J) vocal folds

MUSCLES OF THE SUBMANDIBULAR TRIANGLE
(Questions 174 through 185)

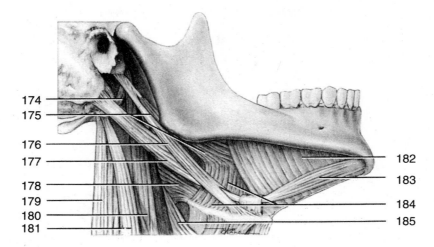

Figure 2–15. Muscles of the submandibular triangle. (Modified and reproduced, with permission, from Montgomery RL: *Head and Neck,* McGraw-Hill, p. 88, 1980.)

Directions: With reference to the diagram, match the numbered structures with their corresponding lettered items.

(A) styloglossus

(B) scalenus medius

(C) inferior pharyngeal constrictor

(D) anterior belly of digastric muscle

(E) rectus capitis

(F) longus capitis

(G) posterior belly of digastric muscle

(H) hyoglossus

(I) middle pharyngeal constrictor

(J) mylohyoid

(K) levator scapulae

(L) stylohyoid

THE SUBLINGUAL GLAND
(Questions 186 through 194)

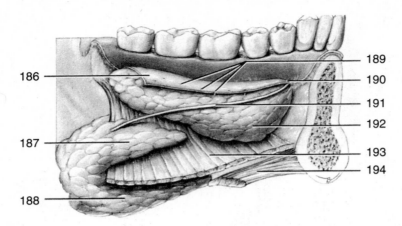

Figure 2–16. The sublingual gland. (Modified and reproduced, with permission, from Montgomery RL: *Head and Neck,* McGraw-Hill, p. 91, 1980.)

Directions: With reference to the diagram, match the numbered structures with their corresponding lettered items.

(A) submandibular gland (superficial portion)

(B) anterior belly of digastric muscle

(C) sublingual gland

(D) sublingual ducts

(E) mylohyoid muscle

(F) oral mucous membrane

(G) submandibular duct

(H) submandibular gland (deep portion)

(I) sublingual caruncle

INNERVATION OF THE SUBMANDIBULAR
AND SUBLINGUAL GLANDS
(Questions 195 through 204)

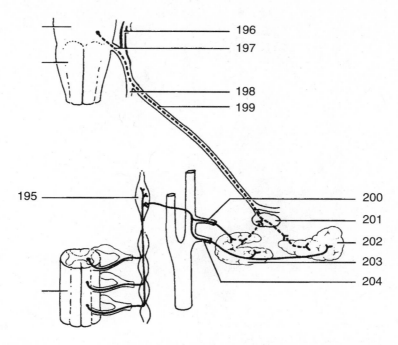

Figure 2–17. Innervation of the submandibular and sublingual glands. (Modified and reproduced, with permission, from Montgomery RL: *Head and Neck,* McGraw-Hill, p. 91, 1980.)

Directions: With reference to the diagram, match the numbered structures with their corresponding lettered items.

(A) chorda tympani

(B) lingual nerve

(C) sublingual gland

(D) lingual artery

(E) mandibular division of trigeminal nerve

(F) superior cervical ganglion

(G) mylohyoid nerve

(H) facial artery

(I) submandibular ganglion

(J) submandibular gland

ANTERIOR VIEW OF THE SKULL
(Questions 205 through 230)

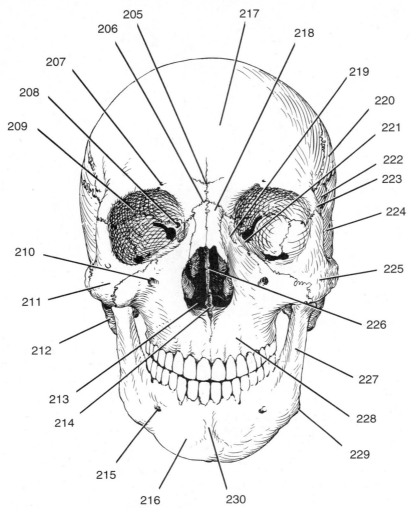

Figure 2–18. Anterior view of the skull. (Modified and reproduced, with permission, from Chusid JG: *Correlative Neuroanatomy & Functional Neurology,* 19th ed. Lange, 1985.)

Directions: With reference to the diagram, match the numbered structures with their corresponding lettered items.

(A) ethmoid bone

(B) ramus of mandible

(C) supraorbital foramen

(D) zygomatic process

(E) lacrimal bone

(F) mental foramen

(G) infraorbital foramen

(H) mastoid process

(I) zygomatic bone

(J) maxilla

(K) zygomatic arch

(L) frontal bone

(M) angle of mandible

(N) glabella

(O) optic foramen

(P) sphenoid bone

(Q) vomer

(R) frontal bone

(S) nasal bone

(T) temporal bone

(U) nasal cavity

(V) orbital cavity

(W) parietal bone

(X) symphysis menti

(Y) nasion

(Z) mandible

LATERAL VIEW OF THE SKULL
(Questions 231 through 256)

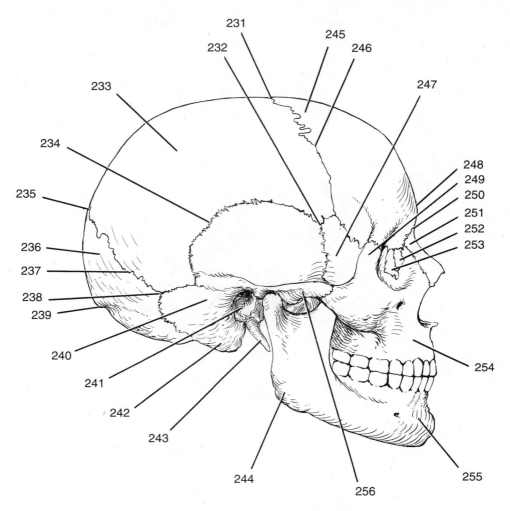

Figure 2–19. Lateral view of the skull. (Modified and reproduced, with permission, from Waxman SG, deGroot J: *Correlative Neuroanatomy,* 22nd ed. Appleton & Lange, 1995.)

Directions: With reference to the diagram, match the numbered structures with their corresponding lettered items.

(A) greater wing of sphenoid

(B) external occipital protuberance

(C) external acoustic meatus

(D) squamosal suture

(E) coronal suture

(F) zygomatic bone

(G) frontal bone

(H) angle of mandible

(I) lambdoidal suture

(J) lacrimal bone

(K) bregma

(L) parietal bone

(M) ethmoid bone

(N) pterion

(O) maxilla

(P) occipital bone

(Q) lambda

(R) glabella

(S) zygomatic arch

(T) nasion

(U) mandible

(V) mastoid process

(W) styloid process

(X) temporal bone

(Y) nasal bone

(Z) asterion

BASAL VIEW OF THE SKULL
(Questions 257 through 283)

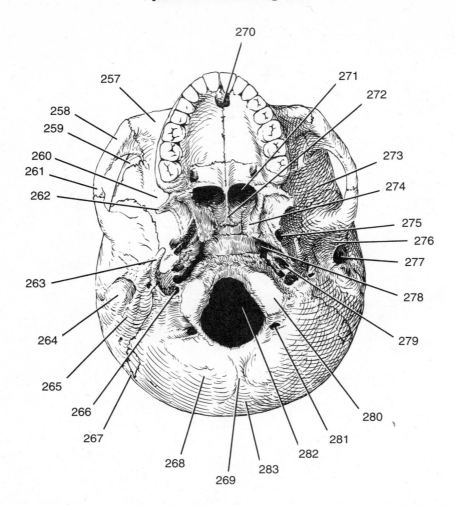

Figure 2–20. Basal view of the skull (external aspect, inferior view). (Modified and reproduced, with permission, from Waxman SG, deGroot J: *Correlative Neuroanatomy,* 22nd ed. Appleton & Lange, 1995.)

Directions: With reference to the diagram, match the numbered structures with their corresponding lettered items.

(A) posterior nasal aperture

(B) external acoustic meatus

(C) inion, or external occipital protuberance

(D) lateral pterygoid plate

(E) condylar canal

(F) medial pterygoid plate

(G) external occipital crest

(H) occipital condyle

(I) zygomatic bone

(J) occipital bone

(K) sphenoid bone

(L) mandibular fossa

(M) jugular foramen

(N) incisive foramen

(O) styloid process

(P) carotid canal

(Q) maxilla

(R) vomer

(S) foramen lacerum

(T) frontal bone

(U) asterion

(V) temporal bone

(W) mastoid process

(X) zygomatic arch

(Y) foramen ovale

(Z) parietal bone

(AA) foramen magnum

BASE OF THE SKULL SHOWING THE FOSSAL AND PRINCIPAL FORAMENS
(Questions 284 through 300)

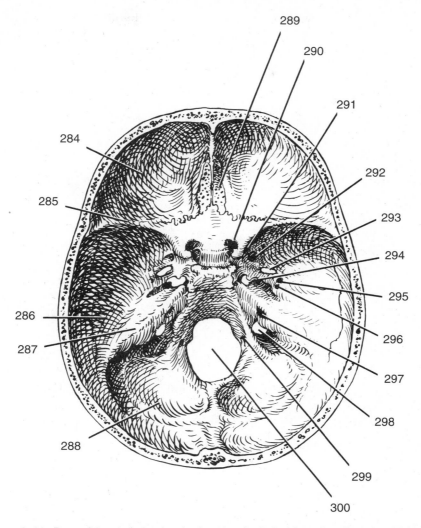

Figure 2–21. Base of the skull showing the fossal and principal foramens (superior view). (Modified and reproduced, with permission, from Waxman SG, deGroot J: *Correlative Neuroanatomy & Functional Neurology,* 22nd ed. Appleton & Lange, 1995.)

Directions: With reference to the diagram, match the numbered structures with their corresponding lettered items.

(A) cribriform plate of ethmoid

(B) anterior cranial fossa

(C) superior orbital fissure

(D) petrous pyramid

(E) innominate canal

(F) foramen ovale

(G) posterior cranial fossa

(H) internal acoustic meatus

(I) middle cranial fossa

(J) optic foramen

(K) sphenoid ridge

(L) foramen magnum

(M) foramen rotundum

(N) jugular foramen

(O) foramen lacerum

(P) hypoglossal canal

(Q) foramen spinosum

FACIAL MUSCULATURE
(Questions 301 through 320)

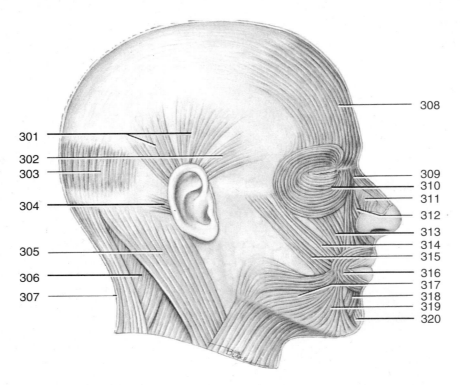

Figure 2–22. Facial musculature. (Modified and reproduced, with permission, from Montgomery RL: *Head and Neck,* McGraw-Hill, p. 182, 1980.)

Directions: With reference to the diagram, match the numbered structures with their corresponding lettered items.

(A) occipitalis

(B) procerus muscle

(C) compressor naris muscle

(D) levator labii superioris alaeque nasi

(E) zygomaticus major

(F) orbicularis oris

(G) sternocleidomastoid muscle

(H) depressor labii inferioris

(I) mentalis

(J) superior auricular muscle

(K) posterior auricular muscle

(L) frontalis

(M) orbicularis oculi

(N) levator labii superioris

(O) zygomaticus minor

(P) platysma

(Q) splenius muscle

(R) depressor anguli oris

(S) trapezius muscle

(T) anterior auricular muscle

PAROTID GLAND AND FACIAL NERVE
(Questions 321 through 330)

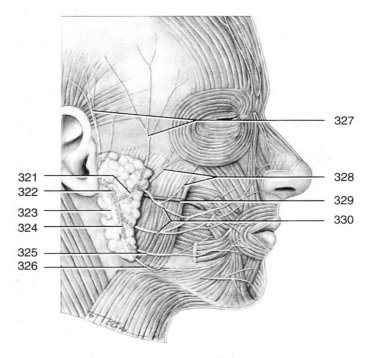

Figure 2–23. Parotid gland and facial nerve. (Modified and reproduced, with permission, from Montgomery RL: *Head and Neck,* McGraw-Hill, p. 192, 1980.)

Directions: With reference to the diagram, match the numbered structures with their corresponding lettered items.

(A) facial nerve

(B) temporal branch

(C) parotid duct

(D) buccal branches

(E) cervical branch

(F) cervicofacial division of facial nerve

(G) parotid gland

(H) zygomatic branches

(I) temporofacial division of facial nerve

(J) marginal mandibular branch of facial nerve

THE PRINCIPAL ARTERIES OF THE HEAD AND NECK
(Questions 331 through 354)

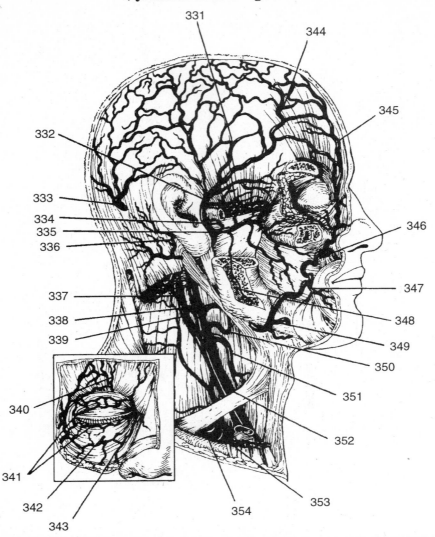

Figure 2–24. The principal arteries of the head and neck. (Modified and reproduced, with permission, from Chusid JG: *Correlative Neuroanatomy & Functional Neurology,* 19th ed. Lange, 1985.)

Directions: With reference to the diagram, match the numbered structures with their corresponding lettered items.

(A) maxillary

(B) internal carotid

(C) parietal branch

(D) frontal branch

(E) subclavian

(F) thyrocervical trunk

(G) common carotid

(H) superficial temporal

(I) superior thyroid

(J) supraorbital

(K) lingual

(L) occipital

(M) posterior auricular

(N) inferior labial

(O) frontal

(P) lateral palpebral

(Q) superior labial

(R) infraorbital

(S) inferior alveolar

(T) angular

(U) occipital

(V) external carotid

(W) middle meningeal

(X) facial

ANTERIOR VIEW OF THE SKULL
(Questions 355 through 371)

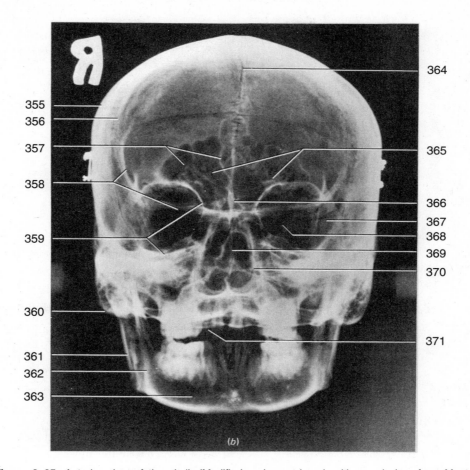

355
356
357
358
359
360
361
362
363

364
365
366
367
368
369
370
371

(b)

Figure 2–25. Anterior view of the skull. (Modified and reproduced, with permission, from Montgomery RL: *Head and Neck,* McGraw-Hill, p. 143, 1980.)

Directions: With reference to the diagram, match the numbered structures with their corresponding lettered items.

(A) orbital rim
(B) external oblique line
(C) mandibular body
(D) lambdoid suture
(E) outer cortex
(F) superior orbital fissure
(G) mastoid process
(H) nasal septum
(I) lateral wall of nasal cavity

(J) crista galli
(K) inner cortex
(L) greater wing of sphenoid
(M) base of skull
(N) sagittal suture
(O) frontal sinus
(P) mandibular ramus
(Q) floor of anterior cranial fossa

THE PALATE
(Questions 372 through 388)

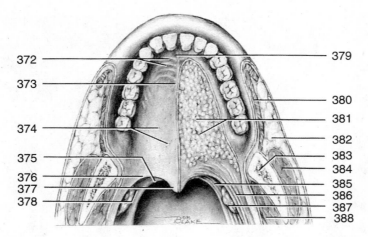

Figure 2–26. The palate. (Modified and reproduced, with permission, from Montgomery RL: *Head and Neck,* McGraw-Hill, p. 240, 1980.)

Directions: With reference to the diagram, match the numbered structures with their corresponding lettered items.

(A) palatoglossal arch

(B) incisive papilla

(C) buccal fat pad

(D) uvula

(E) ramus of mandible

(F) palatopharyngeus muscle

(G) transverse palatine ridges

(H) supratonsillar fossa

(I) palatoglossus muscle

(J) palatine tonsil

(K) palatine raphe

(L) medial pterygoid muscle

(M) masseter muscle

(N) palatine glands

(O) orifice of palatine glands

(P) buccinator muscle

(Q) palatopharyngeal arch

DEEP FASCIA OF THE JAWS
(Questions 389 through 418)

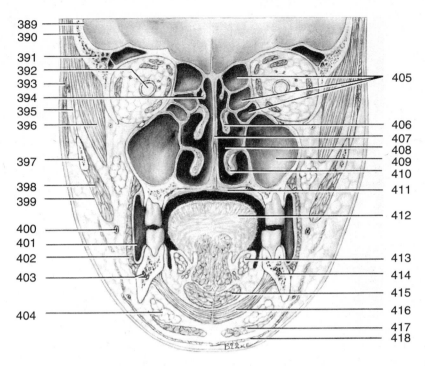

Figure 2–27. Deep fascia of the jaws. (Modified and reproduced, with permission, from Montgomery RL: *Head and Neck,* McGraw-Hill, p. 220, 1980.)

Directions: With reference to the diagram, match the numbered structures with their corresponding lettered items.

(A) temporalis
(B) masseteric fascia
(C) vestibule of mouth
(D) submandibular gland
(E) dura mater
(F) zygoma
(G) maxillary sinus
(H) diploe
(I) mylohyoid muscle
(J) nasal cavity
(K) anterior facial vein
(L) greater wing of sphenoid
(M) masseter muscle
(N) geniohyoid muscle
(O) nasal septum

(P) mandible
(Q) optic nerve
(R) sublingual gland
(S) anterior auricular muscle
(T) middle nasal concha
(U) palate
(V) tongue
(W) anterior belly of digastric muscle
(X) superior nasal concha
(Y) ethmoidal air cells
(Z) platysma
(AA) inferior nasal concha
(AB) buccinator muscle
(AC) temporal fascia
(AD) inferior alveolar artery and nerve

EXTERNAL VIEW OF THE PHARYNX
(Questions 419 through 441)

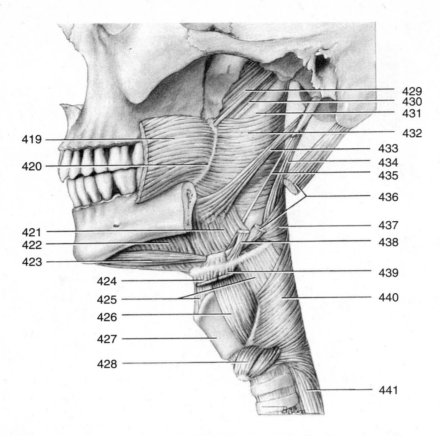

Figure 2–28. External view of the pharynx. (Modified and reproduced, with permission, from Montgomery RL: *Head and Neck,* McGraw-Hill, p. 127, 1980.)

Directions: With reference to the diagram, match the numbered structures with their corresponding lettered items.

(A) thyroid cartilage
(B) cricothyroid muscle
(C) thyrohyoid muscle
(D) esophagus
(E) inferior pharyngeal constrictor
(F) thyrohyoid membrane
(G) superior belly of omohyoid muscle
(H) stylohyoid muscle
(I) sternohyoid muscle
(J) tensor veli palatini muscle
(K) levator veli palatini muscle
(L) anterior belly of digastric muscle

(M) pharyngobasilar fascia
(N) mylohyoid muscle
(O) superior pharyngeal constrictor
(P) hyoglossus muscle
(Q) styloglossus muscle
(R) stylopharyngeus muscle
(S) pterygomandibular raphe
(T) stylohyoid ligament
(U) posterior belly of digastric muscle
(V) buccinator muscle
(W) middle pharyngeal constrictor

PARASAGITTAL VIEW OF SOFT PALATE AND PHARYNX
(Questions 442 through 463)

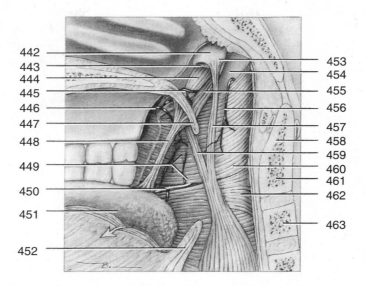

442
443
444
445
446
447
448
449
450
451
452

453
454
455
456
457
458
459
460
461
462
463

Figure 2–29. Parasagittal view of soft palate and pharynx. (Modified and reproduced, with permission, from Montgomery RL: *Head and Neck,* McGraw-Hill, p. 126, 1980.)

Directions: With reference to the diagram, match the numbered structures with their corresponding lettered items.

(A) tonsillar fossa
(B) palatoglossus muscle
(C) glossopharyngeal nerve
(D) muscular uvula
(E) dorsum of tongue
(F) lesser palatine artery
(G) epiglottis
(H) ascending palatine branch of facial artery
(I) torus tubaris
(J) pharyngobasilar fascia
(K) tensor veli palatini muscle
(L) levator veli palatini muscle

(M) salpingopharyngeal muscle
(N) pharyngeal opening of auditory tube
(O) palatine branch of ascending pharyngeal artery
(P) superior pharyngeal constrictor
(Q) axis
(R) middle pharyngeal constrictor
(S) cartilage of auditory tube
(T) third cervical vertebra
(U) palatopharyngeus muscle
(V) dens

THE MOUTH AND ORAL CAVITY
(Questions 464 through 492)

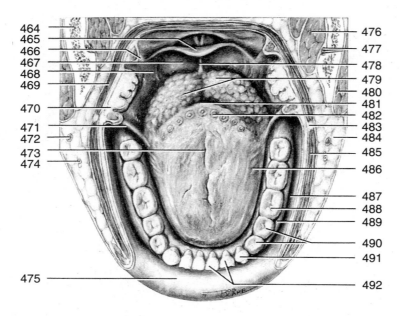

Figure 2–30. The mouth and oral cavity. (Modified and reproduced, with permission, from Montgomery RL: *Head and Neck,* McGraw-Hill, p. 229, 1980.)

Directions: With reference to the diagram, match the numbered structures with their corresponding lettered items.

(A) superior pharyngeal constrictor
(B) palatopharyngeal fold
(C) medial lingual sulcus
(D) ramus of mandible
(E) facial vein
(F) canine teeth
(G) lateral glossoepiglottic fold
(H) premolar teeth
(I) oral vestibule
(J) foliate papilla
(K) buccal fat pad
(L) masseter muscle
(M) median glossoepiglottic fold
(N) medial pterygoid muscle
(O) inferior alveolar artery vein and nerve

(P) lingual tonsil and follicles
(Q) foramen cecum
(R) vallate papilla
(S) buccinator muscle
(T) palatoglossal fold
(U) epiglottis
(V) lower lip
(W) vallecula of epiglottis
(X) incisor teeth
(Y) gingiva
(Z) first molar tooth
(AA) pterygomandibular raphe
(AB) facial artery raphe
(AC) palatine tonsil

THE TONGUE
(Questions 493 through 513)

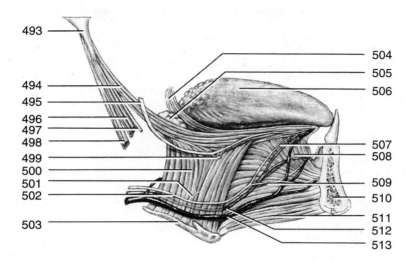

Figure 2–31. The tongue. (Modified and reproduced, with permission, from Montgomery RL: *Head and Neck,* McGraw-Hill, p. 236, 1980.)

Directions: With reference to the diagram, match the numbered structures with their corresponding lettered items.

(A) lingual artery
(B) mandible
(C) styloglossus nerve
(D) dorsum of tongue
(E) hyoid bone
(F) submandibular ganglion
(G) stylohyoid ligament
(H) stylopharyngeus muscle
(I) geniohyoid muscle
(J) genioglossus muscle
(K) palatine tonsil

(L) stylohyoid muscle
(M) lingual vein
(N) lingual nerve
(O) styloglossus muscle
(P) styloid process
(Q) nerve to styloglossus muscle
(R) hyoglossus muscle
(S) palatoglossus muscle
(T) nerve to hyoglossus muscle
(U) hypoglossal nerve
(V) nerve to muscle

POSTERIOR VIEW OF SOFT PALATE AND PHARYNX
(Questions 514 through 543)

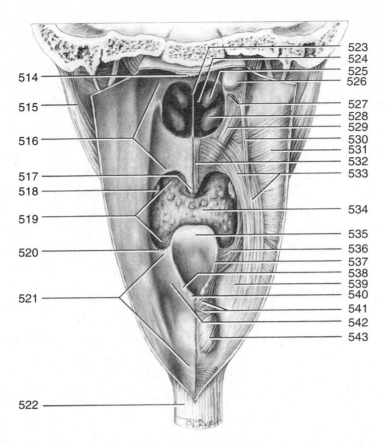

Figure 2–32. Posterior view of soft palate and pharynx. (Modified and reproduced, with permission, from Montgomery RL: *Head and Neck,* McGraw-Hill, p. 125, 1980.)

Directions: With reference to the diagram, match the numbered structures with their corresponding lettered items.

(A) oblique arytenoid muscle

(B) base of tongue

(C) nasal septum

(D) pharyngeal tonsil

(E) cartilage of auditory tube

(F) tensor veli palatini muscle

(G) posterior belly of digastric muscle

(H) superior pharyngeal constrictor

(I) pharyngeal opening of auditory tube

(J) nasal pharynx

(K) pharyngoepiglottic fold

(L) uvula

(M) aryepiglottic fold

(N) palatine tonsil

(O) stylopharyngeus muscle

(P) oral pharynx

(Q) cuneiform tubercle

(R) lateral glossoepiglottic fold

(S) laryngeal pharynx

(T) epiglottis

(U) esophagus

(V) middle nasal concha

(W) inferior nasal concha

(X) salpingopharyngeus muscle

(Y) posterior cricoarytenoid muscle

(Z) posterior nasal aperture

(AA) palatopharyngeus muscle

(AB) corniculate tubercle

(AC) piriform recess

MUSCLES OF THE LARYNX
(Questions 544 through 561)

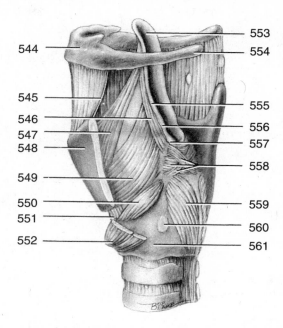

544
545
546
547
548
549
550
551
552

553
554
555
556
557
558
559
560
561

Figure 2–33. Muscles of the larynx. (Modified and reproduced, with permission, from Montgomery RL: *Head and Neck,* McGraw-Hill, p. 117, 1980.)

Directions: With reference to the diagram, match the numbered structures with their corresponding lettered items.

(A) cricothyroid muscle
(B) greater horn of hyoid
(C) median cricothyroid ligament
(D) cuneiform tubercle
(E) thyrohyoid membrane
(F) posterior cricoarytenoid muscle
(G) lateral cricoarytenoid muscle
(H) epiglottis
(I) oblique and transverse arytenoid muscles

(J) thyroarytenoid muscle
(K) thyroid articular surface
(L) corniculate tubercle
(M) thyroid cartilage
(N) cricoid cartilage
(O) aryepiglottic fold
(P) thyroepiglottic muscle
(Q) body of hyoid
(R) aryepiglottic muscle

EXTERNAL, MIDDLE, AND INTERNAL EAR
(Questions 562 through 588)

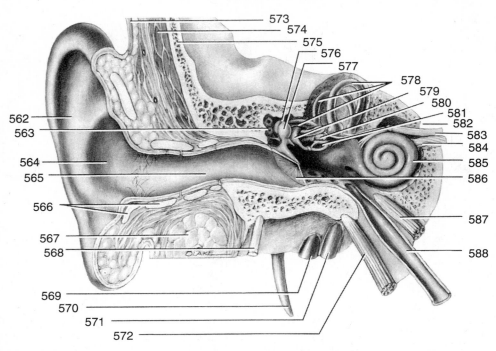

Figure 2–34. External, middle, and internal ear. (Modified and reproduced, with permission, from Montgomery RL: *Head and Neck,* McGraw-Hill, p. 296, 1980.)

Directions: With reference to the diagram, match the numbered structures with their corresponding lettered items.

(A) external acoustic meatus
(B) parotid gland
(C) integument
(D) superior ligament of the malleus
(E) semicircular canals
(F) styloid process
(G) auricle
(H) head of malleus
(I) epitympanic recess
(J) temporalis muscle
(K) auditory tube
(L) concha
(M) incus

(N) levator veli palatine muscle
(O) stapes
(P) internal acoustic meatus
(Q) cartilage of external ear
(R) cochlear nerve
(S) cochlear duct
(T) tympanic membrane
(U) internal carotid artery
(V) vestibular nerve
(W) facial nerve
(X) tensor tympani muscle
(Y) internal jugular vein
(Z) squama of temporal bone

EYEBROW AND EYELIDS
(Questions 589 through 600)

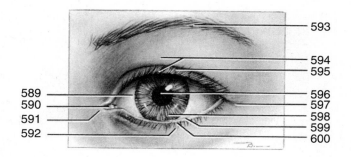

Figure 2–35. Eyebrow and eyelids. (Modified and reproduced, with permission, from Montgomery RL: *Head and Neck,* McGraw-Hill, p. 259, 1980.)

Directions: With reference to the diagram, match the numbered structures with their corresponding lettered items.

(A) lower lid

(B) bulbar conjunctiva over sclera

(C) upper eyelid

(D) lateral angle of eye

(E) posterior border of eyelid

(F) anterior border of eyelid

(G) iris

(H) medial angle of eye

(I) eyebrow

(J) pupil

(K) sulcus of upper eyelid

(L) lacrimal caruncle

THE LACRIMAL DRAINAGE SYSTEM
(Questions 601 through 612)

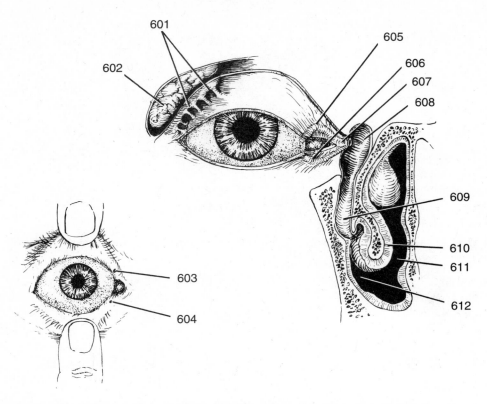

Figure 2–36. The lacrimal drainage system. (Modified and reproduced, with permission, from Thompson J, Elstrom ER: Radiography of the nasolacrimal passageways. *Med Radiog Photogr* 1949;25(3):66.)

Directions: With reference to the diagram, match the numbered structures with their corresponding lettered items.

(A) inferior punctum
(B) lacrimal sac
(C) inferior concha
(D) nasolacrimal duct
(E) secretory ducts
(F) common canalicular duct

(G) lacrimal gland
(H) superior canaliculus
(I) nasal cavity
(J) superior punctum
(K) inferior meatus
(L) inferior canaliculus

INTERNAL STRUCTURES OF THE HUMAN EYE
(Questions 613 through 645)

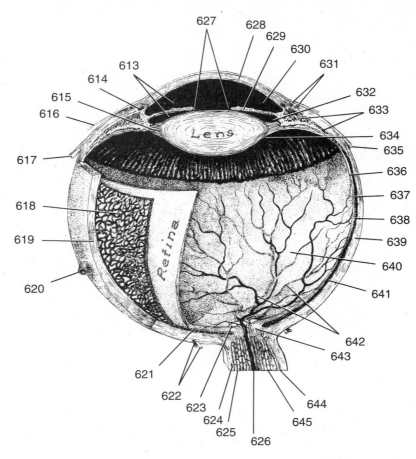

Figure 2–37. Internal structures of the human eye. (Redrawn from an original by Paul Peck. Modified and reproduced, with permission, from *The Anatomy of the Eye*. Courtesy of Lederle Laboratories.)

Directions: With reference to the diagram, match the numbered structures with their corresponding lettered items.

(A) choroid
(B) pupil
(C) anterior chamber angle
(D) aqueous
(E) medial rectus muscle
(F) vitreous
(G) canal of Schlemm
(H) retinal pigment epithelium
(I) retinal arterioles and veins
(J) zonule
(K) pia
(L) conjunctiva
(M) lamina cribrosa
(N) lateral rectus muscle
(O) arachnoid
(P) optic nerve

(Q) vortex vein
(R) long posterior ciliary artery and long ciliary nerve
(S) central retinal artery and vein
(T) sclera
(U) dura
(V) cornea
(W) episcleral vein
(X) ciliary body
(Y) ora serrata
(Z) macula
(AA) iris
(AB) retina
(AC) posterior chamber
(AD) optic disk
(AE) lens capsule

ANTERIOR CHAMBER ANGLE AND SURROUNDING STRUCTURES
(Questions 646 through 667)

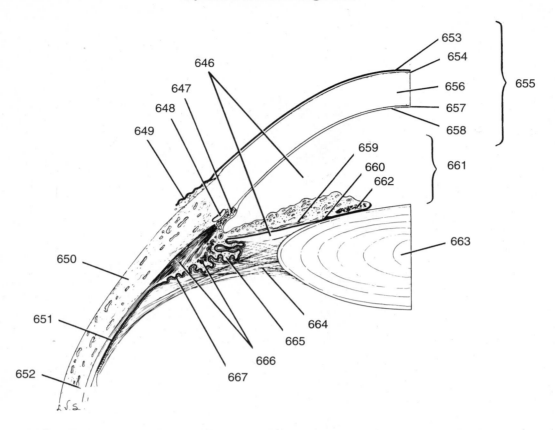

Figure 2–38. Anterior chamber angle and surrounding structures. (Modified and reproduced, with permission, from Vaughan D, Asbury T: *General Ophthalmology,* 11th ed. Appleton & Lange, 1986.)

Directions: With reference to the diagram, match the numbered structures with their corresponding lettered items.

(A) trabecular meshwork
(B) pars plana
(C) Bowman's membrane
(D) endothelium of cornea
(E) dilator muscle
(F) conjunctiva
(G) epithelium of cornea
(H) aqueous
(I) Descemet's membrane
(J) sphincter muscle
(K) lens

(L) canal of Schlemm
(M) stroma of cornea
(N) ciliary epithelium
(O) ciliary muscle
(P) iris
(Q) pigment layer of iris
(R) sclera
(S) cornea
(T) zonular fibers
(U) ciliary process
(V) ora serrata

Answers

SUPERFICIAL VEINS OF THE NECK

1. (H)
2. (C)
3. (E)
4. (A)
5. (F)
6. (B)
7. (D)
8. (G)
9. (K)
10. (J)
11. (I)

TYPICAL CERVICAL VERTEBRAE

12. (E)
13. (H)
14. (K)
15. (A)
16. (D)
17. (F)
18. (J)
19. (G)
20. (I)
21. (L)
22. (B)
23. (C)

INFRAHYOID MUSCLES—LATERAL VIEW

24. (F)
25. (C)
26. (G)
27. (A)
28. (E)
29. (H)
30. (J)
31. (K)
32. (B)
33. (D)
34. (I)
35. (B)

INFRAHYOID MUSCLES—ANTERIOR VIEW

36. (D)
37. (G)
38. (N)
39. (J)
40. (L)
41. (M)
42. (B)
43. (E)
44. (C)
45. (K)
46. (H)
47. (O)
48. (F)
49. (A)
50. (I)

SUBMANDIBULAR TRIANGLE

51. (D)
52. (F)
53. (I)
54. (A)
55. (L)
56. (G)
57. (B)
58. (K)
59. (H)
60. (C)
61. (J)
62. (E)

THYROID GLAND

63. (D)
64. (A)
65. (F)
66. (B)
67. (G)
68. (K)
69. (L)
70. (C)
71. (E)
72. (H)
73. (I)
74. (J)
75. (M)

THYROID GLAND, VENOUS DRAINAGE

76. (F)
77. (D)
78. (B)
79. (A)
80. (G)
81. (C)
82. (E)
83. (H)
84. (M)
85. (I)
86. (J)
87. (N)
88. (L)
89. (K)

PARATHYROID GLANDS

90. (E)
91. (A)
92. (F)
93. (B)
94. (L)
95. (H)
96. (D)
97. (J)
98. (K)
99. (G)
100. (I)
101. (C)

INTERNAL AND EXTERNAL CAROTID ARTERIES

102. (G)	110. (D)
103. (J)	111. (C)
104. (P)	112. (L)
105. (A)	113. (E)
106. (B)	114. (O)
107. (M)	115. (N)
108. (K)	116. (F)
109. (I)	117. (H)

CERVICAL SYMPATHETIC TRUNK

118. (D)	124. (I)
119. (J)	125. (K)
120. (A)	126. (G)
121. (H)	127. (E)
122. (L)	128. (B)
123. (F)	129. (C)

DEEP MUSCULATURE OF THE NECK

130. (E)	134. (F)
131. (C)	135. (B)
132. (A)	136. (D)
133. (H)	137. (G)

ANTERIOR VIEW OF THE CARTILAGES OF THE LARYNX

138. (I)	145. (G)
139. (L)	146. (M)
140. (K)	147. (D)
141. (A)	148. (F)
142. (H)	149. (E)
143. (B)	150. (C)
144. (J)	

POSTERIOR VIEW OF THE CARTILAGES OF THE LARYNX

151. (D)	157. (B)
152. (G)	158. (K)
153. (I)	159. (C)
154. (L)	160. (H)
155. (A)	161. (F)
156. (J)	162. (E)

THE LARYNX

163. (H)	169. (D)
164. (F)	170. (I)
165. (J)	171. (C)
166. (E)	172. (G)
167. (C)	173. (B)
168. (A)	

MUSCLES OF THE SUBMANDIBULAR TRIANGLE

174. (E)	180. (F)
175. (A)	181. (K)
176. (L)	182. (J)
177. (G)	183. (D)
178. (I)	184. (H)
179. (B)	185. (C)

THE SUBMANDIBULAR GLAND

186. (F)	191. (G)
187. (H)	192. (C)
188. (A)	193. (E)
189. (D)	194. (B)
190. (I)	

INNERVATION OF THE SUBMANDIBULAR AND SUBLINGUAL GLANDS

195. (F)	200. (H)
196. (E)	201. (I)
197. (A)	202. (C)
198. (G)	203. (J)
199. (B)	204. (D)

ANTERIOR VIEW OF THE SKULL

205. (N)	218. (S)
206. (Y)	219. (E)
207. (C)	220. (W)
208. (O)	221. (A)
209. (V)	222. (P)
210. (G)	223. (D)
211. (I)	224. (T)
212. (H)	225. (I)
213. (U)	226. (A)
214. (Q)	227. (B)
215. (F)	228. (J)
216. (Z)	229. (M)
217. (R)	230. (X)

LATERAL VIEW OF THE SKULL

231.	(K)	244.	(H)
232.	(N)	245.	(G)
233.	(L)	246.	(E)
234.	(D)	247.	(A)
235.	(Q)	248.	(R)
236.	(P)	249.	(F)
237.	(I)	250.	(T)
238.	(Z)	251.	(Y)
239.	(B)	252.	(J)
240.	(X)	253.	(M)
241.	(C)	254.	(O)
242.	(V)	255.	(U)
243.	(W)	256.	(S)

BASAL VIEW OF THE SKULL

257.	(Q)	271.	(A)
258.	(I)	272.	(R)
259.	(T)	273.	(K)
260.	(K)	274.	(F)
261.	(X)	275.	(Y)
262.	(D)	276.	(L)
263.	(O)	277.	(B)
264.	(W)	278.	(S)
265.	(V)	279.	(P)
266.	(M)	280.	(H)
267.	(U)	281.	(E)
268.	(J)	282.	(AA)
269.	(G)	283.	(C)
270.	(N)		

BASE OF THE SKULL SHOWING THE FOSSAL AND PRINCIPAL FORAMENS

284.	(B)	293.	(F)
285.	(K)	294.	(O)
286.	(I)	295.	(Q)
287.	(D)	296.	(E)
288.	(G)	297.	(H)
289.	(A)	298.	(N)
290.	(J)	299.	(P)
291.	(C)	300.	(L)
292.	(M)		

FACIAL MUSCULATURE

301.	(J)	311.	(C)
302.	(T)	312.	(D)
303.	(A)	313.	(N)
304.	(K)	314.	(O)
305.	(G)	315.	(E)
306.	(Q)	316.	(F)
307.	(S)	317.	(P)
308.	(L)	318.	(H)
309.	(B)	319.	(R)
310.	(M)	320.	(I)

PAROTID GLAND AND FACIAL NERVE

321.	(I)	326.	(E)
322.	(A)	327.	(B)
323.	(G)	328.	(H)
324.	(F)	329.	(C)
325.	(J)	330.	(D)

THE PRINCIPAL ARTERIES OF THE HEAD AND NECK

331.	(C)	343.	(T)
332.	(H)	344.	(D)
333.	(L)	345.	(O)
334.	(W)	346.	(Q)
335.	(A)	347.	(N)
336.	(M)	348.	(S)
337.	(U)	349.	(X)
338.	(V)	350.	(K)
339.	(B)	351.	(I)
340.	(J)	352.	(G)
341.	(P)	353.	(F)
342.	(R)	354.	(E)

ANTERIOR VIEW OF THE SKULL

355.	(E)	364.	(N)
356.	(K)	365.	(D)
357.	(O)	366.	(J)
358.	(Q)	367.	(L)
359.	(A)	368.	(F)
360.	(G)	369.	(H)
361.	(P)	370.	(I)
362.	(B)	371.	(M)
363.	(C)		

THE PALATE

372.	(G)	381.	(N)
373.	(K)	382.	(C)
374.	(O)	383.	(E)
375.	(Q)	384.	(M)
376.	(A)	385.	(F)
377.	(D)	386.	(I)
378.	(H)	387.	(J)
379.	(B)	388.	(L)
380.	(P)		

DEEP FASCIA OF THE JAWS

389.	(E)	404.	(D)
390.	(H)	405.	(Y)
391.	(L)	406.	(T)
392.	(Q)	407.	(O)
393.	(S)	408.	(J)
394.	(X)	409.	(G)
395.	(AC)	410.	(AA)
396.	(A)	411.	(U)
397.	(F)	412.	(V)
398.	(M)	413.	(R)
399.	(B)	414.	(P)
400.	(K)	415.	(N)
401.	(C)	416.	(I)
402.	(AB)	417.	(W)
403.	(AD)	418.	(Z)

EXTERNAL VIEW OF THE PHARYNX

419.	(V)	431.	(M)
420.	(S)	432.	(O)
421.	(P)	433.	(Q)
422.	(N)	434.	(R)
423.	(L)	435.	(T)
424.	(I)	436.	(U)
425.	(F)	437.	(W)
426.	(C)	438.	(H)
427.	(A)	439.	(G)
428.	(B)	440.	(E)
429.	(J)	441.	(D)
430.	(K)		

PARASAGITTAL VIEW OF SOFT PALATE AND PHARYNX

442.	(S)	453.	(I)
443.	(N)	454.	(J)
444.	(K)	455.	(L)
445.	(H)	456.	(O)
446.	(F)	457.	(M)
447.	(D)	458.	(V)
448.	(B)	459.	(U)
449.	(A)	460.	(P)
450.	(C)	461.	(Q)
451.	(E)	462.	(R)
452.	(G)	463.	(T)

THE MOUTH AND ORAL CAVITY

464.	(D)	479.	(P)
465.	(U)	480.	(L)
466.	(B)	481.	(Q)
467.	(W)	482.	(R)
468.	(G)	483.	(AA)
469.	(A)	484.	(K)
470.	(AC)	485.	(S)
471.	(T)	486.	(J)
472.	(AB)	487.	(I)
473.	(C)	488.	(Z)
474.	(E)	489.	(Y)
475.	(V)	490.	(H)
476.	(N)	491.	(F)
477.	(O)	492.	(X)
478.	(M)		

THE TONGUE

493.	(P)	504.	(S)
494.	(O)	505.	(K)
495.	(N)	506.	(D)
496.	(H)	507.	(Q)
497.	(G)	508.	(J)
498.	(L)	509.	(V)
499.	(F)	510.	(B)
500.	(R)	511.	(I)
501.	(T)	512.	(A)
502.	(U)	513.	(M)
503.	(E)		

POSTERIOR VIEW OF SOFT PALATE AND PHARYNX

514.	(D)	529.	(F)
515.	(G)	530.	(X)
516.	(J)	531.	(H)
517.	(L)	532.	(L)
518.	(N)	533.	(AA)
519.	(P)	534.	(B)
520.	(R)	535.	(T)
521.	(S)	536.	(K)
522.	(U)	537.	(M)
523.	(C)	538.	(Q)
524.	(Z)	539.	(O)
525.	(V)	540.	(AB)
526.	(E)	541.	(A)
527.	(I)	542.	(AC)
528.	(W)	543.	(Y)

MUSCLES OF THE LARYNX

544.	(Q)	553.	(H)
545.	(E)	554.	(B)
546.	(R)	555.	(O)
547.	(P)	556.	(D)
548.	(M)	557.	(L)
549.	(J)	558.	(I)
550.	(G)	559.	(F)
551.	(E)	560.	(K)
552.	(A)	561.	(N)

EXTERNAL, MIDDLE, AND INTERNAL EAR

562.	(G)	576.	(D)
563.	(I)	577.	(H)
564.	(L)	578.	(E)
565.	(A)	579.	(M)
566.	(Q)	580.	(W)
567.	(B)	581.	(O)
568.	(W)	582.	(P)
569.	(Y)	583.	(V)
570.	(F)	584.	(R)
571.	(U)	585.	(S)
572.	(N)	586.	(T)
573.	(C)	587.	(X)
574.	(J)	588.	(K)
575.	(Z)		

EYEBROW AND EYELIDS

589.	(B)	595.	(K)
590.	(L)	596.	(J)
591.	(H)	597.	(D)
592.	(A)	598.	(G)
593.	(I)	599.	(E)
594.	(C)	600.	(F)

THE LACRIMAL DRAINAGE SYSTEM

601.	(E)	607.	(F)
602.	(G)	608.	(B)
603.	(J)	609.	(D)
604.	(A)	610.	(C)
605.	(H)	611.	(I)
606.	(L)	612.	(K)

INTERNAL STRUCTURES OF THE HUMAN EYE

613.	(D)	630.	(C)
614.	(G)	631.	(W)
615.	(J)	632.	(AC)
616.	(L)	633.	(X)
617.	(N)	634.	(AE)
618.	(A)	635.	(E)
619.	(T)	636.	(Y)
620.	(Q)	637.	(AB)
621.	(Z)	638.	(A)
622.	(R)	639.	(T)
623.	(AD)	640.	(F)
624.	(U)	641.	(H)
625.	(K)	642.	(I)
626.	(S)	643.	(M)
627.	(B)	644.	(O)
628.	(V)	645.	(P)
629.	(AA)		

ANTERIOR CHAMBER ANGLE AND SURROUNDING STRUCTURES

646.	(H)	657.	(D)
647.	(A)	658.	(S)
648.	(L)	659.	(E)
649.	(F)	660.	(Q)
650.	(R)	661.	(P)
651.	(B)	662.	(J)
652.	(V)	663.	(K)
653.	(G)	664.	(T)
654.	(C)	665.	(U)
655.	(M)	666.	(O)
656.	(I)	667.	(N)

CHAPTER 3

Pelvis and Perineum
Questions

DIRECTIONS (Questions 1 through 85): Each of the numbered items or incomplete statements in this section is followed by answers or by completions of the statement. Select the ONE lettered answer or completion that is BEST in each case.

1. All the following statements concerning the perineum are correct EXCEPT

    (A) it is the entire outlet of the pelvis
    (B) it is diamond-shaped
    (C) it is bounded anteriorly by the pubic symphysis
    (D) it is bounded posterolaterally on either side by the sacrotuberal ligament
    (E) it is bounded anterolaterally on either side by the superior ramus of the pubis

2. Posteriorly, the perineum ends at the

    (A) coccyx
    (B) posterior inferior iliac spine
    (C) posterior superior iliac spine
    (D) sacral spine
    (E) ischial tuberosities

3. The lymphatic drainage of the penis is to which of the following lymph nodes?

    (A) femoral
    (B) popliteal
    (C) superficial inguinal
    (D) sacral
    (E) external iliac

4. All the following statements concerning the vestibule of the vagina are correct EXCEPT

    (A) the mons pubis is part of the vestibule
    (B) the ducts of the greater vestibular glands open into the vestibule
    (C) the urethra opens into the vestibule
    (D) the vaginal opening comes to surface in the vestibule
    (E) it is the cleft between the labia minora

5. All the following statements concerning the penis are correct EXCEPT

    (A) it is composed of four cylindrical masses of cavernous tissue
    (B) the corpus spongiosum penis is traversed by the urethra
    (C) the prominent margin of the glans is the corona
    (D) the superficial dorsal vein of the penis communicates with the superficial external pudendal veins
    (E) the loose areolar tissue of the penis is devoid of fat but reinforced by a prolongation of smooth muscle

6. All the following statements concerning the scrotum are correct EXCEPT

    (A) it is divided into two chambers by the scrotal septum
    (B) the layers of the scrotum are the skin and the tunica dartos
    (C) the posterior scrotal nerves arise from the pudendal nerve
    (D) the posterior scrotal nerves are accompanied by branches of the internal pudendal artery
    (E) the cremaster muscle is located superficial to the tunica dartos *deep*

7. All the following statements concerning the clitoris are correct EXCEPT

    (A) it is the morphological equivalent of the penis
    (B) it contains the female urethra
    (C) it arises by two crura in the superficial space of the urogenital triangle
    (D) the pudendal nerve provides the dorsal nerve
    (E) the internal pudendal artery provides the blood supply

8. All the following statements concerning the bulbospongiosus muscle in males are correct EXCEPT

   (A) it covers the bulb of the penis
   (B) its muscle fibers arise from the central tendinous point of the perineum and from the median raphe anterior to it
   (C) it expels the last of the urine in the urethra
   (D) it expels the semen in ejaculation
   (E) it is the principal muscle of erection

9. All the following statements concerning the ischiocavernosus muscles in males are correct EXCEPT

   (A) they cover the crura of the penis
   (B) they impede the venous return
   (C) they maintain erection of the penis
   (D) they are innervated by the genitofemoral nerve
   (E) the muscle fibers insert into the sides and undersurface of the crus and into the corpus cavernosum

10. All the following statements concerning the pudendal nerve are correct EXCEPT

   (A) it supplies all the perineal musculature
   (B) it is sensory to most of the perineal skin surfaces
   (C) it arises in the pelvis by roots from lumbar nerves 2, 3, and 4
   (D) it passes through the greater sciatic foramen into the gluteal region
   (E) it enters the lesser sciatic foramen between the sacrotuberal and sacrospinal ligaments, accompanied by the internal pudendal vessels

11. The fascial canal formed by a split in the obturator internus fascia is known as the

   (A) inguinal canal
   (B) femoral canal
   (C) adductor canal
   (D) pudendal canal
   (E) obturator canal

12. All the following statements concerning the perineal nerve are correct EXCEPT

   (A) it arises from the pudendal nerve
   (B) it gives rise to the posterior scrotal
   (C) it gives rise to the nerve of the bulb
   (D) it gives rise to the inferior rectal nerves
   (E) it has a deep branch that is mainly muscular

13. All the following statements concerning the inferior rectal artery are correct EXCEPT

   (A) it is a branch of the internal pudendal artery
   (B) it pierces the wall of the pudendal canal
   (C) it anastomoses with the superior rectal artery
   (D) it anastomoses with the perineal artery
   (E) it pierces the wall of the femoral canal

14. Which of the following veins ascends between the arcuate pubic ligament and the transverse ligament of the perineum?

   (A) deep dorsal vein of the clitoris
   (B) superficial dorsal vein of the penis
   (C) external pudendal
   (D) internal pudendal
   (E) internal iliac

15. All the following statements concerning the perineal membrane are correct EXCEPT

   (A) it is rectangular in form
   (B) it fills the interval between the two ischiopubic rami
   (C) it contributes to, and is attached to, the central tendinous point of the perineum
   (D) it gives rise to the transverse ligament of the perineum
   (E) it is perforated by the urethra and the vagina in the female

16. All the following statements concerning the greater vestibule glands are correct EXCEPT

   (A) they are located in the deep perineal space
   (B) they are situated one on either side of the vagina
   (C) they are the homologues of the bulbourethral glands of the male
   (D) their ducts open in the grooves between the hymen and the labia minora
   (E) their ducts are approximately 2 cm long

17. The anal triangle is limited anteriorly by the

   (A) sacrotuberal ligaments
   (B) gluteus medius
   (C) external anal sphincter
   (D) posterior border of the perineal membrane
   (E) tip of the coccyx

18. The pelvis is closed inferiorly by the

   (A) obturator internus
   (B) pelvic diaphragm
   (C) sacrotuberal ligament

(D) sacral promontory

(E) coccyx

19. All the following statements concerning the broad ligament are correct EXCEPT

(A) it is a double-layered sheet of peritoneum

(B) it encloses the uterine tubes

(C) it attaches the uterus to the lateral walls and floor of the pelvis

(D) it gives rise to the mesosalpinx

(E) it assists in the formation of the transverse rectal folds

20. The mesovarium and mesosalpinx are continuous at the pelvic brim with the

(A) rectouterine pouch

(B) external anal sphincter

(C) ischioanal fossa

(D) suspensory ligament of the ovary

(E) retrovaginal septum

21. All the following statements concerning the rectum are correct EXCEPT

(A) the ampullary portion rests on the pelvic diaphragm

(B) it begins at the level of the 3rd sacral vertebra

(C) it ends in front of the tip of the coccyx

(D) it continues as the anal canal below the pelvic diaphragm

(E) it usually has five transverse folds in its interior

22. All the following statements concerning the anal columns are correct EXCEPT

(A) they consist of five to ten vertical folds of mucous membrane

(B) they overlie veins

(C) they are connected by mucosal folds known as anal valves

(D) the anal columns and anal valves characterize the lower 1.5 to 2 cm of the anal canal

(E) the anal columns are separated by grooves

23. The pectinate line is located at the

(A) "white line"

(B) cutaneous zone

(C) intermediate zone

(D) transitional zone

(E) junction of the anal valves and the transitional zone

24. All the following statements concerning the urinary bladder are correct EXCEPT

(A) when filled, it contains approximately 500 cc of urine

(B) it is attached to the base of the prostate gland in males

(C) it lies on the uterus in females

(D) it is enveloped in endopelvic fascia

(E) it is bounded posteriorly by the rectovesical septum in males

25. In spite of its rounded form, the bladder is peaked anteriorly at its apex by the

(A) broad ligament

(B) suspensory ligament

(C) frenulum pudendi

(D) median umbilical ligament

(E) interureteric fold

26. Which of the following structures is included in the female pudendum?

(A) uterus

(B) uterine tubes

(C) bulb of the vestibule

(D) cervix

(E) ovaries

27. The broad ligament encloses the

(A) greater vestibular glands

(B) clitoris

(C) mons pubis

(D) uterine tubes

(E) bulb of the vestibule

28. Bulbourethral glands in males may be located within which of the following muscles?

(A) corpora cavernosus

(B) superficial transverse perineus

(C) bulbospongiosus

(D) ischiocavernosus

(E) sphincter urethrae

29. The vesical trigone is bounded by which of the following structures at its inferior (anterior) angle?

(A) openings of the ureters

(B) urethral aperture

(C) interureteric fold

(D) puboprostatic ligament

(E) uvula

30. The arteries of the bladder are the superior and inferior vesical arteries that arise from which of the following arteries?

    (A) femoral
    (B) obturator
    (C) superior gluteal
    (D) internal iliac
    (E) aorta

31. All the following statements concerning the innervation of the bladder are correct EXCEPT

    (A) the inferior hypogastric plexus contributes to the vesical plexus
    (B) the parasympathetic innervation is provided by the vagus
    (C) the parasympathetic innervation serves the emptying reflex
    (D) afferent impulses are conducted along both the sympathetic and parasympathetic fibers
    (E) impulses of pain due to an overstretched bladder travel with the sympathetic fibers

32. All the following statements concerning the pelvic ureter are correct EXCEPT

    (A) it descends retroperitoneally on the side of the pelvic wall
    (B) it is approximately 12.5 cm long
    (C) it begins at the point where the ureter crosses the bifurcation of the common iliac artery
    (D) the lumen of the ureter is uniform throughout
    (E) it crosses medially the obturator nerve and vessels and the umbilical artery

33. In the female the ureter has several relationships of special significance, including

    (A) it is extraperitoneal
    (B) it forms the anterior and superior limits of the ovarian fossa
    (C) it is crossed obliquely by the uterine artery
    (D) it is in contact with the lateral fornix of the vagina
    (E) it crosses the cervix of the uterus

34. All the following structures are traversed by the male urethra EXCEPT the

    (A) prostate gland
    (B) sphincter urethrae muscle
    (C) superficial transverse perineus muscle
    (D) perineal membrane
    (E) penis

35. Most of the ducts of the prostate gland open into the

    (A) urethral crest
    (B) prostatic sinuses
    (C) seminal colliculus
    (D) prostatic utricle
    (E) ejaculatory duct

36. All the following statements concerning the membranous portion of the urethra in males are correct EXCEPT

    (A) it traverses the annular part of the sphincter urethrae muscle
    (B) it traverses the perineal membrane
    (C) it is the longest part of the urethra
    (D) the bulbourethral glands are located on either side of the membranous portion of the urethra
    (E) the wall of the membranous portion is thin

37. All the following statements concerning the female urethra are correct EXCEPT

    (A) it corresponds to the prostatic and membranous portions of the male
    (B) its external orifice is immediately in front of that of the vagina
    (C) it is behind the glans clitoridis
    (D) it perforates the perineal membrane
    (E) it is characterized by the absence of urethral glands

38. All the following statements concerning the general structure of the testis are correct EXCEPT

    (A) the thick external covering of the testis is the tunica albuginea
    (B) the convoluted seminiferous tubules are located in the compartments between septa
    (C) the convoluted tubes unite to form straight seminiferous tubules
    (D) the straight seminiferous tubules unite to form the rete testis
    (E) the rete testis coalesces to form the ejaculatory duct

39. All the following statements concerning the ductus deferens are correct EXCEPT

    (A) it begins at the head of the epididymis
    (B) it traverses the inguinal canal
    (C) it lies in the center of the other constituents of the spermatic cord
    (D) it can be identified by its hard and cord-like character when rolled between the fingers
    (E) emerging from the deep inguinal ring, the ductus deferens passes on the lateral side of the inferior epigastric artery

40. All the following statements concerning the seminal vesicles are correct EXCEPT

(A) they are lobulated "blind" pouches
(B) they are enclosed by external spermatic fascia
(C) they secrete an alkaline constituent of the seminal fluid
(D) they lie against the fundus of the bladder
(E) the ductus deferentes descend along their medial surface

41. All the following statements concerning the ejaculatory ducts are correct EXCEPT

(A) they lie almost completely outside the prostate
(B) they are formed just above the base of the prostate
(C) they are formed by the union of the seminal vesicle ducts with the ends of the ductus deferentes
(D) they open into the prostatic urethra on the colliculus seminalis
(E) they open at either side of the opening of the prostatic utricle

42. The ovarian artery is a branch of which of the following arteries?

(A) internal iliac
(B) external iliac
(C) femoral
(D) internal pudendal
(E) aorta

43. All the following statements concerning the uterus are correct EXCEPT

(A) it is anteflexed
(B) it is anteverted
(C) in the erect posture, it lies directly on the superior surface of the bladder
(D) the ligaments of the uterus provide the principal supports of the uterus
(E) it has an isthmus located between the body and cervix

44. Lymphatic drainage of the uterus is directed to all the following nodes EXCEPT the

(A) superficial inguinal
(B) femoral
(C) external iliac
(D) internal iliac
(E) lumbar

45. All the following statements concerning the vagina are correct EXCEPT

(A) it extends from the vestibule to the cervix
(B) the upper ends of the vagina clasp the cervix
(C) it has a mucous coat continuous with that of the uterus
(D) a thin layer of erectile tissue exists between the mucosal and muscular coats
(E) the pampiniform plexus of veins drains the vagina

46. The anterior division of the internal iliac artery gives rise to all the following arteries EXCEPT the

(A) obturator
(B) superior gluteal
(C) internal pudendal
(D) middle rectal
(E) inferior vesicle

47. The male genital organs include all the following EXCEPT the

(A) testes
(B) prostate
(C) ductus deferentes
(D) seminal vesicles
(E) penis

48. The pelvic diaphragm includes which of the following muscles?

(A) obturator internus
(B) obturator externus
(C) piriformis
(D) coccygeus
(E) transversus perineus profundus

49. Which of the following muscles is located in the lateral pelvic wall?

(A) piriformis
(B) puborectalis
(C) pubovaginalis
(D) pubococcygeus
(E) iliococcygeus

50. The entire pelvic diaphragm is innervated by which of the following nerves?

(A) pelvic splanchnic
(B) 3rd and 4th sacral
(C) inferior hypogastric plexuses
(D) sciatic
(E) superior gluteal

51. All the following statements concerning male and female pelves are correct EXCEPT

    (A) the female pelvis is more cylindrical than the male

    (B) the female sacrum is shorter and wider than the male

    (C) the female pubic tubercles are farther apart than the male

    (D) the female pubic arch makes a more acute angle than in the male

    (E) the female anterolateral pelvic wall is relatively wider than in the male

52. The pelvic diaphragm is composed of all the following muscles EXCEPT the

    (A) coccygeus

    (B) iliococcygeus

    (C) piriformis

    (D) pubococcygeus

    (E) puborectalis

53. All the following arteries are visceral branches of the internal iliac artery EXCEPT the

    (A) umbilical

    (B) inferior vesical

    (C) middle rectal

    (D) uterine

    (E) iliolumbar

54. Which of the following statements concerning the sacral plexus is correct?

    (A) it takes form on the anterior wall of the pelvis

    (B) its major part lies on the obturator internus muscle

    (C) it gives off the pudendal nerve

    (D) most of its branches pass above the piriformis to appear in the buttock

    (E) it supplies the medial cutaneous area below the knee

55. Which of these nerves is formed by posterior divisions of the sacral plexus?

    (A) common peroneal

    (B) anococcygeal

    (C) pudendal

    (D) nerve to the quadratus femoris

    (E) nerve to the obturator internus and superior gemellus

56. Which of these nerves is formed by anterior divisions of the sacral plexus?

    (A) superior gluteal

    (B) tibial

    (C) inferior gluteal

    (D) nerve to the piriformis

    (E) lateral part of the posterior femoral cutaneous nerve

57. All the following statements concerning pelvic splanchnic nerves are correct EXCEPT

    (A) they contain preganglionic parasympathetic fibers

    (B) they convey visceral afferents from the pelvic plexus to sacral segments of the spinal cord

    (C) they contribute to formation of the inferior hypogastric plexus

    (D) they are branches of the sciatic nerve

    (E) they are known as nervi erigentes

58. Which of these statements correctly describes the obturator nerve?

    (A) it arises from the sacral plexus

    (B) it passes along the lateral pelvic wall

    (C) it supplies abductor muscles of the thigh

    (D) it arises from posterior rami of sacral nerves

    (E) it gives off pelvic splanchnic nerves

59. All the following statements concerning the autonomic plexuses of the pelvis are correct EXCEPT

    (A) the superior rectal plexus consists chiefly of sympathetic fibers

    (B) the ovarian plexus consists chiefly of sympathetic fibers

    (C) parasympathetic components predominate in the inferior hypogastric plexus

    (D) the superior hypogastric plexus is known as the pelvic plexus

    (E) hypogastric nerves help to form the inferior hypogastric plexus

60. A correct description of the rectum includes which of the following statements?

    (A) it begins at the rectosigmoid junction

    (B) it is structurally straight, as its name implies

    (C) the rectal ampulla is at its upper end

    (D) the rectourethral muscle is found only in the female

    (E) its mucosa is identical to that of the sigmoid colon

61. The rectum receives its blood supply primarily by the branches of the

    (A) superior mesenteric artery

    (B) inferior mesenteric artery

    (C) inferior rectal arteries

(D) branches of the external iliac artery

(E) femoral artery

62. All the following statements concerning the inner-vation of the rectum are correct EXCEPT

(A) its motor fibers include sympathetics

(B) its motor fibers are conveyed in the middle rectal plexus

(C) its afferent supply of nerves belongs to the parasympathetic system

(D) pelvic splanchnic nerves are involved in its innervation

(E) the superior rectal plexus may supply rectal blood vessels

63. Which of these structures is not a component of the bladder?

(A) vesical trigone

(B) detrusor muscle

(C) pubovesical muscle

(D) ureteric ostia

(E) vesical sphincter

64. The male urethra traverses all the following struc-tures EXCEPT the

(A) prostate gland

(B) ejaculatory duct

(C) urogenital diaphragm

(D) sphincter urethra

(E) internal urethral orifice

65. Which of the following statements correctly de-scribes the seminal vesicles?

(A) they store sperm

(B) they secrete a seminal fluid component

(C) they lie medial to the ductus deferens

(D) they form the ampulla of the ductus deferens

(E) they empty directly, and alone, into the prostate

66. All the following structures are part of the female internal genital system EXCEPT the

(A) ovary

(B) perineal body

(C) mesovarium

(D) infundibulum

(E) vagina

67. All the following nerves are included in the uterovaginal nerve plexus EXCEPT the

(A) sympathetics

(B) parasympathetics

(C) somatic

(D) afferent

(E) vasomotor

68. Which of the following is characteristic of the vagina?

(A) its anterior fornix is deeper than the posterior fornix

(B) it terminates at the urogenital diaphragm

(C) it fuses around the cervix of the uterus

(D) normally, it is flattened laterally

(E) it allows little distention

69. The superior hypogastric plexus contains all the following types of fibers EXCEPT

(A) preganglionic sympathetic fibers

(B) postganglionic sympathetic fibers

(C) motor fibers to striated muscle

(D) visceral efferent fibers

(E) visceral afferent fibers

70. The greater part of the pelvic diaphragm is formed from the

(A) obturator internus muscle

(B) pelvic fascia

(C) perineal membrane

(D) levator ani

(E) coccygeus

71. Which of the following statements correctly de-scribes the urogenital region of the perineum?

(A) it contains the rectum

(B) it contains the ischiorectal fossa

(C) it includes the coccygeal triangle

(D) it is pierced by the urethra

(E) its floor is the obturator internus muscle

72. Which of the following arteries is the chief blood supply of the perineum?

(A) obturator

(B) superior gluteal

(C) iliolumbar

(D) external iliac

(E) internal pudendal

73. Which of the following nerves is the major inner-vation of the perineum?

(A) sciatic

(B) pudendal

(C) femoral

(D) obturator

(E) inferior gluteal

74. Most perineal structures send their lymphatics to the

    (A) internal iliac nodes
    (B) nodes of the lumbar chain
    (C) superficial inguinal nodes
    (D) external iliac nodes
    (E) inferior mesenteric nodes

75. All the following statements concerning the ischiorectal fossa are correct EXCEPT

    (A) they are spaces on each side of the anal canal
    (B) they contain the pudendal nerve and internal pudendal vessels
    (C) they contain connective tissue and fat
    (D) their inferior walls are formed by the levator ani muscle
    (E) they are bordered laterally by the obturator internus muscle

76. The deep perineal space is described correctly by which of the following statements?

    (A) it is filled completely by the deep perineal muscles
    (B) in the male, it surrounds the scrotum and penis
    (C) it is limited by the superficial fascia
    (D) its fascia is a continuation of abdominal fascia
    (E) it communicates directly with the ischiorectal fossa

77. Nerves required for erection of the penis are the

    (A) pudendals
    (B) inferior rectals
    (C) pelvic splanchnics
    (D) posterior scrotals
    (E) sympathetics

78. The ejaculatory duct opens into the

    (A) prostatic urethra
    (B) bulbourethral gland
    (C) ureter
    (D) penis
    (E) ductus deferens

79. All the following structures attach to the perineal body EXCEPT the

    (A) perineal membrane
    (B) ischiocavernosus
    (C) sphincter ani externus
    (D) transversus perinei superficialis
    (E) bulbospongiosus

80. Which of the following statements correctly describes the bulbourethral glands?

    (A) they are found only in the female
    (B) they open into the membranous urethra
    (C) they are located in the deep perineal pouch
    (D) they are located close to the sides of the anus
    (E) their ducts open into the scrotum

81. Which of the following structures is attached to the posterior aspect of the broad ligament?

    (A) ligament of the ovary
    (B) uterine tube
    (C) round ligament of the uterus
    (D) uterine artery
    (E) ureter

82. All the following statements correctly describe the ovary EXCEPT

    (A) it is covered with cuboidal epithelium
    (B) its anterior border is attached to the broad ligament by the mesovarium
    (C) the suspensory ligament of the ovary suspends its tubal pole
    (D) it has a smooth surface
    (E) the ligament of the ovary attaches it to the lateral margin of the uterus

83. The abdominal orifice of the uterine tube is located at its

    (A) ampulla
    (B) isthmus
    (C) uterine part
    (D) fundus
    (E) infundibulum

84. The part of the uterus that rises above the uterine tubes is the

    (A) external os
    (B) body
    (C) fundus
    (D) cervix
    (E) fornix

85. Correct relations of the female ureters include which of the following?

    (A) they are equidistant from each side of the cervix
    (B) they cross the lateral fornix of the vagina
    (C) they cross above the broad ligament
    (D) they enter the bladder behind the vagina
    (E) they cross above the uterine artery

ANSWERS AND EXPLANATIONS

1. **(E)** The perineum, defined anatomically, is the entire outlet of the pelvis. This diamond-shaped space is bounded anteriorly by the pubic symphysis and anterolaterally, on either side, by the inferior ramus of the pubis and the ramus and tuberosity of the ischium. The posterolateral limit is the sacrotuberal ligament. *(Woodburne, p 509)*

2. **(A)** Posteriorly, the perineum ends at the coccyx, and its posterolateral limit is the sacrotuberal ligament that stretches from the sides of the sacrum and the coccyx to the ischial tuberosity. *(Woodburne, p 509)*

3. **(C)** The lymphatic drainage of the penis is to the superficial inguinal nodes. *(Woodburne, p 510)*

4. **(A)** The vestibule of the vagina is the cleft between the labia minora. In its floor are the openings of the urethra, the vagina, and the ducts of the greater vestibular glands. The labia majora taper anteriorly to form the rounded fatty eminence, the mons pubis. *(Woodburne, pp 511–512)*

5. **(A)** The penis is composed of three cylindrical masses of cavernous tissue bound together by fibrous tissue and covered by skin. The prominent margin of the glans, the corona, projects backward beyond the ends of the corpora cavernosa penis. The corpus spongiosum penis is traversed by the urethra. The subcutaneous connective tissue of the penis is loose areolar tissue devoid of fat but reinforced by a prolongation of smooth muscle fibers from the tunica dartos scroti. The superficial dorsal vein of the penis communicates with the superficial external pudendal veins. *(Woodburne, p 510)*

6. **(E)** The scrotal sac is divided into two chambers by the scrotal septum. The layers of the scrotum are the skin and the tunica dartos. The posterior scrotal nerves arise from the pudendal nerve. The posterior scrotal nerves are accompanied by branches of the internal pudendal artery and vein. The cremaster muscle extends along the spermatic cord. *(Woodburne, pp 510–511)*

7. **(B)** The clitoris is the morphological equivalent of the penis but does not contain the female urethra. The clitoris arises by two crura in the superficial space of the urogenital triangle. The internal pudendal artery provides branches to the clitoris, and the pudendal nerve provides the dorsal nerve of the clitoris. *(Woodburne, p 512)*

8. **(E)** The bulbospongiosus muscle in the male overlies the bulb of the penis. Its muscle fibers arise from the central tendinous point of the perineum and form the median raphe anterior to it. The bulbospongiosus muscle expels the last of the urine in the urethra. It also serves as an accessory muscle of erection for the penis by compressing the bulb and impeding the venous return. It expels the semen in ejaculation. *(Woodburne, pp 513–514)*

9. **(D)** The ischiocavernosus muscles cover the crura of the penis (or clitoris). Its fibers insert into the sides and undersurface of the crus and into the corpus cavernosum. The ischiocavernosus muscles compress the crura, impede the venous return, and maintain erection of the penis (or clitoris). The muscles are supplied by the pudendal nerve, not the genitofemoral. *(Woodburne, p 514)*

10. **(C)** The pudendal nerve is almost the sole somatic nerve of the perineum. It supplies all the perineal musculature and is sensory to most of its skin surfaces. The pudendal nerve arises in the pelvis by roots from sacral nerves 2, 3, and 4. It passes through the greater sciatic foramen into the gluteal region, where it lies medial and inferior to the sciatic nerve. It then crosses the spine of the ischium to enter the lesser sciatic foramen between the sacrotuberal and sacrospinal ligaments, accompanied by the internal pudendal vessels. *(Woodburne, p 514)*

11. **(D)** The pudendal canal is formed by a split in the obturator internus fascia on the lateral wall of the ischioanal fossa. The canal crosses the obturator internus muscle about 4 cm above the lower margin of the ischial tuberosity and conducts the pudendal nerve and the internal pudendal vessels to the urogenital triangle of the perineum. *(Woodburne, p 514)*

12. **(D)** The pudendal nerve has three branches—the inferior rectal, the perineal, and the dorsal nerve of the penis. The perineal branch gives rise to the posterior scrotal and a deep branch that is mainly muscular, supplying branches to the superficial transverse perineus, the bulbospongiosus, the ischiocavernosus, the deep transverse perineus, and the sphincter urethra muscles. *(Woodburne, pp 514–515)*

13. **(E)** The internal pudendal artery traverses the pudendal canal, distributing to the same areas and having essentially the same branches as the pudendal nerve. The inferior rectal branch pierces the wall of the pudendal canal to provide branches across the ischioanal fossa to the muscles and skin of the anal region. The inferior rectal artery anastomoses with the superior rectal, middle rectal, and perineal arteries. *(Woodburne, p 515)*

14. **(A)** The superficial dorsal vein of the penis runs backward immediately under the skin to the pubic symphysis, where it ends in the superficial exter-

nal pudendal veins. The deep dorsal vein of the penis (clitoris) lies in the midline under the deep fascia of the penis. At the root of the penis (clitoris), it passes between the two halves of the suspensory ligament and then ascends between the arcuate pubic ligament and the transverse ligament of the perineum. *(Woodburne, pp 515–516)*

15. **(A)**   The perineal membrane, triangular in form, fills the interval between the two ischiopubic rami. It contributes to, and is attached to, the central tendinous point of the perineum. Its anterior margin forms the transverse ligament of the perineum. The perineal membrane is perforated by the urethra and vagina in the female. *(Woodburne, p 516)*

16. **(A)**   The greater vestibular glands are the homologues of the bulbourethral glands of the male, but they lie in the superficial space of the perineum. They are situated one on either side of the vagina. Their ducts are about 2 cm long and open in grooves between the hymen and the labia minora. *(Woodburne, p 519)*

17. **(D)**   The anal triangle of the perineum is limited behind by the tip of the coccyx and in front by the posterior border of the perineal membrane (line between the anterior parts of the ischial tuberosities). *(Woodburne, p 520)*

18. **(B)**   The pelvis is closed inferiorly by the pelvic diaphragm, reinforced below by the perineal membrane. The inferior aperture, or outlet, is diamond-shaped and is bounded by the back of the pubis, the ischiopubic rami, the ischial tuberosities, the sacrotuberal ligaments, and the tip of the coccyx. *(Woodburne, p 523)*

19. **(E)**   The two layers of peritoneum that cover the two surfaces of the uterus come together at the margins of the uterus and extend laterally toward the side walls of the pelvis. These double-layered sheets are the broad ligaments of the uterus. Enclosed in the free upper edge of each broad ligament that is superior to the mesovarium and surrounds the uterine tube is the mesosalpinx. The broad ligament is not related to the transverse rectal folds located in the interior of the rectum. *(Woodburne, pp 524–525)*

20. **(D)**   The mesovarium and the mesosalpinx are continuous at the pelvic brim with the suspensory ligament of the ovary. The lateral part of the mesosalpinx is free, and the end of the uterine tube curves downward along the posterior border of the ovary. *(Woodburne, p 524)*

21. **(E)**   The ampullary portion of the rectum rests on the pelvic diaphragm. The rectum begins at about the level of the 3rd sacral vertebra and ends about 4 cm below in front of the tip of the coccyx. The side-to-side sinuosity of the rectum is a reflection of the transverse rectal folds in its interior. Three folds are usually present. *(Woodburne, p 525)*

22. **(D)**   The anal columns are from five to ten vertical folds of mucous membrane, separated by grooves, which overlie veins. The columns are connected by mucosal folds, the anal valves. The anal valves and the anal columns characterize the upper 1.5 to 2 cm of the anal canal. *(Woodburne, p 528)*

23. **(E)**   At the underside of the valves, the mucous membrane becomes continuous with the smooth skin of the transitional zone along an irregular line known as the pectinate line. The mucous membrane of the anal canal exhibits differentiation at various levels. The skin of the margin of the anus is pigmented, contains hair follicles and glands, and covers the cutaneous zone of the canal. Internal to it is the intermediate zone (transitional zone), about 1 cm wide, which is characterized by smooth hairless skin. The line of change from the cutaneous zone to the intermediate zone is referred to clinically as the "white line." *(Woodburne, pp 527–528)*

24. **(C)**   The rectovesical septum separates the ampullary portion of the rectum from the fundus of the bladder and from the ductus deferentes, the seminal vesicles, and the posterior surface of the prostate gland. When it is filled, it contains about 500 cc of urine. The bladder rests on, and is firmly attached to, the base of the prostate gland in the male. In the female, it lies on the pelvic diaphragm. The bladder is enveloped in endopelvic fascia. *(Woodburne, pp 525,528–529)*

25. **(D)**   In spite of its rounded form, the bladder is peaked anteriorly at its apex by the remains of its original connection to the allantois, the urachus. In the adult, this is reduced to a fibrous strand that connects the apex of the bladder to the connective tissue of the umbilicus. It is known as the median umbilical ligament. *(Woodburne, p 529)*

26. **(C)**   The female pudendum includes the urethral and vaginal openings, mons pubis, clitoris, bulb of the vestibule, and the greater vestibular glands. The internal female genital organs include the ovaries, uterine tubes, uterus, cervix, and vagina. *(Woodburne, pp 511,537)*

27. **(D)**   Structures located in the pudendum, such as the clitoris, greater vestibular glands, bulb of the vestibule, and mons pubis, are not enclosed by the broad ligament. Internal structures, such as the ovarian ligament, part of the round ligament, the uterine artery and venous plexus, the uterovaginal

plexus of nerves, and part of the ureters, are enclosed by the broad ligament. (Woodburne, pp 538, 540)

28. **(E)** The small bulbourethral glands of the male are embedded in the fibers of the sphincter urethrae muscle. The bulbospongiosus muscle in the male overlies the bulb of the penis. The ischiocavernosus muscle covers the crura of the penis. The superficial transverse perineus muscles arise on the ischial tuberosities and insert into the peroneal body. (Woodburne, pp 513–514)

29. **(B)** In the fundus of the bladder, there is a small triangular area, the vesical trigone, where the mucous membrane is firmly bound to the muscular coat and is always smooth. The vesical trigone is bounded by the openings of the ureters at its posterolateral angles and by the urethral aperture at its inferior (anterior angle). A ridge stands out between the ureteral openings known as the interureteric fold. The uvula of the bladder is a small tongue-like elevation of the trigone above and behind the urethral aperture. It is due to the middle lobe of the prostate. (Woodburne, pp 529–530)

30. **(D)** The arteries of the bladder are the superior and inferior vesical arteries that arise from the anterior trunk of the internal iliac artery. (Woodburne, p 530)

31. **(B)** The vesical plexus is a continuation of the anterior portion of the inferior hypogastric plexus and contains postganglionic sympathetic and preganglionic parasympathetic fibers. The parasympathetic fibers are branches of the pelvic splanchnic nerves that join the inferior hypogastric plexus from sacral nerves 2, 3, and 4. The parasympathetic innervation of the bladder serves the emptying reflex. Afferent impulses are conducted along both the sympathetic and parasympathetic fibers. Impulses of pain due to an overstretched bladder travel with the sympathetic fibers. (Woodburne, p 530)

32. **(D)** The pelvic portion is about 12.5 cm long and begins at the point where the ureter crosses the bifurcation of the common iliac artery or the beginning of the external iliac artery. The pelvic ureter descends retroperitoneally on the pelvic wall. It crosses medially the obturator nerve and vessels and the umbilical artery. The lumen of the ureter is not uniform throughout. It is slightly constricted where it crosses the common iliac artery; it is narrowest in its passage through the bladder wall. (Woodburne, p 531)

33. **(C)** In the female, the ureter has several relationships of special significance. As it descends and then turns forward along the lateral wall of the pelvis, it underlies the parietal peritoneum behind and below the ovary and forms the posterior and inferior limits of the ovarian fossa. It then runs forward and medialward toward the bladder, passing the cervix of the uterus and the lateral fornix of the vagina, at a distance of from 1 to 2 cm. In this portion of its course, the ureter is crossed obliquely by the uterine artery. (Woodburne, p 532)

34. **(C)** The male urethra traverses the prostate gland, the sphincter urethrae muscle, the perineal membrane, and the penis. The superficial transverse perineus muscle is not traversed by the male urethra. (Woodburne, p 532)

35. **(B)** A narrow, longitudinal ridge in the posterior wall of the male urethra, the urethral crest, indents the lumen, so that it is crescentic in cross-section. The grooves on either side of the crest are the prostatic sinuses, and it is here that most of the ducts of the prostate gland open. Beyond the midlength of the crest, there is a rounded eminence, the seminal colliculus. In the median plane of the colliculus, a small slit leads into a pouch that is the prostatic utricle. On each side of the mouth of the prostatic utricle is the more minute opening of the ejaculatory duct. (Woodburne, p 532)

36. **(C)** The membranous portion of the urethra traverses the annular part of the sphincter urethrae muscle and the perineal membrane and is the shortest part of the urethra. The bulbourethral glands lie behind and on either side of the membranous portion of the urethra. The wall of the membranous portion is thin. (Woodburne, p 533)

37. **(E)** The female urethra corresponds to the prostatic and membranous portions of the male urethra. Its external orifice is immediately in front of that of the vagina and is about 2.5 cm behind the glans clitoridis. The tube is characterized by urethral glands and urethral lacunae, as in the male. (Woodburne, p 533)

38. **(E)** The thick external covering of the testis is the tunica albuginea, composed of dense, white, fibrous, connective tissue. The tunica albuginea turns into the substance of the testis to blend with numerous septa. The convoluted seminiferous tubules are situated between the septa compartments. The convoluted seminiferous tubules unite to form a smaller number of straight seminiferous tubules. These anastomose in a network rete testis, which coalesces into twelve to fifteen efferent ducts; these perforate the tunica albuginea and form convoluted masses—the coni epididymis. (Woodburne, p 535)

39. **(A)**   The ductus deferens begins in the tail of the epididymis. It ascends in the spermatic cord and traverses the inguinal canal. The ductus deferens lies in the center of the other constituents of the spermatic cord and can be identified by its hard and cord-like character when rolled between the fingers. Emerging from the deep inguinal ring, the ductus deferens passes on the lateral side of the inferior epigastric artery. *(Woodburne, p 525)*

40. **(B)**   The seminal vesicles are lobulated "blind" pouches which secrete an alkaline constituent of the seminal fluid. They lie against the fundus of the bladder. The ductus deferentes descend along their medial surfaces. They are enclosed by endopelvic fascia and not external spermatic fascia. *(Woodburne, p 535)*

41. **(A)**   The ejaculatory ducts are formed just above the base of the prostate by the union of the ducts of the seminal vesicles with the narrowed ends of the ductus deferentes. The ejaculatory ducts lie almost completely within the prostate. The ducts open by slit-like apertures into the prostatic urethra on the colliculus seminalis at either side of the opening of the prostatic utricle. *(Woodburne, p 536)*

42. **(E)**   The ovarian artery, a branch of the abdominal aorta, reaches the hilum of the ovary by way of its suspensory ligament. Besides branches to the ovary, the vessel gives off a tubal branch that passes medialward in the mesosalpinx for the supply of the tube, and a branch that follows the ovarian ligament to the side of the uterus. *(Woodburne, p 538)*

43. **(D)**   The uterus is not completely straight; there is an angulation between its body and its cervix (anteflexion). It also forms an angle of 100 to 110 degrees with the vagina (anteversion). The isthmus of the uterus is the constricted region between the body and the cervix. The ligaments of the uterus maintain the orientation of the uterus but do not support it. The pelvic floor is the principal support. *(Woodburne, pp 538–540)*

44. **(B)**   The lymphatic drainage of the uterus is directed to the following nodes, principally on a regional basis: The body of the uterus drains to the external and internal iliac nodes; the fundus drains into the lumbar nodes. A few lymph vessels follow the round ligament of the uterus and end in the superficial inguinal nodes. *(Woodburne, p 541)*

45. **(E)**   The veins emerge from the testis and form the dense pampiniform plexus, from which is derived the testicular vein. The vagina extends from the vestibule to the cervix of the uterus. The upper end of the vagina, clasping the cervix, is circular. The vagina has a mucous coat continuous with that of the uterus. A thin layer of erectile tissue exists between the mucosal and muscular coats. The veins form a vaginal plexus along the lateral aspect of the vagina. The efferent vessels of the plexus are tributary to the internal iliac veins. *(Woodburne, pp 535,541,543)*

46. **(B)**   The internal iliac artery commonly divides into a posterior and anterior division. The posterior division gives rise to the iliolumbar, the lateral sacral, and the superior gluteal arteries. The anterior division gives rise to the obturator, internal pudendal, inferior gluteal, umbilical, inferior vesicle, middle rectal, and, in the female, the uterine and vaginal. *(Woodburne, p 543)*

47. **(B)**   The male genital organs include the testes, the ductus deferentes, the seminal vesicles, the ejaculatory ducts, and the penis. The prostate and bulbourethral glands are accessory glandular structures. *(Woodburne, pp 533–534)*

48. **(D)**   The pelvic diaphragm consists of the levator ani and coccygeus muscles and the superior and inferior fasciae. It closes the pelvic cavity posteroinferiorly and assists in the support of the abdominopelvic viscera. The muscles of the lateral pelvic wall are the piriformis and the obturator internus. *(Woodburne, pp 533–554)*

49. **(A)**   The muscles of the lateral pelvic wall are the piriformis and the obturator internus. The levator ani muscle consists of three principal parts—puborectalis, pubococcygeus, and iliococcygeus. These muscles close the pelvic cavity posteroinferiorly and assist in the support of the abdominopelvic viscera. *(Woodburne, pp 553–554)*

50. **(B)**   The entire pelvic diaphragm is innervated by anterior branches of the ventral rami of the 3rd and 4th sacral nerves. The pelvic splanchnic nerves contribute the parasympathetic supply for the pelvic viscera. The inferior hypogastric plexuses may be divided into rectal and vesicle parts in the male. The pudendal nerve is the principal nerve of the perineum. *(Woodburne, pp 551–553,555)*

51. **(D)**   In the male, the pubic arch makes a more acute angle than in the female. As compared to the male, the female pelvis is more cylindrical, shorter, and wider; the pubic tubercles are farther apart, and the anterolateral wall of the pubis is relatively wider. *(Hollinshead, p 740)*

52. **(C)**   The pelvic diaphragm consists of the coccygeus muscle posteriorly and the more extensive levator ani. The named parts of the levator ani are the pubococcygeus, puborectalis, and iliococcygeus. The coccygeus is a small muscle arising from the ischial spine and expanding to insert into the lat-

eral borders of the lower two sacral and upper two coccygeal segments. The piriformis is not a part of the pelvic diaphragm but is a muscle of the lower limb that lines part of the pelvic cavity. *(Hollinshead, pp 740–742)*

53. **(E)** The iliolumbar artery is a branch of the posterior trunk of the internal iliac artery; it branches to the pelvic wall, not to the viscera of the pelvis. The umbilical artery gives off superior vesical arteries to the bladder; the inferior vesical artery is present in the male and reaches the bladder and prostate. The middle rectal artery enters the rectum. The uterine artery, in addition to supplying the uterus, gives rise to the vaginal arteries and terminates in its tubal branch. *(Hollinshead, pp 745–747)*

54. **(C)** The sacral plexus gives off the chief somatic nerve of the perineum, the pudendal nerve. This plexus also sends branches to the pelvic diaphragm. The sacral plexus takes form on the posterior, not the anterior, wall of the pelvis; its major part lies on the anterior surface of the piriformis, not the obturator internus, muscle. All of its larger branches pass through the greater sciatic foramen, most of them below the piriformis, to appear in the buttock. The medial cutaneous area below the knee is supplied by the saphenous nerve, a branch of the femoral nerve, derived from the lumbar, not the sacral plexus. *(Hollinshead, p 749)*

55. **(A)** The common peroneal nerve is the only nerve listed to be formed by posterior divisions of the sacral plexus. The anococcygeal nerve, not considered to be a part of the sacral plexus, contributes to innervation of skin between the anus and tip of the coccyx. The other nerves listed are formed by anterior divisions of the plexus. *(Hollinshead, p 750)*

56. **(B)** The tibial nerve is the only nerve listed formed by anterior divisions of the sacral plexus. All the other nerves cited are formed by posterior divisions of the plexus. *(Hollinshead, p 750)*

57. **(D)** Pelvic splanchnic nerves have no particular relationship to the sciatic nerve; they are not considered to be part of the sacral plexus. The pelvic splanchnics are given off at spinal cord levels S3 and S4 (sometimes S2) and contribute to the formation of the inferior hypogastric or pelvic plexus. Their fibers are preganglionic parasympathetic fibers. These nerves also convey visceral afferents from the pelvic plexus to sacral segments of the spinal cord. They represent parasympathetic outflow and are known as the nervi erigentes because they are the nerves capable of causing erection of the penis or clitoris. *(Hollinshead, pp 751,754)*

58. **(B)** The obturator nerve arises from the anterior divisions of the lumbar plexus (L2, L3, L4). It passes along the lateral pelvic wall to the obturator canal. It supplies adductor, not abductor, muscles of the thigh. Pelvic splanchnic nerves are parasympathetic nerves, not branches of the obturator nerve. *(Hollinshead, pp 385–386,752)*

59. **(D)** The inferior hypogastric plexus is formed by lateral extensions of the superior hypogastric plexus, known as hypogastric nerves, and the pelvic splanchnic nerves. The inferior, not the superior, hypogastric plexus, is known as the pelvic plexus. Both the superior rectal and the ovarian plexuses consist chiefly of sympathetic fibers. Parasympathetic components predominate in the inferior hypogastric plexus. *(Hollinshead, pp 752–753)*

60. **(A)** The rectum begins at the rectosigmoid junction in front of the third sacral vertebra. Contrary to what its name implies, the rectum is not straight but presents the anteroposterior sacral flexure and three lateral curves. The part of the rectum in the region of the middle and lower curves is called the rectal ampulla. As the rectum reaches the pelvic diaphragm, most of its longitudinal muscle fibers continue downward along the anal canal, but a few of the fibers reflect from it. In the male, the anterior fibers are known as the rectourethral muscle; the slips that pass backward to the coccyx form the rectococcygeus muscle. The fluffy, rugose mucosa of the colon becomes smooth mucosa in the rectum. *(Hollinshead, pp 760–761)*

61. **(B)** The rectum is supplied primarily by the inferior mesenteric artery through the branches of its continuation, the superior rectal artery. The lower part of the rectum also receives the middle rectal arteries, branched from the internal iliac artery. They anastomose freely with the superior rectal arteries. The inferior rectal arteries supply the anal canal, rather than the rectum. *(Hollinshead, pp 761–762)*

62. **(A)** The motor fibers to the rectum appear to be entirely parasympathetic. They are conveyed in the middle rectal plexus, derived from the inferior hypogastric plexus. The afferent supply of rectal nerves, both for pain and presence of feces or gas, belongs to the parasympathetic system. Thus, the rectum receives both its afferent and efferent innervation through the pelvic splanchnic nerves in the rectal plexus. *(Hollinshead, p 763)*

63. **(E)** Several surveys have verified that there is no anatomically demonstrable vesical sphincter at the junction of the bladder and urethra. The "internal sphincter of the bladder" is a functional entity that prevents urine from entering the urethra

and ejaculate from entering the bladder; its mechanism is not understood completely. The smooth triangular area outlined by the two ureteric ostia and the internal urethral orifice is called the vesical trigone. The musculature of the bladder as a whole is referred to as the detrusor muscle. The external stratum of the bladder gives rise to the pubovesicle muscle. (*Hollinshead, pp 765–766*)

64. **(B)** The male urethra commences at the internal urethral orifice. It traverses all the structures named except the ejaculatory duct. The ejaculatory ducts enter the prostatic urethra. They are formed by the union of the ampulla of the ductus deferens with the duct of the seminal vesicle. (*Hollinshead, pp 769–770,774,796*)

65. **(B)** The seminal vesicles secrete a fluid that adds fructose to the seminal plasma for maintaining the motility of the spermatozoa. Sperm are stored in the ampulla, the ductus, and the epididymis, but not in the seminal vesicle. The seminal vesicles lie below and lateral, not medial, to the ampulla of the ductus. The distal end of the seminal vesicle becomes narrow and, together with the ductus deferens, forms the ejaculatory duct that opens in the prostatic urethra. (*Hollinshead, p 774*)

66. **(B)** All of the structures listed are parts of the internal female genital system except the perineal body. This structure, called the central tendon of the perineum, is a mass of fibromuscular tissue located between the anal canal and the vagina or bulb of the penis. A number of perineal muscles terminate in it. The perineal body is larger in the female than in the male, and it is of considerable importance in obstetrics and gynecology. (*Hollinshead, pp 744–784,784,796*)

67. **(C)** The uterovaginal autonomic plexus of nerves primarily consists of visceral afferents and sympathetic efferent fibers. It contains only a few, if any, parasympathetic efferents. It includes visceral, but not somatic, fibers. Innervation is not necessary to functions of the uterus. (*Hollinshead, p 787*)

68. **(C)** The vagina terminates by fusing around the cervix of the uterus. At the upper end, its lumen forms recesses (fornices), the posterior fornix being deeper than the anterior and lateral fornices. Normally, the vagina is flattened anteroposteriorly, not laterally. It is greatly distensible. (*Hollinshead, p 784*)

69. **(C)** No somatic motor fibers appear in the superior hypogastric nerve plexus, an autonomic plexus. It is a direct continuation of the aortic plexus below the aortic bifurcation. The visceral afferents found in the plexus mediate pain from the uterus and follow the course of sympathetic efferents. (*Hollinshead, p 753*)

70. **(D)** The pelvic diaphragm consists of the coccygeus muscle posteriorly and the more extensive and complex levator ani anterolaterally. The levator ani muscle originates along a semicircular line that skirts the pelvic walls from the pelvic surface of the body of the pubis to the ischial spine. In between these bony points, the levator ani is attached to a band-like reinforcement in the obturator fascia, the arcus tendineus. (*Hollinshead, pp 741–742*)

71. **(D)** The perineal area can be divided into two triangular regions by a line connecting the two ischial tuberosities—anteriorly, the urogenital region, and posteriorly, the anal region. The anal region contains the rectum, the anal canal, and the ischiorectal fossae on each side of the anal canal. In the urogenital region, a muscular shelf stretches between the conjoint ischiopubic rami of the two sides; this is the urogenital diaphragm. It is pierced by the urethra and, in the female, also by the vagina. The diaphragm serves for attachment of the external genitalia. The obturator internus muscle is not in the urogenital region. (*Hollinshead, p 789*)

72. **(E)** The chief blood supply of the perineum is provided by the internal pudendal artery. It is a large branch of the anterior trunk of the internal iliac artery. It leaves the pelvis between the piriformis and coccygeus muscles and descends vertically on the exterior of the levator ani into the perineum. (*Hollinshead, pp 747,790*)

73. **(B)** The pudendal nerve is the sole somatic motor nerve of the perineum; also, it is sensory to most of the perineal skin. The pudendal nerve conducts sensations from the prepuce and penis, from the glans penis or clitoris, from the vestibule of the vagina, from parts of the anal canal, and from the perineal skin, as well as from posterior parts of the labia majora and the scrotum. The areas on the periphery of the perineum are supplied by other cutaneous nerves. (*Hollinshead, pp 810–812*)

74. **(C)** Most perineal structures send their lymphatics along the branches of the external pudendal vessels to the superficial inguinal nodes. Lymphatics of the lower anal canal, the perineal skin, the spongy urethra, and the entire vulva drain to the inguinal nodes. (*Hollinshead, p 810*)

75. **(D)** The levator ani forms not the inferior walls of the ischiorectal fossae, but their sloping superomedial walls. These fossae are spaces on each side of the anal canal. They contain fat and connective tissue and also the pudendal canal. This canal is a fascial sheath, in which the pudendal nerve and the internal pudendal artery reach the perineum, and the internal pudendal veins leave it. The more

or less vertical wall of each ischiorectal fossa is formed by the obturator internus muscle. *(Hollinshead, pp 738,793–794)*

76. (A) The superior and inferior fasciae of the urogenital diaphragm enclose what is called the deep perineal space or pouch. In fact, it is not a space at all (not even a partial one) since it is filled completely by the deep perineal muscles. The deep perineal space is closed completely, and it does not communicate with the ischiorectal fossa or other perineal or pelvic spaces. Choices B, C, and D are characteristic of the superficial, not the deep, perineal space. *(Hollinshead, pp 797–798)*

77. (C) The visceral efferents required for erection of the penis are derived from the pelvic splanchnic nerves, which represent the sacral parasympathetic outflow. They are also known as nervi erigentes because they are capable of causing erection. Arteries of the penis, in response to excitation of the cavernous nerves (derived from the nervi erigentes), pour arterial blood into the cavernae at a faster rate than it can leave through the cavernous veins. Erection is thus achieved by tumescence of the corpora with arterial blood. *(Hollinshead, pp 754,800,812)*

78. (A) The ejaculatory duct is formed by union of the distal end of the duct of the seminal vesicle together with the ductus deferens. The ejaculatory ducts converge toward each other as they run through the prostate. They open into the prostatic urethra close together on the colliculus seminalis just lateral to the utriculus. *(Hollinshead, pp 770–771,774)*

79. (B) The perineal body is a small, fibrous mass at the center of the perineum. Attached here are the base of the perineal membrane and several muscles. The ischiocavernosus muscle surrounds the free surface of each crus of the penis. It is attached to the ischiopubic ramus, but not to the perineal body. *(Basmajian, pp 198,202; Hollinshead, p 803)*

80. (C) The bulbourethral glands are found in the male. They are two small glands, each the size of a pea, that lie deep to the urogenital diaphragm in the deep perineal pouch. Their long ducts travel in the wall of the urethra for 2 to 3 cm before opening into the spongy urethra. *(Basmajian, p 203)*

81. (A) The ligament of the ovary stands out in relief from the back of the broad ligament. It joins the lower pole of the ovary to the angle between the side of the uterus and the uterine tube. A similar cord, the round ligament of the uterus, stands out from the front of the broad ligament. It passes from the angle between the uterus and tube across the pelvic brim to the deep inguinal ring. *(Basmajian, p 229)*

82. (D) The ovary does not have a smooth surface. It has pits and scars on its surface that mark the sites of the absorbed corpora lutea (corpus luteum). These scars occur monthly from shedding of the ova. All other statements are correct. *(Basmajian, p 229)*

83. (E) The abdominal orifice of the uterine tube lies at the bottom of a funnel-shaped depression—the infundibulum. Fringes, or fimbria, lined with ciliated epithelium project from the infundibulum and encourage ova, when shed, into the tube. One fimbria is attached to the ovary. Listed choices A, B, and C are other parts of the uterine tube. *(Basmajian, p 230)*

84. (C) The fundus of the uterus is the part that rises above the uterine tubes. The fundus and the body form the upper 5 cm, the cervix the lower 3 cm of the uterus. The uterine tubes enter at its widest part. *(Basmajian, p 230)*

85. (B) In the female, the ureter crosses the lateral fornix of the vagina. Because of the obliquity of the uterine axis, the ureter lies closer to the cervix on one side (generally the left). The ureter crosses below, not above, the broad ligament and the uterine artery. It enters the bladder in front of the vagina. *(Basmajian, pp 233–234)*

Clinical Pelvis and Perineum Questions

DIRECTIONS (Questions 1 through 15): Each of the numbered items or incomplete statements in this section is followed by answers or by completions of the statement. Select the ONE lettered answer or completion that is BEST in each case.

1. Infection may reach the ischiorectal fossa from all of the following EXCEPT

   (A) inflammation of the anal sinuses
   (B) downward extension of a perirectal abscess
   (C) following a tear in the anal mucous membrane
   (D) a penetrating wound in the anal region
   (E) a ruptured urethra

2. Embryologically, which of these structures in the female is homologous to the scrotum in the male?

   (A) labia majora
   (B) labia minora
   (C) mons pubis
   (D) vestibule of the vagina
   (E) hymen

3. Some obstetricians are reluctant to perform a median episiotomy because it may

   (A) injure the baby's head
   (B) involve the external anal sphincter
   (C) enlarge the distal end of the birth canal
   (D) injure the urethral sphincter
   (E) lacerate the labia minora

4. The diagonal conjugate diameter of the pelvis is a measurement of the superior pelvic aperture between which of the following points?

   (A) the midpoint of the inferior border of the symphysis pubis to the midpoint of the sacral promontory
   (B) the midpoint of the superior border of the symphysis pubis to the midpoint of the sacral promontory

superior

   (C) transversely from the linea terminalis on one side to this line on the opposite side
   (D) from one iliopubic eminence to the opposite sacroiliac joint
   (E) from one ischial spine to the opposite ischial spine

5. A pelvis in which the anteroposterior (AP) diameter of the superior pelvic aperture is short and the transverse diameter is long is called

   (A) gynecoid
   (B) anthropoid
   (C) platypelloid
   (D) android
   (E) piriform

6. The nerve most likely to be injured during removal of cancerous lymph nodes from the side wall of the pelvis is the

   (A) femoral
   (B) lumbosacral trunk
   (C) sciatic
   (D) pudendal
   (E) obturator

7. In the male, obstruction of the ureter by ureteric stones occurs most often at which of the following portions of this structure?

   (A) nearest the kidney
   (B) on the side wall of the pelvis
   (C) just superior to the ischial spine
   (D) just lateral to the ductus deferens
   (E) where it crosses the external iliac artery and the brim of the pelvis

8. All the following statements are characteristics of a gynecoid pelvis EXCEPT

   (A) a circular superior aperture
   (B) a wide subpubic arch
   (C) widely spaced ischial spines
   (D) resemblance to a shallow, flat bowl
   (E) usually associated with a reasonably uneventful delivery

9. All of the following statements concerning pelvic venous plexuses are important clinically EXCEPT

   (A) the rectal venous plexuses drain into the superior, middle, and inferior rectal veins
   (B) cancer cells may metastasize from the prostatic venous plexus
   (C) veins from the internal rectal plexus may become varicose
   (D) frequently, portal obstruction results in rectal varicosities
   (E) they contain valves

10. All the following are correct concerning benign prostatic hypertrophy EXCEPT

    (A) nocturia
    (B) dysuria
    (C) urgency
    (D) extravasation of urine into the superficial perineal pouch
    (E) common in older men

11. All the following statements concerning hemorrhoids are correct EXCEPT

    (A) they may be associated with portal hypertension
    (B) internal hemorrhoids are varicosities of the superior rectal vein
    (C) thrombus formation is more common in external than in internal hemorrhoids
    (D) external hemorrhoids are varicosities of the inferior rectal veins
    (E) surgery is not considered with internal hemorrhoids

12. The structure or structures that usually rupture during the first stage of labor include the

    (A) placenta
    (B) amniotic sac
    (C) perineal membrane
    (D) broad ligament
    (E) mesosalpinx

13. All the following statements concerning the pectinate line are correct EXCEPT

    (A) the line separates the lymphatics of the anal canal
    (B) the line separates the vascular supply ✓
    (C) the line separates the nerve supply to the anal canal ✓
    (D) characteristics of carcinomas differ above and *adeno* below the line *SCC*
    (E) internal hemorrhoids occur below the line

14. All the following statements concerning benign prostatic hyperplasia are correct EXCEPT

    all correct

    (A) it usually affects the "middle" lobe
    (B) it occurs with increasing frequency beyond the 5th decade of life
    (C) it frequently causes urethral obstruction
    (D) it is the second leading cause of death in men after age 75
    (E) it can be readily palpated digitally

15. All the following statements concerning cancer of the bladder are correct EXCEPT it

    (A) originates in the muscular coat
    (B) tends to be superficial
    (C) tends to be multiple
    (D) can be examined with a cystoscope
    (E) develops in the lining epithelium

ANSWERS AND EXPLANATIONS

1. **(E)** Infection may reach the ischiorectal fossae from any of the sources listed except from a ruptured urethra. A ruptured urethra into the superficial perineal space allows urine to pass into the areolar tissue in the scrotum, around the penis, and upward into the anterior abdominal wall. *(Moore, p 303)*

2. **(A)** Embryologically, the labia majora are homologous to the scrotum of the male. The labia majora are two large folds of skin, filled largely with subcutaneous fat, that run downward and backward from the mons pubis, a rounded eminence lying anterior to the symphysis pubis. The labia minora are two thin, delicate folds of skin lying between the labia majora. The space between the labia minora is the vestibule of the vagina. The hymen is a thin, incomplete fold of mucous membrane surrounding the vaginal opening. *(Moore, pp 325–327)*

3. **(B)** Some obstetricians are reluctant to perform a median episiotomy, fearing that it may tear or extend posteriorly and involve the external anal sphincter or the rectum. In this type of episiotomy, the cut is in the midline of the perineum, beginning at the frenulum of the labia minora and passing posteriorly through the skin, the vaginal mu-

cosa, and the central perineal tendon. The incision stops well short of the external anal sphincter. *(Moore, pp 331–333)*

4. **(A)** The diagonal conjugate diameter of the pelvis is the measurement from the midpoint of the inferior border of the symphysis pubis to the midpoint of the sacral promontory. Choice B measures the anteroposterior diameter of the superior pelvic aperture. Choice C describes the transverse diameter of the superior pelvic aperture, its greatest width. Choice D measures the oblique diameter of the superior pelvic aperture. Choice E, the midplane (interspinous) diameter of the pelvis between the ischial spines, cannot be measured but may be estimated by palpating the sacrospinous ligament during a vaginal examination. *(Moore, pp 337–339)*

5. **(C)** The platypelloid pelvis is a flattened type of pelvis that is present in about 2.5% of females. It resembles a shallow, flat bowl. In patients with this type of pelvis, there may be difficulty with the fetal head engaging in the superior pelvic aperture, which may necessitate a cesarean section. Other items listed are various shapes of pelves found in the female. Piriform is not a type of pelvic shape. *(Moore, pp 341–343)*

6. **(E)** The obturator nerve is the only nerve supplying the lower limb, which lies on the side wall of the pelvis in the extraperitoneal fat. Here, it is vulnerable to injury during removal of cancerous lymph nodes from the side wall of the pelvis. Injury to this nerve results in deficient adduction power of the thigh on the affected side. *(Moore, p 357)*

7. **(E)** Ureteric stones may cause complete or intermittent obstruction of urinary flow anywhere along the ureter. It occurs most often, however, at either of two points: (1) where the ureter crosses the external iliac artery and the brim of the pelvis, and (2) where it passes obliquely through the wall of the urinary bladder. *(Moore, p 369)*

8. **(D)** A gynecoid pelvis has the characteristics noted in the first three choices. Usually, a woman with a gynecoid pelvis has a reasonably uneventful delivery. A platypelloid pelvis is broad or flat and is described as resembling a shallow, flat bowl. In patients with this type of pelvis, there may be difficulty with the fetal head engaging in the superior pelvic aperture. *(Moore, pp 341–343)*

9. **(E)** The superior rectal vein drains into the inferior mesenteric vein and forms one of the clinically important communications between the portal and

systemic venous systems. Portal obstruction, associated with cirrhosis of the liver, frequently results in development of rectal varicosities. In some people, veins forming the internal rectal plexus become varicose and form internal hemorrhoids. The prostatic venous plexus may drain, via the sacral veins, into the vertebral venous plexus. Thus, these large, valveless veins may transport cancer cells to the vertebral column, where they metastasize to the vertebrae. *(Moore, pp 365–367)*

10. **(D)** Benign prostatic hypertrophy is a common condition in older males. The condition results in varying degrees of obstruction of the neck of the bladder. In most males, the prostate progressively undergoes hypertrophy. It is a common cause of urethral obstruction leading to nocturia (need to urinate during the night), dysuria (difficulty and pain on urination), and urgency (sudden desire to void). *(Moore, p 379)*

11. **(E)** Internal hemorrhoids are varicosities of the tributaries of the superior rectal vein. External hemorrhoids are varicosities of the inferior rectal vein. Thrombus formation is more common in external than in internal hemorrhoids. The anastomosis between the superior and middle rectal veins forms a clinically important communication between the portal and systemic systems. In portal hypertension, as in hepatic cirrhosis, the tiny anastomotic veins in the anal canal and elsewhere become varicose and may rupture. *(Moore, p 402)*

12. **(B)** The amniotic and chorionic sacs (amniochorionic membrane) rupture, permitting the amniotic fluid to escape. Usually, this rupture occurs during the first stage of labor or at the end of it. The amniotic and chorionic sacs protrude into the cervical canal during the first stage of labor and help to dilate the cervix. *(Moore, pp 411,416)*

13. **(E)** The characteristics of carcinomas differ above and below the pectinate line, and the line also separates the lymphatic, vascular, and nerve supply of the anal canal. Afferent nerves are visceral above the line and somatic below. The lymphatic drainage ascends above the line but, from the terminal canal, follows the genitofemoral sulcus to the superficial inguinal nodes. Internal hemorrhoids may form above the line and external hemorrhoids below. *(Woodburne, p 528)*

14. **(D)** The prostate is the site of two clinical conditions of much importance—benign prostatic hyperplasia and carcinoma. The hyperplasia commonly affects the "middle" lobe and occurs with increasing frequency beyond the 5th decade of life. Pro-

static carcinoma is the second leading cause of death from cancer in men after age 75. Both benign prostatic hyperplasia and carcinoma can be readily palpated digitally. Both tend to cause urethral obstruction and this may be the first indication of their presence. *(Woodburne, p 537)*

15. **(A)** The interior of the bladder and its three orifices can be examined with a cystoscope inserted through the urethra. Cancer of the bladder develops in its lining epithelium; it tends to be superficial and multiple. In advanced stages, it invades the bladder's muscular coat. *(Moore, p 227)*

Developmental Pelvis and Perineum Questions

Questions 1 through 10

Associate each of the following structures with one of the embryonic structures listed below.

(A) mesonephric duct
(B) paramesonephric duct
(C) genital ridges

1. Appendix testes

2. Uterine tube

3. Seminal vesicle

4. Uterus

5. Epoophoron

6. Cervix

7. Paroophoron

8. Ductus deferens

9. Testes

10. Ovaries

Questions 11 through 15

Associate each of the following phrases with one of the conditions listed below.

(A) hypospadias
(B) epispadias
(C) Klinefelter's syndrome
(D) Turner's syndrome
(E) ectopia of the bladder

11. The most common major abnormality of sexual differentiation

12. Gonadal dysgenesis

13. Seen frequently in combination with epispadias

14. The urethra is located on the inferior aspect of the penis

15. The urethra is located on the dorsal aspect of the penis

ANSWERS AND EXPLANATIONS

1. **(B)** The paramesonephric duct in the male degenerates, except for a small portion at the cranial end, the appendix testis. *(Sadler, p 278)*

2. **(B)** The paramesonephric duct develops into the main genital duct of the female. The first two parts develop into the uterine tube. *(Sadler, p 278)*

3. **(A)** The mesonephric duct persists (except for its most cranial portion—the appendix epididymis) and forms the main genital duct. The seminal vesicles develop from the mesonephric ducts. *(Sadler, p 277)*

4. **(B)** The second portion of the paramesonephric ducts fuse in the midline. The fused paramesonephric ducts give rise to the uterus. *(Sadler, p 279)*

5. **(A)** In the female, the mesonephric duct disappears except for a small cranial portion found in the mesovarium, where it forms the epoophoron. *(Sadler, p 282)*

6. **(B)** The second portion of the paramesonephric ducts fuses in the midline. The fused paramesonephric ducts give rise to the uterus and cervix. *(Sadler, p 279)*

7. **(A)** Some remnants of the cranial end of the mesonephric may be located in the mesovarium, where they form the epoophoron and paroophoron. *(Sadler, p 282)*

8. **(A)** From the tail of the epididymis to the outbudding of the seminal vesicle, the mesonephric duct obtains a thick, muscular coat and is known as the ductus deferens. *(Sadler, p 277)*

9. **(C)** The gonads appear initially as a pair of longitudinal ridges—the genital, or gonadal, ridges. Under the influence of the Y chromosome, which encodes the testis-determining factor (TDF), the primitive sex cords continue to proliferate and penetrate deep into the medulla to form the testis. *(Sadler, pp 271–273)*

10. **(C)** The gonadal ridges give rise to the ovary and testis. It may be stated that the sex of an embryo is determined at the time of fertilization and depends on whether the spermatocyte carries an X or Y chromosome. *(Sadler, pp 271–273)*

11. **(C)** Klinefelter's syndrome, with a karyotype of 47,XXY (or XXXY) is the most common major abnormality of sexual differentiation, occurring with a frequency of 1 in 500 males. Patients are characterized by infertility, gynecomastia, varying degrees of impaired sexual maturation. *(Sadler, p 287)*

12. **(D)** Gonadal dysgenesis (Turner's syndrome) is found in patients with 44 autosomes and one X chromosome. Since the Y chromosome is absent, the placental and maternal estrogens will influence development of the paramesonephric duct system and external genitalia, as in the normal female. Since the gonad does not produce any hormones after birth, differentiation of the paramesonephric duct and external genitalia ceases following birth and the sex characteristics remain infantile. *(Sadler, pp 287–288)*

13. **(E)** Ectopia of the bladder, seen frequently in combination with epispadias, is a condition in which the posterior wall of the bladder is exposed to the outside. *(Sadler, p 286)*

14. **(A)** When fusion of the urethral folds is incomplete, abnormal openings of the urethra may be found along the inferior aspect of the penis. Most frequently, the abnormal orifices are near the glands, along the shaft or near the base of the penis. *(Sadler, p 284)*

15. **(B)** In this abnormality, the urethral meatus is found on the dorsum of the penis. Instead of having developed at the cranial margin of the cloacal membrane, the genital tubercle seems to have formed in the region of the urogenital septum. Hence, a portion of the cloacal membrane is then found cranial to the genital tubercle, and when this membrane ruptures, the outlet of the urogenital sinus comes to lie on the cranial aspect of the penis. *(Sadler, pp 285–286)*

Nervous Pelvis and Perineum
Questions

DIRECTIONS (Questions 1 through 10): Each group of items in this section consists of lettered headings followed by a set of numbered words or phrases. For each numbered word or phrase, select the ONE lettered heading that is most closely associated with it. Each lettered heading may be selected once, more than once, or not at all.

(A) pelvic splanchnic nerve
(B) pudendal nerve
(C) inferior hypogastric plexus
(D) vagus nerve

1. Pain fibers from the pelvic portion of the ureter

2. The dorsal nerve of the penis

3. The posterior scrotal nerve

4. Serves the emptying reflex of the bladder

5. Impulses of pain due to an overstretched bladder

6. Parasympathetic innervation to the testes

7. Parasympathetic innervation to the ovaries

8. Sympathetic innervation to the prostate gland

9. Somatic innervation to the clitoris

10. Erection depends on stimuli through these nerves

ANSWERS AND EXPLANATIONS

1. **(C)** The nerve supply of the lower portions of the ureters comes from the hypogastric nerves and the inferior hypogastric plexuses. *(Woodburne, p 298)*

2. **(B)** The terminal end of the pudendal nerve is the dorsal nerve of the penis (or clitoris). The pudendal nerve is almost the sole somatic nerve of the perineum. *(Woodburne, pp 514–515)*

3. **(B)** The perineal nerve arises from the pudendal nerve within the pudendal canal, and leaves it toward the posterior border of the perineal membrane. Its posterior scrotal (or posterior labial) branches become superficial and distribute to the skin and fascia of the perineum and the scrotum (or labium majus). *(Woodburne, p 514)*

4. **(A)** The pelvic splanchnic nerves represent the sacral portion of the parasympathetic division of the autonomic nervous system, and its distribution is largely pelvic. The more important proprioceptive impulses from the muscular wall, initiated by normal stretching of the muscle layers as the viscus fills, travel over the parasympathetic fibers. Their stimulation results in reflex emptying of the bladder. *(Woodburne, pp 530,549)*

5. **(C)** The abdominal aortic plexus continues over the sacral promontory as the superior hypogastric plexus and divides into the hypogastric nerves for the sympathetic supply of the pelvic viscera. Afferent impulses are conducted along both the sympathetic and parasympathetic sets of nerves; impulses of pain are due to the overstretched bladder traveling with the sympathetic fibers. *(Woodburne, pp 530,549)*

6. **(D)** The testicular plexus contains vagal parasympathetic fibers and sympathetic neurons from the 10th thoracic segment of the spinal cord. *(Woodburne, p 535)*

7. **(D)** The ovarian plexus supplies the ovary, the broad ligament, and the uterine tubes, and communicates with the uterine plexus. It may be predicted, on embryologic and reflex grounds, that the parasympathetic fibers of the testicular and ovarian plexuses are vagal in origin. *(Woodburne, p 499)*

8. **(C)** Sympathetic and parasympathetic fibers pass to the structures of the perineum from the prostatic plexus in the male. The nerve fibers concerned are derived from the upper three lumbar

segments (inferior hypogastric plexus, the principal sympathetic roots of the latter) and from the pelvic splanchnic nerves (sacral segments 2 to 4). *(Woodburne, pp 514,522)*

9. **(B)** The pudendal nerve is almost the sole somatic nerve of the perineum. It supplies all the perineal musculature and is sensory to most of its skin surface. The terminal end of the pudendal nerve forms the dorsal nerve of the clitoris. *(Woodburne, pp 514–515)*

10. **(A)** Erection depends on stimuli through the parasympathetic nerves, leading to engorgement of the corpora cavernosa by dilatation of their arteries or, possibly, by relaxation of their vasculature tone. *(Woodburne, p 520)*

Illustrations
Questions

THE COXAL BONE
(Questions 1 through 19)

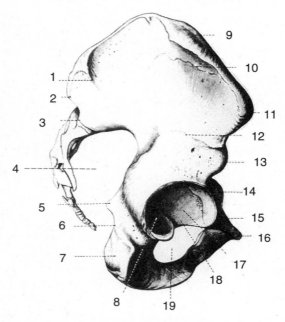

Figure 3–1. Coxal bone. (Modified and reproduced, with permission, from Montgomery RL: *Basic Anatomy,* Urban & Schwarzenberg, p. 63, 1980.)

Directions: With reference to the diagram, match the numbered structures with their corresponding lettered items.

(A) greater sciatic notch

(B) iliac crest

(C) anterior inferior iliac spine

(D) superior gluteal line

(E) iliopubic eminence

(F) acetabular labrium

(G) obturator foramen

(H) ischial spine

(I) acetabular notch

(J) pubic tubercle

(K) posterior inferior iliac spine

(L) acetabular fossa

(M) pecten pubis

(N) ischial tuberosity

(O) inferior gluteal line

(P) lesser sciatic notch

(Q) anterior superior iliac spine

(R) posterior superior iliac spine

URINARY SYSTEM (MALE)
(Questions 20 through 28)

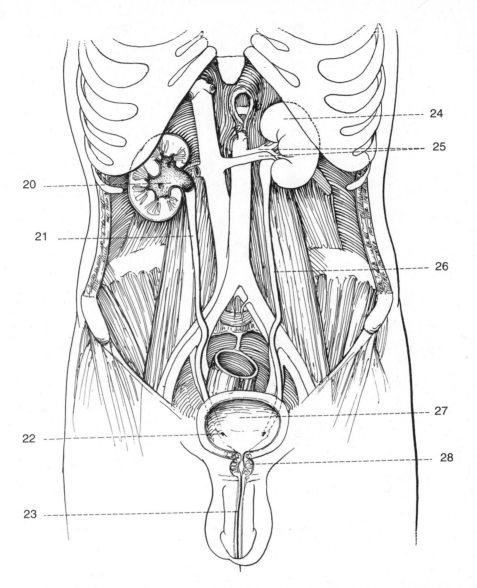

Figure 3–2. Urinary system (diagrammatic view). (Modified and reproduced, with permission, from Montgomery RL: *Basic Anatomy,* Urban & Schwarzenberg, p. 389, 1980.)

Directions: With reference to the diagram, match the numbered structures with their corresponding lettered items.

(A) left ureter
(B) left kidney
(C) pelvis of kidney
(D) ureteral orifice
(E) right ureter

(F) urinary bladder
(G) prostate
(H) urethra
(I) renal vessels

PARASAGITTAL VIEW OF MALE PELVIS
(Questions 29 through 53)

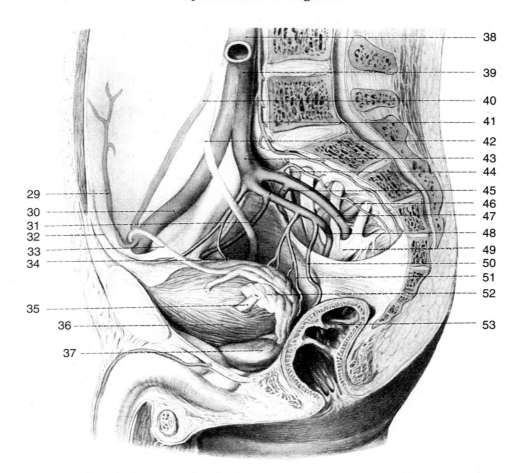

Figure 3–3. Parasagittal view of male pelvis. (Modified and reproduced, with permission, from Montgomery RL: *Basic Anatomy,* Urban & Schwarzenberg, p. 394, 1980.)

Directions: With reference to the diagram, match the numbered structures with their corresponding lettered items.

(A) internal pudendal artery

(B) lateral sacral artery

(C) deep circumflex iliac artery

(D) median sacral artery

(E) inferior gluteal artery

(F) prostate

(G) right ureter

(H) urinary bladder

(I) internal iliac artery

(J) left ureter

(K) iliolumbar artery

(L) superior vesical artery

(M) superior gluteal artery

(N) ductus deferens

(O) sciatic nerve

(P) median umbilical ligament

(Q) middle rectal artery

(R) obturator artery

(S) seminal vesicle

(T) external iliac artery

(U) inferior vesical artery

(V) rectum

(W) inferior epigastric artery

(X) abdominal aorta

(Y) common iliac artery

BLADDER AND URETHRA
(Questions 54 through 66)

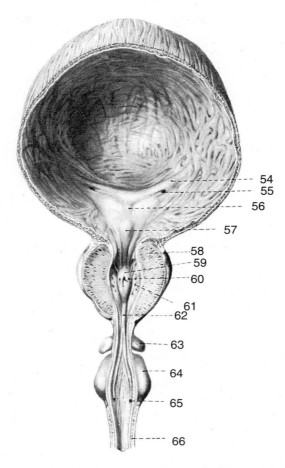

Figure 3–4. Bladder and urethra (internal view). (Modified and reproduced, with permission, from Montgomery RL: *Basic Anatomy,* Urban & Schwarzenberg, p. 395, 1980.)

Directions: With reference to the diagram, match the numbered structures with their corresponding lettered items.

(A) prostate

(B) prostatic utricle

(C) bulb of penis

(D) corpus cavernosum urethra

(E) interureteric fold

(F) urethral crest

(G) duct of bulbourethral gland

(H) opening of ureter

(I) vesical trigone

(J) uvula

(K) ejaculatory duct

(L) bulbourethral gland

(M) seminal colliculus

MALE REPRODUCTIVE SYSTEM
(Questions 67 through 85)

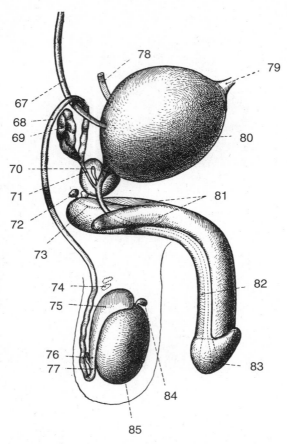

Figure 3–5. Male reproductive system (diagrammatic view). (Modified and reproduced, with permission, from Montgomery RL: *Basic Anatomy,* Urban & Schwarzenberg, p. 398, 1980.)

Directions: With reference to the diagram, match the numbered structures with their corresponding lettered items.

(A) ductus deferens
(B) paradidymis
(C) right ureter
(D) bulbourethral gland
(E) tail of epididymis
(F) ejaculatory duct
(G) urachus
(H) corpus cavernosum penis
(I) prostatic utricle
(J) corpus cavernosum urethra

(K) glans penis
(L) left ureter
(M) bulbourethral duct
(N) epididymis
(O) testis
(P) appendix testis
(Q) urinary bladder
(R) head of epididymis
(S) seminal vesicle

MALE REPRODUCTIVE SYSTEM
(Questions 86 through 98)

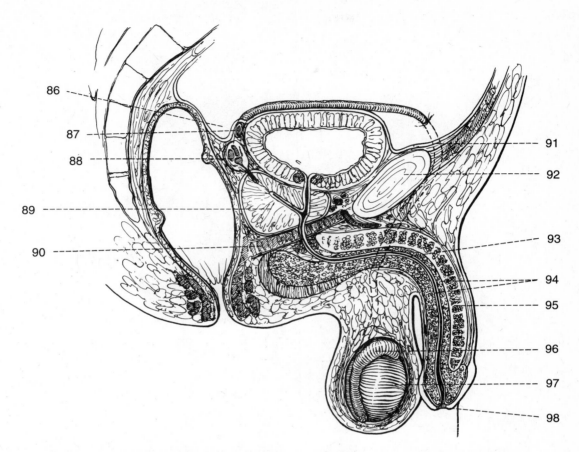

Figure 3–6. Male reproductive system (sagittal view). (Modified and reproduced, with permission, from Montgomery RL: *Basic Anatomy,* Urban & Schwarzenberg, p. 399, 1980.)

Directions: With reference to the diagram, match the numbered structures with their corresponding lettered items.

(A) seminal vesicle

(B) urogenital diaphragm

(C) urethral orifice

(D) ductus deferens

(E) corpus cavernosum penis

(F) urethra

(G) epididymis

(H) pubis

(I) testis

(J) corpus cavernosum urethra

(K) rectovesical pouch

(L) prostate

PELVIC VISCERA
(Questions 99 through 129)

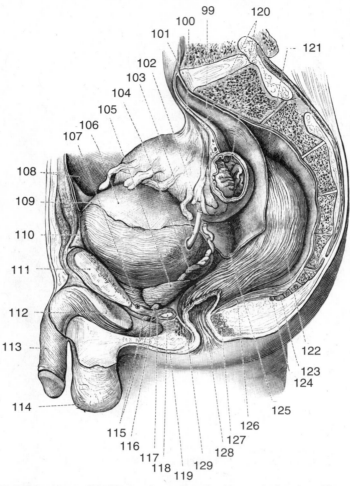

Figure 3–7. Pelvic viscera. (Modified and reproduced, with permission, from Montgomery RL: *Basic Anatomy,* Urban & Schwarzenberg, p. 400, 1980.)

Directions: With reference to the diagram, match the numbered structures with their corresponding lettered items.

(A) pelvic diaphragm
(B) symphysis pubis
(C) parietal peritoneum
(D) scrotum
(E) bulb of penis
(F) sigmoid colon
(G) retroperitoneal space
(H) ureter
(I) crus corpus cavernosum penis
(J) sacral rectal flexure
(K) apex of coccyx
(L) perineum
(M) membranous portion of urethra
(N) sigmoid mesocolon
(O) coccyx

(P) visceral peritoneum
(Q) seminal vesicle
(R) pelvic diaphragm
(S) prostate
(T) perineal rectal flexure
(U) anus
(V) ductus deferens
(W) external anal sphincter
(X) retrovesical pouch
(Y) promontorium
(Z) retropubic space
(AA) corpus cavernosum penis
(AB) bulbourethral gland
(AC) urinary bladder
(AD) urogenital diaphragm

ANTERIOR ABDOMINAL WALL AND SCROTAL HOMOLOGUES
(Questions 130 through 147)

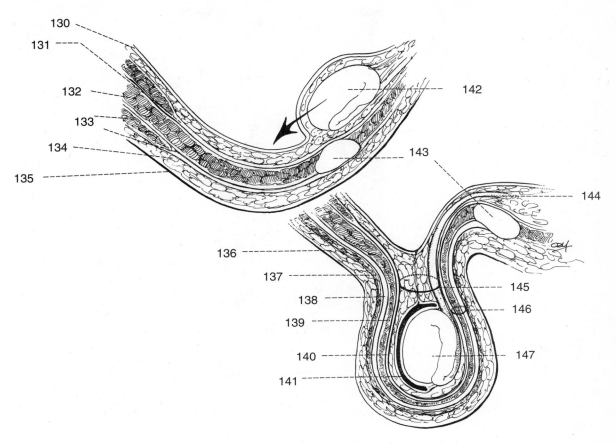

Figure 3–8. Anterior abdominal wall and scrotal homologues. (Modified and reproduced, with permission, from Montgomery RL: *Basic Anatomy,* Urban & Schwarzenberg, p. 401, 1980.)

Directions: With reference to the diagram, match the numbered structures with their corresponding lettered items.

(A) external abdominal oblique muscle

(B) skin

(C) cremasteric fascia and muscle

(D) descending testis

(E) superficial fascia

(F) ductus deferens

(G) fascia transversalis

(H) testis

(I) internal abdominal oblique muscle

(J) external spermatic fascia

(K) pubis

(L) peritoneum

(M) tunica vaginalis testis

(N) spermatic cord

(O) internal spermatic fascia

(P) cord coverings

(Q) tunica dartos

TESTIS, EPIDIDYMIS, AND SPERMATIC CORD
(Questions 148 through 159)

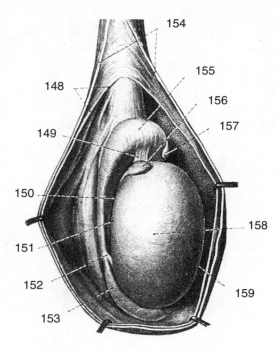

Figure 3–9. Testis, epididymis, and spermatic cord. (Modified and reproduced, with permission, from Montgomery RL: *Basic Anatomy,* Urban & Schwarzenberg, p. 403, 1980.)

Directions: With reference to the diagram, match the numbered structures with their corresponding lettered items.

(A) inferior epididymal ligament

(B) internal spermatic fascia

(C) appendix testis

(D) lateral side of testis

(E) tunica vaginalis testis

(F) head of epididymis

(G) superior epididymal ligament

(H) appendix epididymis

(I) anterior margin of testis

(J) sinus of epididymis

(K) tail of epididymis

(L) posterior margin of testis

TUBULAR NETWORK OF THE TESTIS AND EPIDIDYMIS
(Questions 160 through 167)

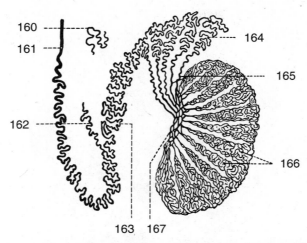

Figure 3–10. Tubular network of the testis and epididymis. (Modified and reproduced, with permission, from Montgomery RL: *Basic Anatomy,* Urban & Schwarzenberg, p. 403, 1980.)

Directions: With reference to the diagram, match the numbered structures with their corresponding lettered items.

(A) ductus deferens

(B) head of epididymis

(C) rete testis

(D) efferent ductules

(E) paradidymis

(F) ductus epididymis

(G) seminiferous tubules

(H) aberrant ductule

DUCTUS DEFERENS AND SEMINAL VESICLES
(Questions 168 through 180)

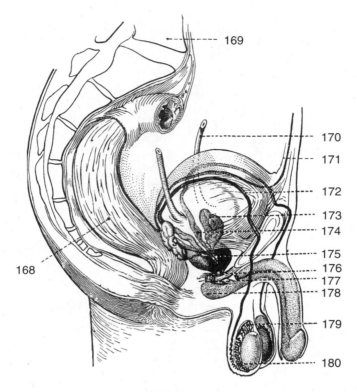

Figure 3–11. Ductus deferens and seminal vesicles. (Modified and reproduced, with permission, from Montgomery RL: *Basic Anatomy,* Urban & Schwarzenberg, p. 406, 1980.)

Directions: With reference to the diagram, match the numbered structures with their corresponding lettered items.

(A) ureter

(B) ductus deferens

(C) ampulla of ductus deferens

(D) peritoneum

(E) membranous portion of urethra

(F) bulbourethral gland

(G) tail of epididymis

(H) rectum

(I) ejaculatory duct

(J) head of epididymis

(K) bulb of penis

(L) seminal vesicle

(M) lumbar vertebra

DUCTUS DEFERENS
(Questions 181 through 199)

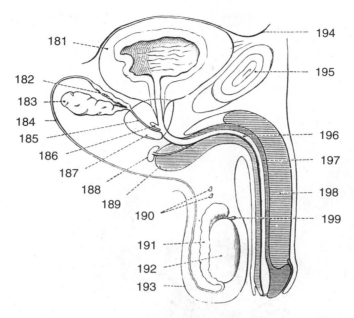

Figure 3–12. Ductus deferens (diagrammatic view). (Modified and reproduced, with permission, from Montgomery RL: *Basic Anatomy,* Urban & Schwarzenberg, p. 406, 1980.)

Directions: With reference to the diagram, match the numbered structures with their corresponding lettered items.

(A) ejaculatory duct

(B) paradidymis

(E) epididymis

(C) head of epididymis

(D) urinary bladder

(E) appendix testis

(F) ampulla of ductus deferens

(G) prostatic utricle

(H) seminal vesicle

(I) bulb of penis

(J) bulbourethral glands

(K) scrotum

(L) ductus deferens

(M) symphysis pubis

(N) corpus cavernosum urethra

(O) prostate

(P) urethra

(Q) corpus cavernosum penis

(R) peritoneum

(S) testis

FEMALE REPRODUCTIVE SYSTEM
(Questions 200 through 211)

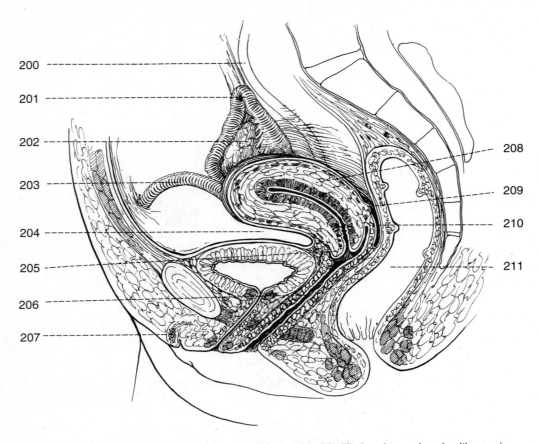

Figure 3–13. Female reproductive system (sagittal view). (Modified and reproduced, with permission, from Montgomery RL: *Basic Anatomy,* Urban & Schwarzenberg, p. 414, 1980.)

Directions: With reference to the diagram, match the numbered structures with their corresponding lettered items.

(A) vagina

(B) cervix

(C) clitoris

(D) uterovesical pouch

(E) uterus

(F) round ligament

(G) rectouterine fold

(H) ovary

(I) rectouterine pouch

(J) uterine tube

(K) rectum

(L) ureter

UTERINE TUBES AND UTERUS
(Questions 212 through 229)

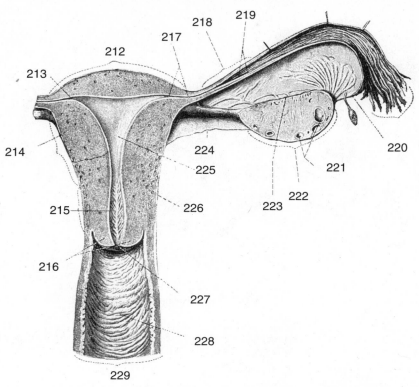

Figure 3–14. Uterine tubes and uterus (internal view). (Modified and reproduced, with permission, from Montgomery RL: *Basic Anatomy,* Urban & Schwarzenberg, p. 416, 1980.)

Directions: With reference to the diagram, match the numbered structures with their corresponding lettered items.

(A) uterine tube opening

(B) epimetrium body of uterus

(C) ovarian follicle

(D) mesosalpinx

(E) uterine cavity

(F) fundus

(G) rugae of vagina

(H) cervix of uterine

(I) vagina

(J) ovary

(K) isthmus of uterine tube

(L) infundibulum with fimbria of uterine tube

(M) external cervical opening

(N) myometrium

(O) ovarian ligament

(P) uterine tube

(Q) cervix of uterine

(R) uterine tube

UTERUS
(Questions 230 through 255)

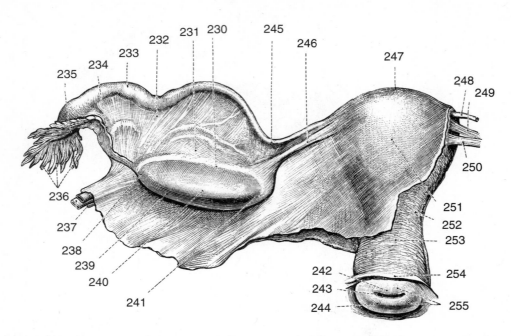

Figure 3–15. Uterus (external view). (Modified and reproduced, with permission, from Montgomery RL: *Basic Anatomy,* Urban & Schwarzenberg, p. 419, 1980.)

Directions: With reference to the diagram, match the numbered structures with their corresponding lettered items.

(A) ampulla of uterine tube

(B) lateral margin of ovary

(C) external os

(D) isthmus of uterine tube

(E) fundus of uterus

(F) margin of mesovarium

(G) posterior labium

(H) mesosalpinx

(I) tubal end of ovarian ligament

(J) ovarian ligament

(K) fimbria of uterine tube

(L) mesovarium

(M) uterine tube

(N) round ligament of uterus

(O) ovarian artery and vein

(P) body of uterus

(Q) isthmus of uterus

(R) ostium of uterine tube

(S) cervix of uterus

(T) free margin of ovary

(U) fornix of uterus

(V) vaginal portion of cervix

(W) anterior labium

(X) uterine end of ovarian ligament

UROGENITAL AND ANORECTAL TRIANGLES
(Questions 256 through 259)

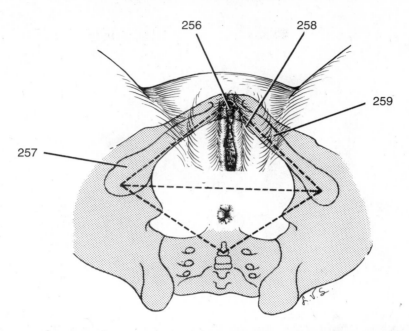

Figure 3–16. Urogenital and anorectal triangles. (Modified and reproduced, with permission, from deCherney AH, Pernoll ML [editors]: *Current Obstetric & Gynecologic Diagnosis & Treatment,* 8th ed. Appleton & Lange, 1994.)

Directions: With reference to the diagram, match the numbered structures with their corresponding lettered items.

(A) lateral border of pubic bones
(B) clitoris
(C) ischiopubic rami
(D) ischial tuberosity

UTERUS
(Questions 260 through 278)

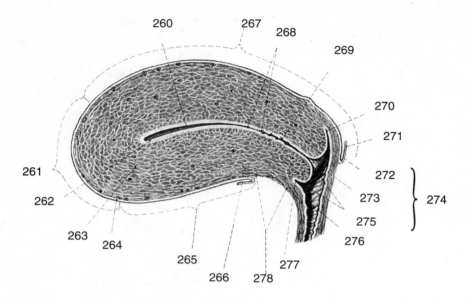

Figure 3–17. Uterus (sagittal view). (Modified and reproduced, with permission, from Montgomery RL: *Basic Anatomy,* Urban & Schwarzenberg, p. 420, 1980.)

Directions: With reference to the diagram, match the numbered structures with their corresponding lettered items.

(A) peritoneum

(B) fundus of uterus

(C) posterior aspect of cervix (vaginal portion)

(D) anterior aspect of cervix (vaginal portion)

(E) endometrium

(F) external opening of cervix

(G) intestinal surface of uterus

(H) cervix

(I) myometrium

(J) anterior fornix of vagina

(K) cervical canal

(L) urinary bladder surface of uterus

(M) posterior fornix of vagina

(N) isthmus of uterus

(O) vagina

(P) epimetrium

(Q) cavity of uterus

(R) vaginal portion of cervix

LIGAMENTS OF THE UTERUS
(Questions 279 through 290)

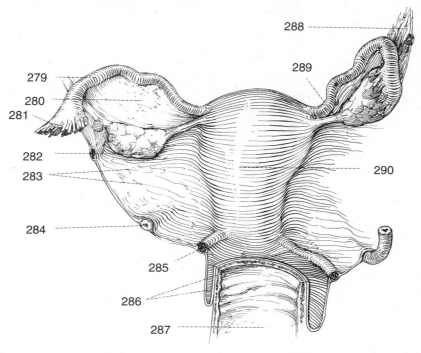

Figure 3–18. Ligaments of the uterus. (Modified and reproduced, with permission, from Montgomery RL: *Basic Anatomy,* Urban & Schwarzenberg, p. 420, 1980.)

Directions: With reference to the diagram, match the numbered structures with their corresponding lettered items.

(A) fimbria

(B) left ureter

(C) suspensory ligament of ovary

(D) body of uterus

(E) ovarian ligament

(F) mesosalpinx

(G) uterine tube

(H) rectouterine fold and pouch

(I) broad ligament of uterus

(J) rectum

(K) rectouterine ligament and muscle

(L) ovary

EXTERNAL GENITALIA (FEMALE)
(Questions 291 through 301)

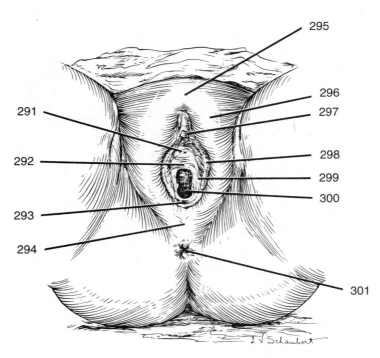

Figure 3–19. External genitalis of the adult female (parous). Note labium are spread laterally. (Modfied and reproduced with permission from deCherney AH, Pernoll ML [editor]: *Current Obstetric & Gynecologic Diagnosis & Treatment,* 7th ed. Appleton & Lange, 1994.)

Directions: With reference to the diagram, match the numbered structures with their corresponding lettered items.

(A) mons pubis

(B) glans clitoris

(C) vaginal orifice

(D) labium majora

(E) external urethral orifice

(F) hymen

(G) perineal body

(H) vestibule

(I) anus

(J) labium minora

(K) fossa navicularis

FEMALE PERINEUM
(Questions 302 through 322)

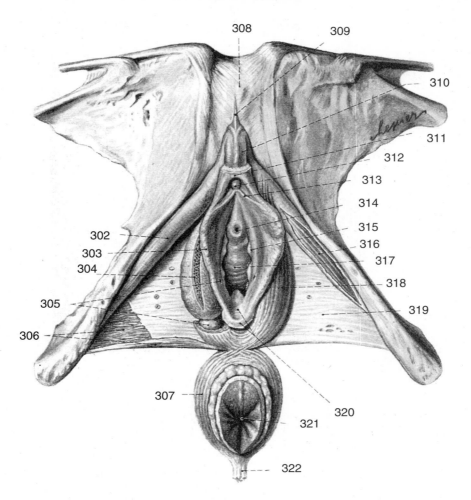

Figure 3–20. Superficial perineum of the female. (Modified and reproduced, with permission, from Montgomery RL: *Basic Anatomy,* Urban & Schwarzenberg, p. 425, 1980.)

Directions: With reference to the diagram, match the numbered structures with their corresponding lettered items.

(A) deep transverse perineus muscle

(B) body of clitoris

(C) opening of greater vestibular glands and greater vestibular gland

(D) anus

(E) bulb of vestibule

(F) posterior commissure

(G) external anal sphincter

(H) external urethral meatus

(I) labium minus

(J) carunculae hymenale

(K) suspensory ligament of clitoris

(L) crus of clitoris

(M) bulbocavernosus muscle

(N) frenulum of clitoris

(O) prepuce of clitoris

(P) symphysis pubis

(Q) inferior fascia of urogenital diaphragm

(R) vagina

(S) ischiocavernosus muscle

(T) glans of clitoris

PELVIC MUSCULATURE (FEMALE)
(Questions 323 through 332)

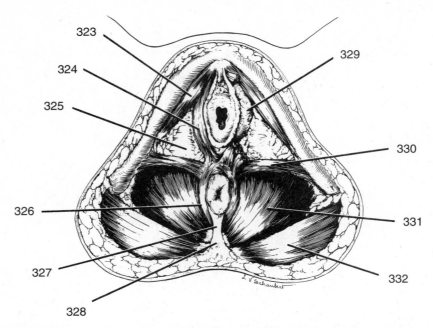

Figure 3–21. Pelvic musculature in the female (inferior view). (Modfied and reproduced with permission from deCherney AH, Pernoll ML [editor]: *Current Obstetric & Gynecologic Diagnosis & Treatment,* 8th ed. Appleton & Lange, 1994.)

Directions: With reference to the diagram, match the numbered structures with their corresponding lettered items.

(A) anococcygeal ligament

(B) bulbocavernosus muscle

(C) bulb of vestibule

(D) superficial transverse perineal muscle

(E) adipose tissue

(F) levator ani muscle

(G) gluteus maximus muscle

(H) coccyx

(I) ischiocavernosus muscle

(J) external anal sphincter

RELATIONSHIP OF THE BLADDER, PROSTATE, SEMINAL VESICLES, PENIS, URETHRA, AND SCROTAL CONTENTS
(Questions 333 through 350)

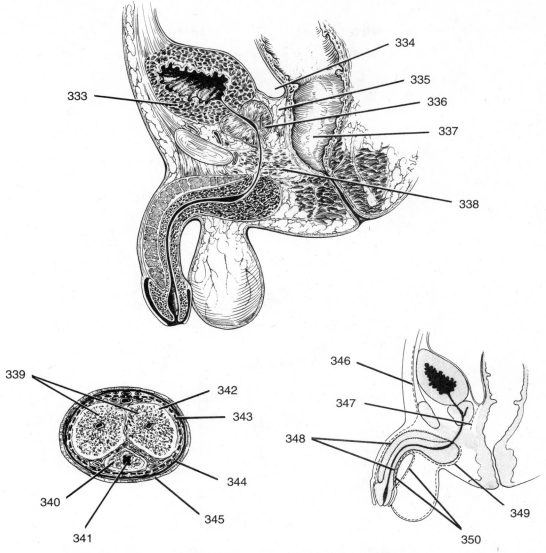

Figure 3–22. *Top:* Relations of the bladder, prostate, seminal vesicles, penis, urethra, and scrotal contents. *Lower left:* Transverse section through the penis. The paired upper structures are the corpora cavernosa. The single lower structure surrounding the urethra is the corpus spongiosum. *Lower right:* Fascial planes of the lower genitourinary tract. (Modified and reproduced, with permission, from Tanagho EA, McAninch JW: *Smith's General Urology,* 14th ed. Appleton & Lange, 1995.)

Directions: With reference to the diagram, match the numbered structures with their corresponding lettered items.

(A) rectum

(B) tunica albuginea

(C) urinary bladder

(D) Buck's fascia

(E) urogenital diaphragm

(F) rectovesical pouch

(G) corpus cavernosum urethra

(H) fascia of Denovilliers

(I) Colles' fascia

(J) prostate

(K) skin

(L) Scarpa's fascia

(M) corpus cavernosum penis

(N) urethra

(O) Dartos fascia

FEMALE REPRODUCTION SYSTEM
(Questions 351 through 380)

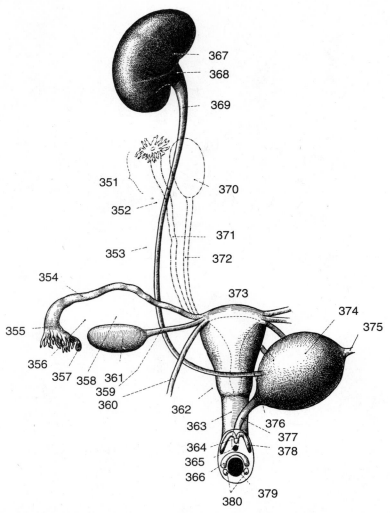

Figure 3–23. Female reproduction system (diagrammatic view). (Modified and reproduced, with permission, from Montgomery RL: *Basic Anatomy,* Urban & Schwarzenberg, p. 413, 1980.)

Directions: With reference to the diagram, match the numbered structures with their corresponding lettered items.

(A) pelvis of ureter

(B) mesonephros

(C) infundibulum of uterine tube

(D) vagina

(E) vestibular bulb

(F) urinary bladder

(G) ureter

(H) crus of clitoris

(I) ovarian ligament

(J) opening of vagina

(K) epoophoron tube

(L) mesonephros tubules

(M) urachus

(N) greater vestibular gland

(O) urethra

(P) uterine tube

(Q) appendix vesicle

(R) glans of clitoris

(S) uterus

(T) Müllerian duct

(U) wolffian duct

(V) ovary

(W) external urethral opening

(X) round ligament of uterus

(Y) kidney

(Z) paroophoron

TRANSFORMATION OF THE UNDIFFERENTIATED GENITAL SYSTEM INTO THE DEFINITIVE MALE SYSTEM
(Questions 381 through 394)

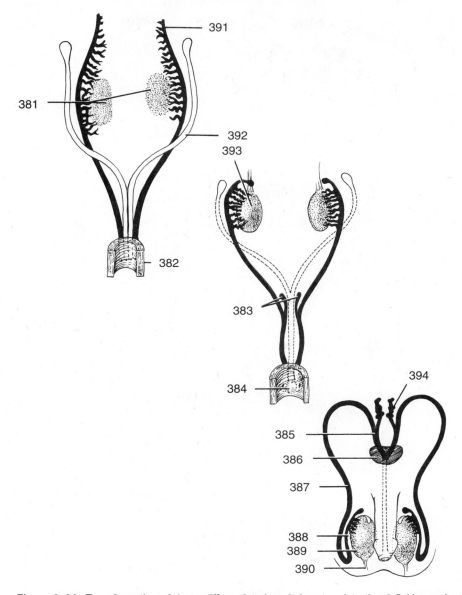

Figure 3–24. Transformation of the undifferentiated genital system into the definitive male system. (Modified and reproduced, with permission, from Tanagho EA, McAninch JW: *Smith's General Urology,* 14th ed. Appleton & Lange, 1995.)

Directions: With reference to the diagram, match the numbered structures with their corresponding lettered items.

(A) urogenital sinus

(B) ejaculatory duct

(C) epididymis

(D) gubernaculum testis

(E) mesonephric ducts

(F) undifferentiated gonads

(G) seminal vesicles

(H) primitive testis

(I) Müllerian ducts

(J) buds to form seminal vesicles

(K) prostate

(L) vas deferens

(M) Müller's tubercle

(N) testis

INNERVATION OF THE URINARY BLADDER AND URETHRA
(Questions 395 through 406)

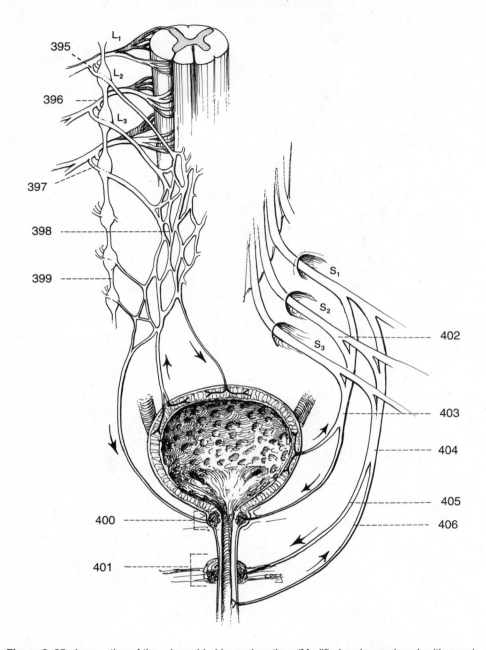

Figure 3–25. Innervation of the urinary bladder and urethra. (Modified and reproduced, with permission, from Montgomery RL: *Basic Anatomy,* Urban & Schwarzenberg, p. 396, 1980.)

Directions: With reference to the diagram, match the numbered structures with their corresponding lettered items.

(A) parasympathetic

(B) sympathetic trunk

(C) motor branch of pudendal

(D) white rami communicantes

(E) sensory branch of pudendal

(F) pudendal nerve

(G) pelvic splanchnic

(H) external sphincter

(I) lumbar nerve

(J) hypogastric plexus

(K) sympathetic

(L) internal sphincter (physiological—functional)

RELATIONSHIP OF THE DUCTUS DEFERENS, SEMINAL VESICLES, PROSTATE, AND URETERS
(Questions 407 through 419)

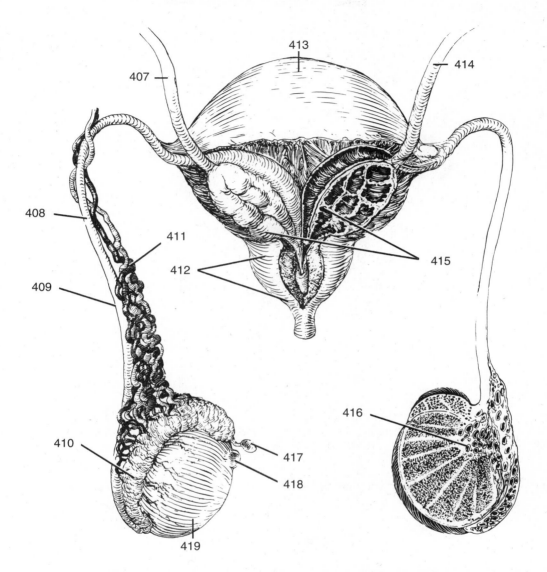

Figure 3–26. Relationships of the ductus deferens, seminal vesicles, prostate, and ureters to the posterior base of the bladder. (Modified and reproduced, with permission, from Tanagho EA, McAninch JW: *Smith's General Urology,* 12th ed. Appleton & Lange, 1988.)

Directions: With reference to the diagram, match the numbered structures with their corresponding lettered items.

(A) epididymis
(B) spermatic vessels
(C) seminal vesicles
(D) left ureter
(E) appendix epididymis
(F) testicle
(G) prostate

(H) right ureter
(I) appendix testis
(J) urinary bladder
(K) region of deep inguinal ring
(L) mediastinum testis
(M) ductus deferens

URINARY SYSTEM (MALE)
(Questions 420 through 426)

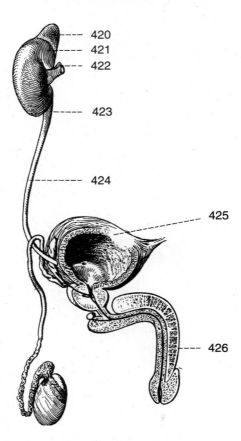

Figure 3–27. Urinary system (male). (Modified and reproduced, with permission, from Montgomery RL: *Basic Anatomy,* Urban & Schwarzenberg, p. 390, 1980.)

Directions: With reference to the diagram, match the numbered structures with their corresponding lettered items.

(A) ureter

(B) renal artery

(C) suprarenal gland

(D) urethra

(E) kidney

(F) renal pelvis

(G) bladder

MIDSAGITTAL VIEW OF THE FEMALE PELVIC ORGANS
(Questions 427 through 437)

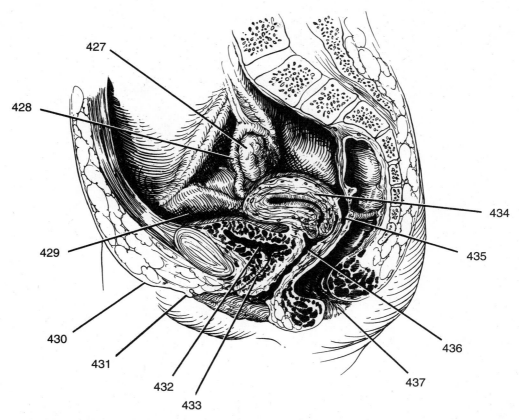

Figure 3–28. Midsaggital view of the female pelvic organs. (Modified and reproduced, with permission, from Benson RC: *Handbook of Obstetrics & Gynecology,* 8th ed. Lange, 1983.)

Directions: With reference to the diagram, match the numbered structures with their corresponding lettered items.

(A) bladder

(B) rectovesical pouch

(C) vagina

(D) clitoris

(E) anus

(F) rectouterine pouch

(G) mons pubis

(H) ovary

(I) uterus

(J) uterine tube

(K) urethra

FASCIAL PLANES OF THE FEMALE PELVIS
(Questions 438 through 445)

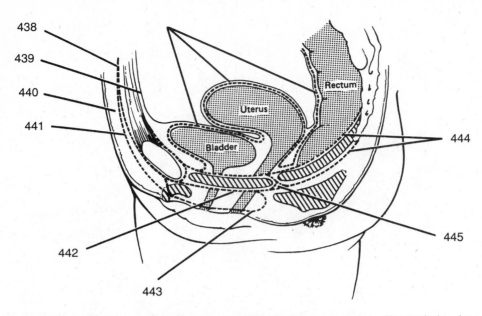

Figure 3–29. Fascial planes of the female pelvis. (Modified and reproduced, with permission, from deCherney AH, Pernoll ML [editors]: *Current Obstetric & Gynecologic Diagnosis & Treatment,* 8th ed. Appleton & Lange, 1994.)

Directions: With reference to the diagram, match the numbered structures with their corresponding lettered items.

(A) Scarpa's fascia

(B) inferior fascia of urogenital diaphragm

(C) Colles' fascia

(D) rectus sheath

(E) central perineal tendon

(F) peritoneum

(G) fascia of levator ani

(H) Camper's fascia

FEMALE PELVIC ORGANS
(Questions 446 through 461)

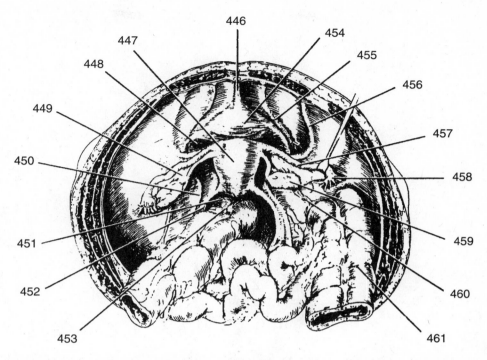

Figure 3–30. The female pelvis organs (superior view). (Modified and reproduced, with permission, from deCherney AH, Pernoll ML [editors]: *Current Obstetric & Gynecologic Diagnosis & Treatment,* 8th ed. Appleton & Lange, 1994.)

Directions: With reference to the diagram, match the numbered structures with their corresponding lettered items.

(A) uterus
(B) bladder
(C) median umbilical fold
(D) ascending colon
(E) median umbilical ligament
(F) suspensory ligament of ovary
(G) ovary
(H) rectouterine pouch

(I) uterovesical pouch
(J) fimbria
(K) rectouterine fold
(L) mesosalpinx
(M) lateral umbilical fold
(N) uterine tube
(O) ureter
(P) rectum

BLOOD SUPPLY TO THE FEMALE PELVIS
(Questions 462 through 470)

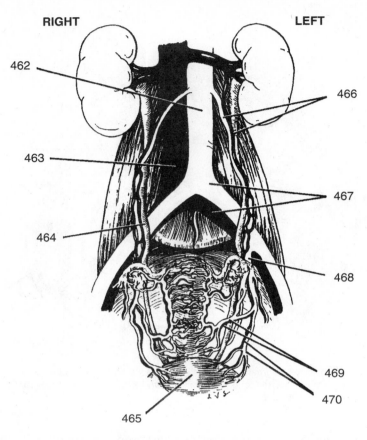

RIGHT **LEFT**

462
466
463
467
464
468
465
469
470

Figure 3–31. Blood supply to the female pelvis. (Modified and reproduced, with permission, from deCherney AH, Pernoll ML [editors]: *Current Obstetric & Gynecologic Diagnosis & Treatment,* 8th ed. Appleton & Lange, 1994.)

Directions: With reference to the diagram, match the numbered structures with their corresponding lettered items.

(A) ovarian artery and vein

(B) ureter

(C) common iliac artery and vein

(D) inferior vena cava

(E) uterine artery and vein

(F) hypogastric artery

(G) aorta

(H) inferior vesical artery and vein

(I) bladder

Answers

THE COXAL BONE

1. (D)
2. (R)
3. (K)
4. (A)
5. (H)
6. (P)
7. (N)
8. (F)
9. (B)
10. (D)

11. (Q)
12. (O)
13. (C)
14. (E)
15. (M)
16. (J)
17. (L)
18. (I)
19. (G)

URINARY SYSTEM (MALE)

20. (C)
21. (E)
22. (D)
23. (H)
24. (B)

25. (I)
26. (A)
27. (F)
28. (G)

PARASAGITTAL VIEW OF THE MALE PELVIS

29. (W)
30. (T)
31. (R)
32. (P)
33. (N)
34. (L)
35. (J)
36. (H)
37. (F)
38. (X)
39. (Y)
40. (C)
41. (D)

42. (G)
43. (I)
44. (K)
45. (M)
46. (B)
47. (E)
48. (A)
49. (O)
50. (Q)
51. (U)
52. (S)
53. (V)

BLADDER AND URETHRA

54. (E)
55. (H)
56. (I)
57. (J)
58. (A)
59. (M)
60. (K)

61. (B)
62. (F)
63. (L)
64. (C)
65. (G)
66. (D)

MALE REPRODUCTIVE SYSTEM (DIAGRAMMATIC VIEW)

67. (C)
68. (A)
69. (S)
70. (I)
71. (F)
72. (D)
73. (M)
74. (B)
75. (R)
76. (N)

77. (E)
78. (L)
79. (G)
80. (Q)
81. (H)
82. (J)
83. (K)
84. (P)
85. (O)

MALE REPRODUCTIVE SYSTEM (SAGITTAL VIEW)

86. (K)
87. (D)
88. (A)
89. (L)
90. (B)
91. (D)
92. (H)

93. (F)
94. (J)
95. (E)
96. (G)
97. (I)
98. (C)

PELVIC VISCERA

99.	(C)	115.	(M)
100.	(N)	116.	(E)
101.	(Y)	117.	(AD)
102.	(V)	118.	(AB)
103.	(H)	119.	(L)
104.	(Q)	120.	(F)
105.	(S)	121.	(G)
106.	(P)	122.	(J)
107.	(A)	123.	(O)
108.	(C)	124.	(K)
109.	(AC)	125.	(X)
110.	(Z)	126.	(R)
111.	(B)	127.	(W)
112.	(I)	128.	(U)
113.	(AA)	129.	(T)
114.	(D)		

ANTERIOR ABDOMINAL WALL AND SCROTAL HOMOLOGUES

130.	(L)	139.	(C)
131.	(G)	140.	(O)
132.	(I)	141.	(M)
133.	(A)	142.	(D)
134.	(E)	143.	(K)
135.	(B)	144.	(F)
136.	(B)	145.	(N)
137.	(Q)	146.	(P)
138.	(J)	147.	(H)

TESTIS, EPIDIDYMIS, AND SPERMATIC CORD

148.	(E)	154.	(B)
149.	(G)	155.	(F)
150.	(J)	156.	(C)
151.	(L)	157.	(H)
152.	(A)	158.	(D)
153.	(K)	159.	(I)

TUBULAR NETWORK OF THE TESTIS AND EPIDIDYMIS

160.	(E)	164.	(B)
161.	(A)	165.	(D)
162.	(H)	166.	(G)
163.	(F)	167.	(C)

DUCTUS DEFERENS AND SEMINAL VESICLES

168.	(H)	175.	(I)
169.	(M)	176.	(E)
170.	(A)	177.	(F)
171.	(D)	178.	(K)
172.	(B)	179.	(J)
173.	(L)	180.	(G)
174.	(C)		

DUCTUS DEFERENS

181.	(D)	191.	(C)
182.	(F)	192.	(S)
183.	(H)	193.	(K)
184.	(L)	194.	(R)
185.	(A)	195.	(M)
186.	(G)	196.	(P)
187.	(O)	197.	(N)
188.	(J)	198.	(Q)
189.	(I)	199.	(E)
190.	(B)		

FEMALE REPRODUCTIVE SYSTEM

200.	(L)	206.	(A)
201.	(J)	207.	(C)
202.	(H)	208.	(E)
203.	(F)	209.	(G)
204.	(D)	210.	(I)
205.	(B)	211.	(K)

UTERINE TUBES AND UTERUS

212.	(F)	221.	(C)
213.	(A)	222.	(J)
214.	(B)	223.	(D)
215.	(H)	224.	(O)
216.	(Q)	225.	(E)
217.	(R)	226.	(N)
218.	(K)	227.	(M)
219.	(P)	228.	(G)
220.	(L)	229.	(I)

UTERUS

230.	(F)	243.	(C)
231.	(L)	244.	(G)
232.	(H)	245.	(D)
233.	(M)	246.	(J)
234.	(A)	247.	(E)
235.	(R)	248.	(M)
236.	(K)	249.	(J)
237.	(O)	250.	(N)
238.	(I)	251.	(P)
239.	(B)	252.	(Q)
240.	(T)	253.	(S)
241.	(X)	254.	(U)
242.	(W)	255.	(V)

UROGENITAL AND ANORECTAL TRIANGLES

256.	(B)	258.	(A)
257.	(D)	259.	(C)

UTERUS

260.	(Q)	270.	(M)
261.	(B)	271.	(A)
262.	(E)	272.	(C)
263.	(I)	273.	(F)
264.	(P)	274.	(R)
265.	(L)	275.	(D)
266.	(A)	276.	(O)
267.	(G)	277.	(J)
268.	(N)	278.	(H)
269.	(K)		

LIGAMENTS OF THE UTERUS

279.	(G)	285.	(K)
280.	(F)	286.	(H)
281.	(A)	287.	(J)
282.	(L)	288.	(C)
283.	(I)	289.	(E)
284.	(B)	290.	(D)

EXTERNAL GENITALIA (FEMALE)

291.	(E)	297.	(B)
292.	(H)	298.	(J)
293.	(K)	299.	(F)
294.	(G)	300.	(C)
295.	(A)	301.	(I)
296.	(D)		

FEMALE PERINEUM

302.	(L)	313.	(N)
303.	(I)	314.	(H)
304.	(E)	315.	(J)
305.	(C)	316.	(S)
306.	(A)	317.	(R)
307.	(G)	318.	(M)
308.	(P)	319.	(Q)
309.	(K)	320.	(F)
310.	(B)	321.	(D)
311.	(O)	322.	(G)
312.	(T)		

PELVIC MUSCULATURE (FEMALE)

323.	(I)	328.	(H)
324.	(B)	329.	(C)
325.	(E)	330.	(D)
326.	(J)	331.	(F)
327.	(A)	332.	(G)

RELATIONSHIP OF THE BLADDER, PROSTATE, SEMINAL VESICLES, PENIS, URETHRA, AND SCROTAL CONTENTS

333.	(C)	342.	(B)
334.	(F)	343.	(D)
335.	(H)	344.	(I)
336.	(J)	345.	(K)
337.	(A)	346.	(L)
338.	(E)	347.	(H)
339.	(M)	348.	(D)
340.	(G)	349.	(I)
341.	(N)	350.	(O)

FEMALE REPRODUCTIVE SYSTEM

351.	(B)	366.	(E)
352.	(L)	367.	(Y)
353.	(U)	368.	(A)
354.	(P)	369.	(G)
355.	(C)	370.	(V)
356.	(K)	371.	(T)
357.	(Q)	372.	(I)
358.	(Z)	373.	(S)
359.	(I)	374.	(F)
360.	(X)	375.	(M)
361.	(V)	376.	(G)
362.	(S)	377.	(O)
363.	(D)	378.	(H)
364.	(R)	379.	(J)
365.	(W)	380.	(N)

TRANSFORMATION OF THE UNDIFFERENTIATED GENITAL SYSTEM INTO THE DEFINITIVE MALE SYSTEM

381. (F)	388. (C)
382. (A)	389. (N)
383. (J)	390. (D)
384. (M)	391. (F)
385. (B)	392. (I)
386. (K)	393. (H)
387. (L)	394. (G)

INNERVATION OF THE URINARY BLADDER AND URETHRA

395. (K)	401. (H)
396. (I)	402. (A)
397. (D)	403. (G)
398. (J)	404. (F)
399. (B)	405. (C)
400. (L)	406. (E)

RELATIONSHIP OF THE DUCTUS DEFERENS, SEMINAL VESICLES, PROSTATE, AND URETERS

407. (D)	414. (H)
408. (M)	415. (C)
409. (K)	416. (L)
410. (A)	417. (E)
411. (B)	418. (I)
412. (G)	419. (F)
413. (J)	

URINARY SYSTEM (MALE)

420. (C)	424. (A)
421. (E)	425. (G)
422. (B)	426. (D)
423. (F)	

MIDSAGITTAL VIEW OF THE FEMALE PELVIC ORGANS

427. (H)	433. (K)
428. (J)	434. (I)
429. (B)	435. (F)
430. (G)	436. (C)
431. (D)	437. (E)
432. (A)	

FASCIAL PLANES OF FEMALE PELVIS

438. (D)	442. (B)
439. (F)	443. (C)
440. (H)	444. (G)
441. (A)	445. (E)

FEMALE PELVIS ORGANS

446. (E)	454. (B)
447. (A)	455. (C)
448. (I)	456. (M)
449. (L)	457. (N)
450. (O)	458. (J)
451. (H)	459. (G)
452. (K)	460. (F)
453. (P)	461. (D)

BLOOD SUPPLY TO THE FEMALE PELVIS

462. (G)	467. (C)
463. (D)	468. (F)
464. (B)	469. (E)
465. (I)	470. (H)
466. (A)	

CHAPTER 4

Vertebral Canal and Cranial Cavity
Questions

DIRECTIONS (Questions 1 through 27): Each of the numbered items or incomplete statements in this section is followed by answers or by completions of the statement. Select the ONE lettered answer or completion that is BEST in each case.

1. The spinal cord extends from the foramen magnum to which of the following vertebral levels?

    (A) T6
    (B) L2
    (C) L5
    (D) S2
    (E) S5

2. All the following statements concerning the spinal cord are correct EXCEPT

    (A) it has both a cervical and lumbosacral enlargement
    (B) the spinal cord segments correspond with the vertebral levels
    (C) the thoracic region of the spinal cord is the longest part of the cord
    (D) the spinal cord occupies only the superior two-thirds of the vertebral canal
    (E) the sacral region is the shortest

3. The inferior end of the spinal cord tapers rather abruptly into the

    (A) cauda equina
    (B) filum terminalis
    (C) conus medullaris
    (D) lumbosacral enlargement
    (E) anococcygeal ligament

4. Cell bodies of axons making up the ventral roots are located in the

    (A) spinal root ganglion
    (B) posterior gray column
    (C) anterior gray column
    (D) lateral funiculus
    (E) anterior funiculus

5. The spinal ganglia are located

    (A) in the vertebral canal
    (B) in the foramen magnum
    (C) medial to the anterior longitudinal ligament
    (D) dorsal to the laminae
    (E) in the intervertebral foramina

6. The anterior spinal artery is formed by the union of two small branches from which of the following arteries?

    (A) deep cervical
    (B) intercostal
    (C) lumbar
    (D) vertebral
    (E) thyrocervical

7. The anterior spinal artery is usually smallest in which of the following cord segments?

    (A) T4 to T8
    (B) C2 to C6
    (C) T12 to L4
    (D) L5 to S4
    (E) S5 to 1st coccygeal

8. The cavity between the bony and ligamentous walls of the ventral canal and the dura contains all of the following structures EXCEPT

    (A) fat
    (B) anterior vertebral venous plexus
    (C) posterior vertebral venous plexus
    (D) capillary layer of fluid
    (E) loose connective tissue

9. Cerebrospinal fluid circulates in which of the following areas?

    (A) below the pia
    (B) subarachnoid space
    (C) subdural space
    (D) epidural space
    (E) central canal

10. The spinal cord is suspended in the dural sac by a saw-toothed structure known as the

   (A) filum terminale
   (B) cauda equina
   (C) denticulate ligament
   (D) anococcygeal ligament
   (E) coccygeal ligament

11. All the following statements concerning the falx cerebri are correct EXCEPT

   (A) it is sickle-shaped
   (B) it is located in the longitudinal fissure
   (C) it attaches anteriorly to the crista galli
   (D) it attaches posteriorly to the internal occipital protuberance
   (E) it separates the occipital lobes of the cerebral hemispheres from the cerebellum

12. The occipital venous sinus is located in the base of the

   (A) falx cerebelli
   (B) falx cerebri
   (C) tentorium cerebelli
   (D) cavernous sinus
   (E) diaphragma sellae

13. All the following statements concerning the middle meningeal artery are correct EXCEPT

   (A) it is the largest of the meningeal arteries
   (B) it is a branch of the maxillary artery
   (C) it is embedded in the external layer of the dura
   (D) it enters the cranial cavity through the foramen spinosum
   (E) it passes through the diaphragma sellae

14. The middle meningeal veins empty into which of the following veins?

   (A) vertebral
   (B) pterygoid plexus
   (C) hypophyseal plexus
   (D) external jugular
   (E) facial

15. The rich, sensory nerve supply to the dura is provided by which of the following nerves?

   (A) cervical sympathetic trunk
   (B) cervical plexus
   (C) trigeminal nerve
   (D) glossopharyngeal nerve
   (E) 7th cranial nerve

16. All the following statements concerning the pia mater are correct EXCEPT

   (A) it is poorly vascularized
   (B) it is the innermost layer of the meninges
   (C) it dips into the sulci
   (D) it follows penetrating cerebral vessels for a short distance into the brain
   (E) it is thicker than the arachnoid

17. All the following statements concerning the confluence of sinuses are correct EXCEPT

   (A) it is located at the internal occipital protuberance
   (B) it is the termination of the superior sagittal sinus
   (C) five sinuses often communicate at the confluence
   (D) it begins at the cavernous sinus
   (E) it may be referred to as the torcular Herophili

18. The main site of passage of cerebrospinal fluid into venous blood is through the

   (A) pterygoid plexus
   (B) arachnoid villi
   (C) cerebral veins
   (D) parietal foramina
   (E) meningeal veins

19. All of the following statements concerning the inferior sagittal sinus are correct EXCEPT

   (A) it is smaller than the superior sagittal sinus
   (B) it occupies the entire free edge of the falx cerebri
   (C) it ends by joining the great cerebral vein
   (D) it receives cortical veins
   (E) it joins another vein to form the straight sinus

20. The lateral wall of each cavernous sinus contains all the following nerves EXCEPT the

   (A) oculomotor
   (B) abducens
   (C) trochlear
   (D) ophthalmic nerve
   (E) maxillary nerve

21. Which of the following fissures and sulci separates the precentral gyrus from the postcentral gyrus?

   (A) central sulcus
   (B) calcarine sulcus
   (C) parieto-occipital sulcus

(D) transverse cerebral fissure

(E) longitudinal cerebral fissure

22. Which of the following lobes of the cerebral hemispheres is associated with the visual area?

    (A) parietal
    (B) insular
    (C) temporal
    (D) occipital
    (E) frontal

23. The main lobes of the cerebral hemispheres include all the following EXCEPT the

    (A) insular
    (B) frontal
    (C) temporal
    (D) occipital
    (E) parietal

24. The diencephalon surrounds the

    (A) cingulate gyrus
    (B) third ventricle
    (C) corpora quadrigemina
    (D) cerebral aqueduct
    (E) fornix

25. The cerebral aqueduct is located in the

    (A) thalamus
    (B) hypothalamus
    (C) midbrain
    (D) pineal gland
    (E) pituitary

26. Which of the following structures contains the pyramids?

    (A) pons
    (B) medulla
    (C) midbrain
    (D) thalamus
    (E) cerebral peduncles

27. Which of the following structures contain the cardiovascular and respiratory center?

    (A) diencephalon
    (B) midbrain
    (C) pons
    (D) medulla
    (E) cerebellum

DIRECTIONS (Questions 28 through 50): Each group of items in this section consists of lettered headings followed by a set of numbered words or phrases. For each numbered word or phrase, select the ONE lettered heading that is most closely associated with it. Each lettered heading may be selected once, more than once, or not at all.

Questions 28 through 36

    (A) thalami
    (B) cerebellum
    (C) internal capsule
    (D) precentral gyrus
    (E) midbrain

28. Located at the junction of the middle and posterior cranial fossae

29. Motor functions that regulate posture

30. Makes up four-fifths of the diencephalon

31. Muscle tone

32. Separates the thalamus and caudate nucleus from the lentiform nucleus

33. Muscular coordination

34. Occupies most of the posterior cranial fossa

35. "Little brain"

36. Primary motor area

Questions 37 through 45

    (A) pontine cistern
    (B) interpeduncular cistern
    (C) cistern of the lateral fissure
    (D) superior cistern
    (E) cerebellomedullary cistern

37. Contains the great cerebral vein

38. Contains the middle cerebral artery

39. Contains the pineal body

40. Contains the posterior part of the cerebral arterial circle of Willis

41. Often referred to clinically as the quadrigeminal cistern

42. Contains the basilar artery

43. The median aperture opens into this cistern

44. Also known as the cisterna magna

45. Lies between the splenium of the corpus callosum and the superior surface of the cerebellum

Questions 46 through 50

   (A) ophthalmic artery
   (B) basilar artery
   (C) anterior cerebral artery
   (D) posterior cerebral artery
   (E) middle cerebral artery

46. Supplies the temporal lobe

47. Supplies the occipital pole

48. Supplies the eye

49. Formed by the union of the two vertebral arteries

50. Divides into the two posterior cerebral arteries

ANSWERS AND EXPLANATIONS

1. **(B)** The spinal cord extends from the foramen magnum in the occipital bone to the level of the L2 vertebra. It ranges from 42 to 45 cm in length. *(Moore, p 359)*

2. **(B)** The spinal cord has a cervical and lumbosacral enlargement. The spinal cord segments do not correspond with the vertebral levels. The thoracic region of the spinal cord is the longest part of the cord, and the sacral region is the shortest part. *(Moore, p 359)*

3. **(C)** The inferior end of the spinal cord tapers rather abruptly into the conus medullaris. From its inferior end, a slender fibrous strand called the filum terminale, descends among the nerve rootlets comprising the cauda equina. The filum terminale blends with the superior end of the anococcygeal ligament. *(Moore, p 359)*

4. **(C)** The cell bodies of axons making up the ventral roots are in the ventral (anterior) gray horn (column) of the spinal cord, whereas the cell bodies of axons making up the dorsal roots are outside the spinal cord in the spinal ganglia (dorsal root ganglia). *(Moore, p 360)*

5. **(E)** The spinal ganglia are located in the intervertebral foramina, where they rest on the pedicles of the vertebral arches. Just outside the intervertebral foramina, the dorsal and ventral nerve roots unite to form a spinal nerve. *(Moore, p 360)*

6. **(D)** The anterior spinal artery is formed by the union of two small branches from the vertebral arteries. It runs the length of the spinal cord in the anterior median fissure and supplies the anterior two-thirds of the spinal cord. *(Moore, p 364)*

7. **(A)** The caliber of the anterior spinal artery varies according to its proximity to a major radicular artery. It is usually smallest in the T4 to T8 region of the cord. *(Moore, p 362)*

8. **(D)** The cavity between the bony and ligamentous walls of the vertebral canal and the dura is called the extradural (epidural) space. It contains fat, loose connective tissue, and the anterior and posterior vertebral venous plexuses. *(Moore, p 366)*

9. **(B)** Between the dura and arachnoid, there is a potential space, called the subdural space, containing only a capillary layer of fluid. Between the arachnoid and pia, there is an actual space, called the subarachnoid space, which contains cerebrospinal fluid and the vessels of the spinal cord. *(Moore, p 366)*

10. **(C)** The spinal cord is suspended in this dural sac by a saw-toothed denticulate ligament on each side. This ribbon-like ligament, composed of pia mater, is attached along the lateral surface of the spinal cord, midway between the dorsal and ventral nerve roots. The lateral edges of the denticulate ligament are notched or serrated. *(Moore, p 366)*

11. **(E)** The falx cerebri is a large, sickle-shaped, vertical partition in the longitudinal fissure between the two cerebral hemispheres. This thick, tough dural fold is attached in the median plane to the internal surface of the calvaria from the frontal bone and the crista galli of the ethmoid bone anteriorly to the internal occipital protuberance posteriorly. The tentorium cerebelli separates the occipital lobes of the cerebral hemispheres from the cerebellum. *(Moore, p 686)*

12. **(A)** Falx cerebelli is a small sickle-shaped median dural fold in the posterior part of the posterior cranial fossa. It extends almost vertically, inferior to the inferior surface of the tentorium cerebelli. Its free edge projects slightly between the cerebellar hemispheres. The occipital venous sinus is located in the base of the falx cerebelli. *(Moore, p 687)*

13. **(E)** The middle meningeal artery is the largest of the meningeal arteries. It is a branch of the maxillary artery and is embedded in the external layer of the dura. It enters the cranial cavity through the foramen spinosum in the floor of the middle cranial fossa. It does not enter the diaphragma sellae. *(Moore, p 687)*

14. **(B)**   The middle meningeal veins leave the skull through the foramen spinosum and foramen ovale to join the pterygoid plexus. *(Moore, p 687)*

15. **(C)**   The rich, sensory nerve supply to the dura is largely through the three divisions of the trigeminal nerve. Most of the supratentorial part of the dura is supplied by branches of the mandibular division of the trigeminal nerve. Sensory branches are also received from the vagus nerve and the three superior cervical nerves through the hypoglossal nerve. *(Moore, p 687)*

16. **(A)**   The pia mater is a thin membrane, but it is thicker than the arachnoid. The pia mater is the innermost of the three layers of meninges and is a highly vascularized, loose connective tissue membrane that adheres closely to the surface of the brain. It dips into all sulci and fissures and carries small blood vessels with it. When branches of cerebral vessels penetrate the brain, the pia follows them for a short distance, forming a sleeve of pia. *(Moore, p 688)*

17. **(D)**   At the terminal end of the superior sagittal sinus is a dilation known as the confluence of the sinuses. Occasionally this dilation is referred to as the sinus confluens or the torcular Herophili. Five sinuses often communicate at the confluence. It begins at the crista galli, not at the cavernous sinus. *(Moore, p 689)*

18. **(B)**   The main site of passage of cerebrospinal fluid into venous blood is through the arachnoid villi, especially those projecting into the superior sagittal sinus and the adjacent lateral venous lacunae. *(Moore, p 689)*

19. **(B)**   The inferior sagittal sinus is much smaller than the superior sagittal sinus. It occupies the posterior two-thirds of the free inferior edge of the falx cerebri. It ends by joining the great cerebral vein to form the straight sinus. The inferior sagittal receives cortical veins from the medial aspects of the cerebral hemispheres. *(Moore, p 690)*

20. **(B)**   The lateral wall of each cavernous sinus contains—from superior to inferior—oculomotor, trochlear, ophthalmic, and maxillary divisions of the trigeminal nerve. Inside each cavernous sinus is the internal carotid artery with its sympathetic plexus and the abducens nerve. *(Moore, p 690)*

21. **(A)**   The central sulcus runs inferoanteriorly from the middle of the superior margin of the cerebral hemisphere, stopping just short of the lateral sulcus. The central sulcus is an important landmark of the cerebral cortex because the motor area (precentral gyrus) lies anterior to it and the general sensory cortex (postcentral gyrus) posterior to it. *(Moore, p 693)*

22. **(D)**   The occipital lobes are located posterior to the parieto-occipital sulci. They rest on the tentorium cerebelli, superior to the posterior cranial fossa. Although they are relatively small, these lobes are very important because they contain the visual area. *(Moore, p 693)*

23. **(A)**   The main lobes of the cerebral hemispheres include the frontal, parietal, temporal, and occipital. *(Moore, p 693)*

24. **(B)**   The cavity of the diencephalon surrounds the third ventricle of the brain and forms the central core of the brain. It is surrounded by the cerebral hemispheres. *(Moore, p 696)*

25. **(C)**   The cavity of the midbrain is represented by a narrow canal called the cerebral aqueduct. It conducts cerebrospinal fluid from the lateral and third ventricles to the fourth ventricle. *(Moore, p 696)*

26. **(B)**   The medulla is continuous with the spinal cord at the foramen magnum. The distinctive characteristics of its ventral surface are the elongated pyramids. *(Moore, p 696)*

27. **(D)**   The medulla contains the cardiovascular and respiratory centers for the automatic control of heartbeat and respiration, respectively. *(Moore, p 696)*

28. **(E)**   The midbrain is the smallest part of the brain stem, and it is located at the junction of the middle and posterior cranial fossae, lying partly in each. *(Moore, p 696)*

29. **(B)**   The cerebellum is mainly concerned with motor functions that regulate posture. The cerebellum consists of a midline portion—the vermis—and two lateral hemispheres. *(Moore, pp 696–697)*

30. **(A)**   The diencephalon is composed of the thalamus, hypothalamus, epithalamus, and subthalamus. The two thalami make up four-fifths of the diencephalon. *(Moore, p 696)*

31. **(B)**   The cerebellum is concerned with muscle tone. *(Moore, p 697)*

32. **(C)**   The internal capsule separates the thalamus and the caudate nucleus from the lentiform nucleus, which lies deep to the insula in the depth of the lateral sulcus. *(Moore, p 697)*

33. **(B)**   The cerebellum is concerned with muscular coordination. *(Moore, p 697)*

34. (B) The cerebellum occupies most of the posterior cranial fossa. *(Moore, p 697)*

35. (B) The cerebellum is known as the "little brain." It overlies the posterior aspect of the pons and medulla and extends laterally beneath the tentorium cerebelli. *(Moore, p 696)*

36. (D) The primary motor area is located in the precentral gyrus, including the anterior wall of the central sulcus. *(Moore, p 694)*

37. (D) The superior cistern contains the great cerebral vein. *(Moore, p 700)*

38. (C) The cistern of the lateral fissure contains the middle cerebral artery and is located anterior to each temporal lobe, where the arachnoid covers the lateral sulcus. *(Moore, p 700)*

39. (D) The superior cistern contains the pineal body. *(Moore, p 700)*

40. (B) The interpeduncular cistern is located between the cerebral peduncles and contains the posterior part of the cerebral arterial circle of Willis. *(Moore, p 700)*

41. (D) The superior cistern lies dorsal to the colliculi of the midbrain and, therefore, is often referred to clinically as the quadrigeminal cistern. *(Moore, p 700)*

42. (A) The pontine cistern is an extensive space along the ventral and lateral surfaces of the pons, containing the basilar artery and some of the cranial nerves. *(Moore, p 700)*

43. (E) The cerebellomedullary cistern receives cerebrospinal fluid from the median aperture of the fourth ventricle and is continuous with the large subarachnoid space around the brain and spinal cord. *(Moore, p 699)*

44. (E) The cerebellomedullary cistern is also known as the cisterna magna. *(Moore, p 699)*

45. (D) The superior cistern lies between the splenium of the corpus callosum and the superior surface of the cerebellum. *(Moore, p 700)*

46. (E) The middle cerebral artery supplies the lateral surface of the cerebral hemispheres, which includes the temporal bone. *(Moore, pp 701–702)*

47. (D) The posterior cerebral artery supplies the inferior surface and the occipital pole. *(Moore, p 702)*

48. (A) The cerebral part of the internal carotid artery immediately gives off the important ophthalmic artery, which supplies the eye. *(Moore, p 700)*

49. (B) The basilar artery is formed by the union of the two vertebral arteries. *(Moore, p 701)*

50. (B) The basilar artery ends by dividing into the two posterior cerebral arteries. *(Moore, p 701)*

Clinical Vertebral Canal and Cranial Cavity Questions

DIRECTIONS (Questions 1 through 10): Each group of items in this section consists of lettered headings followed by a set of numbered words or phrases. For each numbered word or phrase, select the ONE lettered heading that is most closely associated with it. Each lettered heading may be selected once, more than once, or not at all.

(A) craniopharyngioma
(B) spina bifida
(C) anencephalus
(D) meningocele
(E) meningomyelocele
(F) hydrocephalus
(G) meningoencephalocele
(H) meningohydroencephalocele

1. Failure of the cephalic part of the neural tube to close

2. Abnormal accumulation of cerebrospinal fluid within the ventricular system or between the brain and dura mater

3. Almost always continuous with an open cord in the cervical region

4. Vault of the skull is absent

5. Thought to be due to an obstruction of the aqueduct of Sylvius in the majority of cases

6. Only the meninges bulge through the opening

7. Both meninges and brain bulge through the opening

8. Meninges, brain, and ventricle bulge through the opening

9. Usually localized in the sacrolumbar region

10. Sometimes contains the meninges and the spinal cord and its nerves

ANSWERS AND EXPLANATIONS

1. **(C)** Anencephalus is characterized by failure of the cephalic part of the neural tube to close, and, at birth, the brain is represented by a mass of degenerated tissue exposed to the surface. *(Sadler, p 378)*

2. **(F)** Hydrocephalus is characterized by an abnormal accumulation of cerebrospinal fluid within the ventricular system or, as in the case of external hydrocephalus, between the brain and dura mater. *(Sadler, p 378)*

3–4. **(C)** Anencephalus is almost always continuous with an open cord in the cervical region. The vault of the skull is absent, giving the head a characteristic appearance, with the eyes bulging forward and the surfaces of the face and chest forming a continuous plane. *(Sadler, p 378)*

5. **(F)** In the majority of cases, hydrocephalus in the newborn is thought to be due to an obstruction of the aqueduct of Sylvius. This prevents the cerebrospinal fluid of the lateral and third ventricles from passing into the fourth ventricle and from there into the subarachnoid space. *(Sadler, p 378)*

6. **(D)** If more than one or two vertebrae are involved, the meninges of the spinal cord bulge through the opening, and a sac covered with skin, known as a meningocele, is visible on the surface. *(Sadler, pp 362–363)*

7. **(G)** If both meninges and brain bulge through the defect, it is called meningoencephalocele. *(Sadler, p 377)*

8. **(H)** If meninges, brain, and ventricle penetrate the opening, it is then called meningohydroencephalocele. *(Sadler, p 377)*

9. **(B)** A spina bifida usually occurs in the sacrolumbar region and is covered by skin. It is not noticeable on the surface except for the pressure of a small tuft of hair over the affected area (spina bifida occulta). *(Sadler, p 362)*

10. **(E)** Sometimes the defect in the vertebral column is so large it contains meninges and the spinal cord and its nerves. *(Sadler, p 363)*

Developmental Vertebral Canal and Cranial Cavity
Questions

DIRECTIONS (Question 1): Each of the numbered items or incomplete statements in this section is followed by answers or by completions of the statement. Select the ONE lettered answer or completion that is BEST in each case.

1. Closure of the cranial neuropore occurs approximately at which of the following somite stages?

    (A) 5th
    (B) 10th
    (C) 20th
    (D) 30th
    (E) 40th

DIRECTIONS (Questions 2 through 20): Each group of items in this section consists of lettered headings followed by a set of numbered words or phrases. For each numbered word or phrase, select the ONE lettered heading that is most closely associated with it. Each lettered heading may be selected once, more than once, or not at all.

Questions 2 through 5

    (A) prosencephalon
    (B) mesencephalon
    (C) rhombencephalon

2. Telencephalon

3. Diencephalon

4. Metencephalon

5. Myelencephalon

Questions 6 through 12

    (A) basal plate
    (B) alar plate
    (C) intermediate horn
    (D) neural crest cells

6. Anterior horn cells

7. Present only at thoracic and upper lumbar levels

8. Sensory cell bodies of the spinal cord

9. Dorsal root ganglia

10. Trigeminal ganglion

11. Geniculate ganglion

12. Jugular ganglion

Questions 13 through 20

    (A) microglia cells
    (B) oligodendroglia cells
    (C) Schwann cells
    (D) ependymal cells
    (E) protoplasmic astrocytes

13. Form the myelin sheaths around the ascending and descending axons in the marginal layer

14. Are highly phagocytic

15. Accomplish myelination of the peripheral nerves

16. Originate from the neural crest

17. Differentiate in the mantle layer

18. Differentiate into these cells when the neuroepithelial cells cease to produce neuroblasts and gliablasts

19. Derived from mesenchyme

20. Found mainly in the marginal layer

ANSWERS AND EXPLANATIONS

1. **(C)** Closure of the cranial neuropore occurs at the 18 to 20 somite stage (25th day). The closure of the caudal neuropore occurs about 2 days later. *(Sadler, p 352)*

2–3. **(A)** When the embryo is 5 weeks old, the prosencephalon consists of two parts: (1) the telencephalon or endbrain, formed by a midportion and two lateral outpocketings—the primitive cerebral hemispheres—and (2) the diencephalon, characterized by the outgrowth of the optic vesicles. *(Sadler, p 354)*

4–5. **(C)** The rhombencephalon consists of two parts: (1) the metencephalon, which later forms the pons and cerebellum, and (2) the myelencephalon, which later forms the medulla. *(Sadler, p 354)*

6. **(A)** The basal plates contain the ventral motor horn cells and form the motor areas of the spinal cord. *(Sadler, p 356)*

7. **(C)** In addition to the ventral motor horn and the dorsal sensory horn, a group of neurons accumulates between the two areas and causes the formation of a small intermediate horn that contains mainly neurons of the sympathetic portion of the autonomic nervous system and is present only in the thoracic and upper lumbar levels. *(Sadler, p 356)*

8. **(B)** The dorsal thickenings—the alar plates—form the sensory areas of the spinal cord. *(Sadler, p 356)*

9–12. **(D)** During the invagination of the neural plate, a group of cells appears along each edge of the neural groove. These cells, ectodermal in origin and known as the neural crest cells, temporarily form an intermediate zone between the tube and the surface ectoderm. Here the cells give rise to the sensory ganglia or dorsal root ganglia of the spinal and cranial nerves (5th, 7th, 9th, and 10th). *(Sadler, p 359)*

13. **(B)** Another type of supporting cell possibly derived from the gliablasts is the oligodendroglia cell, which forms the myelin sheaths around the ascending and descending axons in the marginal layer. *(Sadler, p 358)*

14. **(A)** The microglia cell appears in the central nervous system and is highly phagocytic. *(Sadler, p 359)*

15–16. **(C)** Myelination of the peripheral nerves is accomplished by the cells of Schwann. They migrate peripherally and wrap themselves around the axons, thus forming the neurilemma sheath. These cells originate from the neural crest. *(Sadler, p 360)*

17. **(E)** The majority of the primitive supporting cells, the gliablasts, are formed by the neuroepithelial cells after the production of neuroblasts has ceased. From the neuroepithelial layer, the gliablasts migrate to the mantle and marginal layers. In the mantle layer, they differentiate into the protoplasmic and fibrillar astrocytes. *(Sadler, p 358)*

18. **(D)** When the neuroepithelial cells cease to produce neuroblasts and gliablasts, they finally differentiate into the ependymal cells. *(Sadler, p 359)*

19. **(A)** The microglia cell is derived from mesenchyme, not neuroepithelial cells. *(Sadler, p 358)*

20. **(B)** The oligodendroglia cell is mainly found in the marginal layer to form myelin around the ascending and descending tracts in the marginal layer. *(Sadler, p 359)*

Illustrations
Questions

LATERAL VIEW OF LEFT CEREBRAL HEMISPHERE
(Questions 1 through 19)

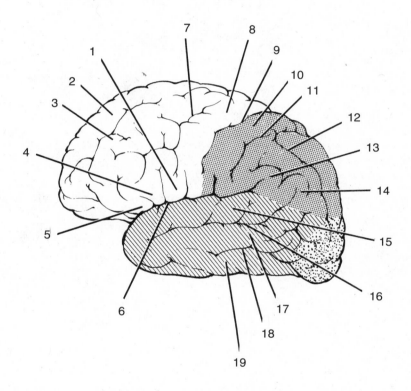

Figure 4–1. Lateral view of the left cerebral hemisphere. (Modified and reproduced, with permission, from Waxman SG, deGroot J: *Correlative Neuroanatomy*, 22nd ed. Lange, 1995.)

Directions: With reference to the diagram, match the numbered structures with their corresponding lettered items.

(A) central sulcus (fissure of Rolando)
(B) lateral cerebral fissure (fissure of Sylvius)
(C) opercular portion of inferior frontal gyrus
(D) orbital portion of inferior frontal gyrus
(E) triangular portion of inferior frontal gyrus
(F) posterior central gyrus
(G) angular gyrus
(H) precentral sulcus
(I) superior temporal gyrus
(J) inferior temporal gyrus

(K) superior frontal gyrus
(L) middle temporal gyrus
(M) precentral gyrus
(N) middle frontal gyrus
(O) superior temporal sulcus
(P) supramarginal gyrus
(Q) postcentral sulcus
(R) intraparietal sulcus
(S) middle temporal sulcus

MEDIAL VIEW OF RIGHT CEREBRAL HEMISPHERE
(Questions 20 through 32)

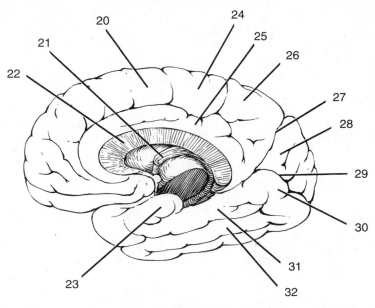

Figure 4–2. Medial view of right cerebral hemisphere. (Modified and reproduced, with permission, from Waxman SG, deGroot J: *Correlative Neuroanatomy,* 22nd ed. Lange, 1995.)

Directions: With reference to the diagram, match the numbered structures with their corresponding lettered items.

(A) occipitotemporal gyrus

(B) superior frontal gyrus

(C) parahippocampal gyrus

(D) calcarine fissure

(E) corpus callosum

(F) paracentral lobule

(G) uncus

(H) parieto-occipital fissure

(I) fornix

(J) lingual gyrus

(K) cingulate gyrus

(L) precuneus

(M) cuneus

CORONAL SECTION THROUGH CEREBRUM
AT LEVELS OF ANTERIOR COMMISSURE
(Questions 33 through 46)

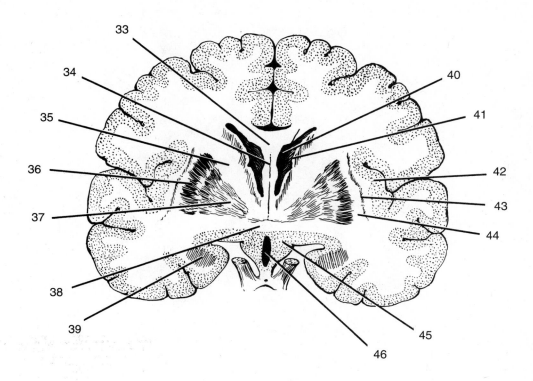

Figure 4–3. Coronal section through cerebrum at levels of anterior commissure. (Modified and reproduced, with permission, from Chusid JG: *Correlative Neuroanatomy & Functional Neurology,* 19th ed. Lange, 1985.)

Directions: With reference to the diagram, match the numbered structures with their corresponding lettered items.

(A) anterior commissure

(B) lateral ventricle

(C) septum pellucidum

(D) external capsule

(E) hypothalamus

(F) caudate nucleus

(G) corpus callosum

(H) insula

(I) internal capsule

(J) claustrum

(K) putamen

(L) third ventricle

(M) globus pallidus

(N) amygdaloid body

HORIZONTAL SECTIONS THROUGH CEREBRUM AT 2 LEVELS
TO SHOW BASAL GANGLIA
(Questions 47 through 56)

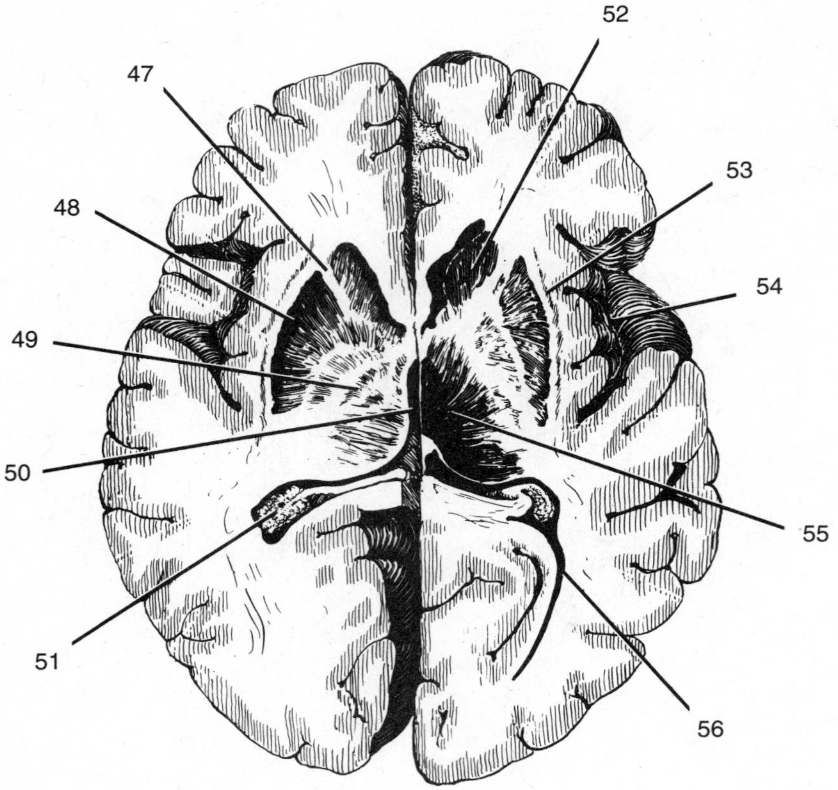

Figure 4–4. Horizontal sections through cerebrum at 2 levels to show basal ganglia. (Modified and reproduced, with permission, from Chusid JG: *Correlative Neuroanatomy & Functional Neurology,* 19th ed. Lange, 1985.)

Directions: With reference to the diagram, match the numbered structures with their corresponding lettered items.

(A) posterior horn of lateral ventricle

(B) caudate nucleus

(C) insula

(D) internal capsule (anterior limb)

(E) choroid plexus

(F) claustrum

(G) putamen

(H) thalamus

(I) globus pallidus

(J) third ventricle

SAGITTAL SECTION THROUGH BRAIN
SHOWING THE DIENCEPHALON
(Questions 57 through 72)

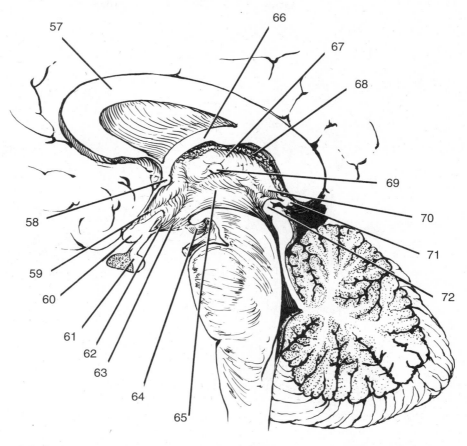

Figure 4–5. Sagittal section through brain showing the diencephalon. (Modified and reproduced, with permission, from Chusid JG: *Correlative Neuroanatomy & Functional Neurology,* 19th ed. Lange, 1985.)

Directions: With reference to the diagram, match the numbered structures with their corresponding lettered items.

(A) choroid plexus of third ventricle
(B) supraoptic recess
(C) interthalamic adhesion
(D) corpus callosum
(E) posterior commissure
(F) hypothalamic sulcus
(G) anterior commissure
(H) neurohypophysis

(I) fornix (corpus)
(J) habenular nuclei
(K) optic chiasm
(L) pineal body
(M) infundibulum
(N) thalamus
(O) mamillary body
(P) tuber cinereum

EXTERNAL ANATOMY OF THE BRAIN STEM
(Questions 73 through 82)

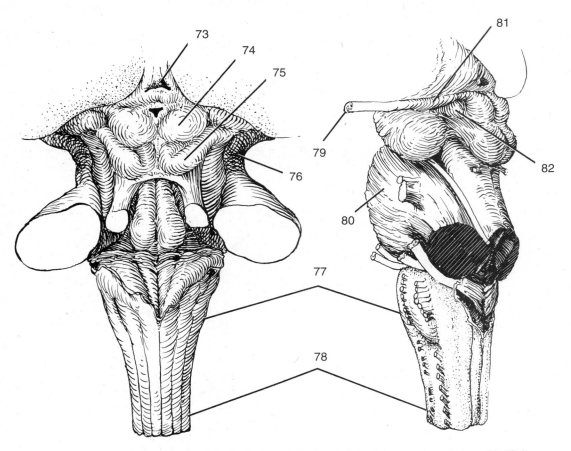

Figure 4–6. External anatomy of the brain stem. *Left:* dorsal view; *right:* dorsolateral view. (Modified and reproduced, with permission, from Chusid JG: *Correlative Neuroanatomy & Functional Neurology,* 19th ed. Lange, 1985.)

Directions: With reference to the diagram, match the numbered structures with their corresponding lettered items.

(A) lateral geniculate body

(B) cerebral peduncle

(C) medial geniculate body

(D) superior colliculus

(E) medulla oblongata

(F) third ventricle

(G) spinal cord

(H) inferior colliculus

(I) pons

(J) optic tract

DORSAL ASPECT OF THE BRAIN STEM
(Questions 83 through 101)

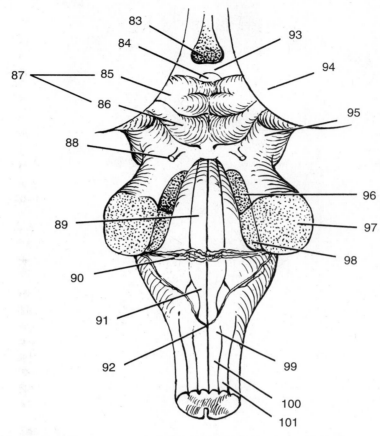

Figure 4–7. Dorsal aspect of the brain stem. (Modified and reproduced, with permission, from Chusid JG: *Correlative Neuroanatomy & Functional Neurology,* 19th ed. Lange, 1985.)

Directions: With reference to the diagram, match the numbered structures with their corresponding lettered items.

(A) superior cerebellar peduncle (brachium conjunctivum)

(B) rhomboid fossa (superior portion)

(C) middle cerebellar peduncle (brachium pontis)

(D) third ventricle

(E) rhomboid fossa (inferior portion)

(F) inferior cerebellar peduncle (corpus restiforme)

(G) fasciculus gracilis

(H) superior colliculus

(I) habenular commissure

(J) pineal body

(K) clava

(L) thalamus

(M) trochlear nerve

(N) corpora quadrigemina

(O) cerebral peduncle

(P) inferior colliculus

(Q) obex

(R) medullary stria

(S) fasciculus cuneatus

THE VENTRICULAR SYSTEM
(Questions 102 through 109)

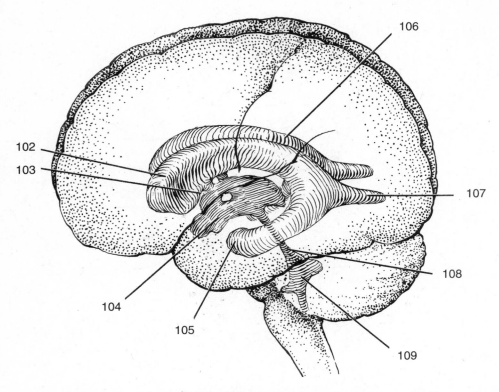

Figure 4–8. The ventricular system. (Modified and reproduced, with permission, from Chusid JG: *Correlative Neuroanatomy & Functional Neurology,* 19th ed. Lange, 1985.)

Directions: With reference to the diagram, match the numbered structures with their corresponding lettered items.

(A) cerebral aqueduct (aqueduct of Sylvius)
(B) interventricular foramen (Monro)
(C) posterior horn
(D) lateral ventricle

(E) fourth ventricle
(F) anterior horn
(G) third ventricle
(H) inferior horn

CIRCULATION OF CEREBROSPINAL FLUID
(Questions 110 through 123)

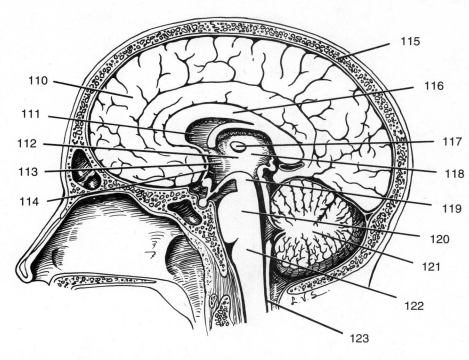

Figure 4–9. Circulation of cerebrospinal fluid. (Modified and reproduced, with permission, from Junqueira LC, Carneiro J: *Basic Histology,* 4th ed. Lange, 1983.)

Directions: With reference to the diagram, match the numbered structures with their corresponding lettered items.

(A) interthalamic adhesions

(B) hypothalamic sulcus

(C) spinal cord

(D) cerebral hemisphere

(E) corpus callosum

(F) medulla

(G) septum pellucidum

(H) skull

(I) cerebellum

(J) lamina terminalis

(K) pons

(L) thalamus

(M) midbrain

(N) hypothalamus

CIRCLE OF WILLIS AND PRINCIPAL ARTERIES
OF THE BRAIN
(Questions 124 through 139)

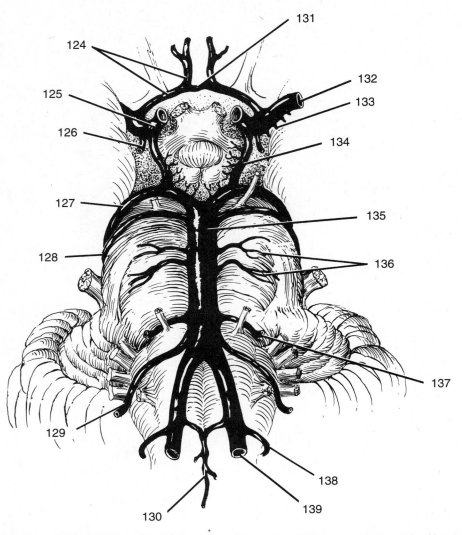

Figure 4–10. Circle of Willis and principal arteries of the brain. (Modified and reproduced, with permission, from Chusid JG: *Correlative Neuroanatomy & Functional Neurology,* 19th ed. Lange, 1985.)

Directions: With reference to the diagram, match the numbered structures with their corresponding lettered items.

(A) anterior communicating artery

(B) internal carotid artery

(C) internal auditory artery

(D) posterior inferior cerebellar artery

(E) anterior cerebral artery

(F) posterior communicating artery

(G) anterior inferior cerebellar artery

(H) middle cerebral artery

(I) anterior spinal artery

(J) anterior choroidal artery

(K) lenticulostriate artery

(L) posterior cerebral artery

(M) vertebral artery

(N) basilar artery

(O) superior cerebellar artery

(P) pontine arteries

EMERGENCE OF CRANIAL NERVES FROM THE BRAIN
(Questions 140 through 160)

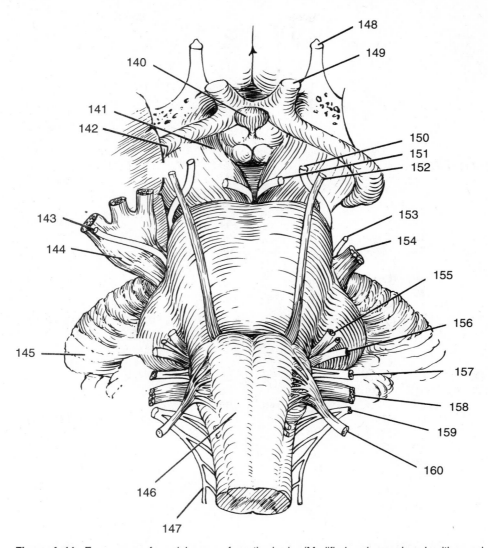

Figure 4–11. Emergence of cranial nerves from the brain. (Modified and reproduced, with permission, from Waxman SG, deGroot J: *Correlative Neuroanatomy,* 22nd ed. Lange, 1995.)

Directions: With reference to the diagram, match the numbered structures with their corresponding lettered items.

(A) spinal root of accessory nerve

(B) oculomotor nerve

(C) glossopharyngeal nerve

(D) pituitary gland

(E) olfactory tract

(F) vestibulocochlear nerve

(G) cerebral peduncle

(H) hypoglossal nerve

(I) motor root of trigeminal nerve

(J) semilunar ganglion

(K) sensory root of trigeminal nerve

(L) optic tract

(M) abducens nerve

(N) vagus nerve

(O) trochlear nerve

(P) medulla

(Q) spinal accessory nerve

(R) facial nerve

(S) cerebellum

(T) motor root of V

(U) optic nerve

Answers

LATERAL VIEW OF LEFT CEREBRAL HEMISPHERE

1. (C)	11. (Q)
2. (K)	12. (R)
3. (N)	13. (P)
4. (E)	14. (G)
5. (D)	15. (I)
6. (B)	16. (O)
7. (H)	17. (L)
8. (M)	18. (S)
9. (A)	19. (J)
10. (F)	

MEDIAL VIEW OF RIGHT CEREBRAL HEMISPHERE

20. (B)	27. (H)
21. (I)	28. (M)
22. (E)	29. (D)
23. (G)	30. (J)
24. (F)	31. (C)
25. (K)	32. (A)
26. (L)	

CORONAL SECTION THROUGH CEREBRUM AT LEVELS OF ANTERIOR COMMISSURE

33. (G)	40. (B)
34. (C)	41. (F)
35. (I)	42. (H)
36. (K)	43. (J)
37. (M)	44. (D)
38. (A)	45. (E)
39. (N)	46. (L)

HORIZONTAL SECTIONS THROUGH CEREBRUM AT 2 LEVELS TO SHOW BASAL GANGLIA

47. (D)	52. (B)
48. (G)	53. (F)
49. (I)	54. (C)
50. (J)	55. (H)
51. (E)	56. (A)

SAGITTAL SECTION THROUGH BRAIN SHOWING THE DIENCEPHALON

57. (D)	65. (F)
58. (G)	66. (I)
59. (B)	67. (N)
60. (K)	68. (A)
61. (H)	69. (C)
62. (M)	70. (J)
63. (P)	71. (L)
64. (O)	72. (E)

EXTERNAL ANATOMY OF THE BRAIN STEM

73. (F)	78. (G)
74. (D)	79. (J)
75. (H)	80. (I)
76. (B)	81. (A)
77. (E)	82. (C)

DORSAL ASPECT OF THE BRAIN

83.	(D)	93.	(I)
84.	(J)	94.	(L)
85.	(H)	95.	(O)
86.	(P)	96.	(A)
87.	(N)	97.	(C)
88.	(M)	98.	(F)
89.	(B)	99.	(K)
90.	(R)	100.	(G)
91.	(E)	101.	(S)
92.	(Q)		

THE VENTRICULAR SYSTEM

102.	(F)	106.	(D)
103.	(B)	107.	(C)
104.	(G)	108.	(A)
105.	(H)	109.	(E)

CIRCULATION OF CEREBROSPINAL FLUID

110.	(D)	117.	(A)
111.	(G)	118.	(L)
112.	(B)	119.	(M)
113.	(N)	120.	(K)
114.	(J)	121.	(I)
115.	(H)	122.	(F)
116.	(E)	123.	(C)

CIRCLE OF WILLIS AND PRINCIPAL ARTERIES OF THE BRAIN

124.	(E)	132.	(H)
125.	(B)	133.	(K)
126.	(J)	134.	(F)
127.	(L)	135.	(N)
128.	(O)	136.	(P)
129.	(G)	137.	(C)
130.	(I)	138.	(D)
131.	(A)	139.	(M)

EMERGENCE OF CRANIAL NERVES FROM THE BRAIN

140.	(D)	151.	(B)
141.	(G)	152.	(M)
142.	(L)	153.	(I)
143.	(T)	154.	(K)
144.	(J)	155.	(R)
145.	(S)	156.	(F)
146.	(P)	157.	(C)
147.	(A)	158.	(N)
148.	(E)	159.	(Q)
149.	(U)	160.	(H)
150.	(O)		

─────────────────────────── CHAPTER 5 ───────────────────────────

The Back
Questions

DIRECTIONS (Questions 1 through 17): Each of the numbered items or incomplete statements in this section is followed by answers or by completions of the statement. Select the ONE lettered answer or completion that is BEST in each case.

1. All the following statements concerning the middle cluneal nerves are correct EXCEPT

   (A) they are dorsal primary rami
   (B) they become cutaneous at the anterior superior iliac spine
   (C) they supply the skin and subcutaneous tissues over the back of the sacrum
   (D) they are lateral branches of dorsal rami
   (E) they arise from the 1st, 2nd, and 3rd sacral nerves

2. All the following structures provide origins for the trapezius muscle EXCEPT the

   (A) distal one-third of the superior nuchal line
   (B) external occipital protuberance
   (C) ligamentum nuchae
   (D) spine of the 7th cervical vertebra
   (E) spines of all thoracic vertebrae

3. The latissimus dorsi inserts into which of the following structures?

   (A) acromion
   (B) coracoid process
   (C) floor of the intertubercular groove of the humerus
   (D) supraglenoid tubercle
   (E) greater tubercle of the humerus

4. All the following statements concerning the erector spinae are correct EXCEPT the

   (A) they extend the vertebral column
   (B) the muscle is innervated serially by branches of the dorsal rami of all spinal nerves
   (C) they are deep to the semispinalis and multifidus muscles of the transversospinal group

(D) they occupy the vertebrocostal groove of the back
(E) they are surrounded by thoracolumbar fasciae

5. All the following muscles have attachments with the skull EXCEPT

   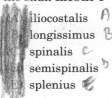
   iliocostalis A
   longissimus B
   spinalis C
   semispinalis D
   splenius E

6. The vertebral arch includes the

   (A) transverse processes
   (B) spinous processes
   (C) vertebral bodies
   (D) pedicles
   (E) intervertebral disks

7. All the following characteristics of thoracic vertebrae are correct EXCEPT

   (A) they exhibit costal facets
   (B) they have circular vertebral foramina
   (C) they have long spinous processes
   (D) they have superior articular processes that face directly forward
   (E) the articular facets favor lateral bending and rotation of the column

8. All the following movements are permitted at the auricular surfaces of the lumbar vertebrae EXCEPT

   (A) flexion
   (B) extension
   (C) side-to-side bending
   (D) rotation
   (E) sliding

9. All the following characteristics of cervical vertebrae are correct EXCEPT

   (A) the spinous process is short and bifid
   (B) the transverse process is perforated by the
   transverse foramen
   (C) the vertebral foramen is small and oval-
   shaped
   (D) they are the smallest of the vertebrae
   (E) the 1st, 2nd, and 7th cervical vertebrae are
   atypical

10. All the following statements concerning the 2nd
cervical vertebra are correct EXCEPT

    (A) it is known as the atlas
    (B) it has a bifid spine
    (C) its transverse processes contain transverse
    foramina
    (D) the bodies of the 1st and 2nd cervical verte-
    brae are fused
    (E) it is considered to be atypical

11. The laminae of the 5th sacral, and sometimes the
4th, fail to meet, and thus produce the

    (A) sacral promontory
    (B) sacral hiatus
    (C) sacral ala
    (D) dorsal sacral foramina
    (E) pelvic sacral foramina

12. All the following statements concerning the vertebral column are correct EXCEPT

    (A) the majority of vertebral columns range be-
    tween 72 and 75 cm in length
    (B) one-fourth of the vertebral column length is
    accounted for by the intervertebral disks
    (C) the adult vertebral column has four curva-
    tures
    (D) two primary curvatures exist in fetal life
    (E) the center of gravity of the body is located at
    the dens

13. All the following statements concerning the intervertebral disks are correct EXCEPT

    (A) they are of uniform thickness at thoracic lev-
    els
    (B) they are thickest in the lumbar region
    (C) they are important shock absorbers
    (D) they are attached ventrally and dorsally to
    the anterior and posterior longitudinal liga-
    ments
    (E) they are thinner in front than behind in the
    cervical and lumbar regions

14. All the following statements concerning the posterior longitudinal ligament are correct EXCEPT

    (A) it is located in the vertebral canal
    (B) it is continuous with the tectorial membrane
    (C) it is attached to the occipital bone
    (D) it ends below in the sacral canal
    (E) it extends along the anterior surfaces of the
    bodies of the vertebrae

15. All the following statements concerning the ligamenta flava are correct EXCEPT

    (A) they connect the laminae of adjacent verte-
    brae
    (B) they extend lateralward as far as the articu-
    lar capsules
    (C) they assist in maintaining the upright pos-
    ture
    (D) they are fibrocartilaginous ligaments
    (E) the two portions of the two sides meet at the
    root of the spine

16. Which of the following nerves provide the innervation for the facet joints?

    (A) medial branches of the dorsal primary rami
    (B) lateral cutaneous branches of the ventral pri-
    mary rami
    (C) medial branch of the anterior cutaneous
    (D) lateral branch of the dorsal primary rami
    (E) posterior branch of the lateral cutaneous

17. The tectorial membrane is the continuation of
which of the following ligaments?

    (A) anterior longitudinal
    (B) posterior longitudinal
    (C) supraspinous
    (D) ligamentum nuchae
    (E) ligamenta flava

DIRECTIONS (Questions 18 through 37): Each group of items in this section consists of lettered headings followed by a set of numbered words or phrases. For each numbered word or phrase, select the ONE lettered heading that is most closely associated with it. Each lettered heading may be selected once, more than once, or not at all.

Questions 18 through 25

(A) splenius capitis
(B) iliocostalis
(C) longissimus
(D) spinalis
(E) semispinalis capitis
(F) multifidus
(G) rotators
(H) inferior capitis oblique

18. Takes origin from the spinal process of the C2 vertebra and runs obliquely and anteriorly to insert on the inferior surface of the transverse process of the C1 vertebra

19. Arises from the transverse processes of the T1 to T6 vertebrae and inserts on the medial half of the area between the superior and inferior nuchal lines on the occipital bone

20. Forms the largest muscle mass in the posterior aspect of the neck

21. Passes superomedially from the vertebral arches to the spinous processes, spanning one to three vertebrae

22. Arises from the transverse process of one vertebra and inserts into the base of the spinous process of the vertebra superior to it

23. Inserts into the angles of the ribs

24. Inserts into the transverse processes of the thoracic and cervical vertebrae and the mastoid process of the temporal bone of the skull

25. Takes origin on the inferior half of the ligamentum nuchae and the spinous processes of the T1 to T6 vertebrae

Questions 26 through 29

For each vertebra listed below, select the statement that applies to it.

(A) it is called the vertebra prominens
(B) it is the largest of all movable vertebrae
(C) the spinous process is long and slender
(D) it has no spinous processes
(E) its distinguishing feature is the blunt tooth-like dens

26. 1st cervical

27. 2nd cervical

28. 5th lumbar

29. 3rd thoracic

Questions 30 through 33

For each ligament listed below, select the statement that applies to it.

(A) it is the upward continuation of the posterior longitudinal ligament
(B) it extends from the tip of the dens to the axis
(C) it is an adult derivative of the notochord
(D) it holds the dens of the axis against the anterior arch of the atlas
(E) it extends from the dens to the lateral margins of the foramen magnum

30. Transverse ligament of the atlas

31. Alar ligaments

32. Tectorial membrane

33. Apical ligament

Questions 34 through 37

For each muscle listed below, select the statement that applies to it.

(A) it inserts into the mastoid process of the temporal bone
(B) it is a suboccipital muscle
(C) it is the lateral column of the erector spinae muscle
(D) it is an extrinsic back muscle
(E) it extends the vertebral column and rotates it toward the opposite side

34. Trapezius

35. Longissimus capitis

36. Multifidus

37. Inferior capitis obliquus

DIRECTIONS (Questions 38 and 39): Each of the numbered items or incomplete statements in this section is followed by answers or by completions of the statement. Select the ONE lettered answer or completion that is BEST in each case.

38. Which of the following statements correctly applies to the medial column of the erector spinae muscle?

(A) it is known as the longissimus muscle

(B) it arises from spinous processes

(C) it inserts into transverse processes

(D) it is a flexor of the vertebral column

(E) it is a superficial muscle

39. Which of the following muscles is concerned with the maintenance of posture and movements of the vertebral column?

(A) serratus posterior inferior

(B) trapezius

(C) latissimus dorsi

(D) levator scapulae

(E) longissimus

ANSWERS AND EXPLANATIONS

1. (B) The lateral branches of dorsal rami of the 1st, 2nd, and 3rd sacral nerves form the middle cluneal nerves. These become cutaneous on a line connecting the posterior superior iliac spine and the tip of the coccyx to supply the skin and subcutaneous tissues over the back of the sacrum and the adjacent area of the gluteal region. *(Woodburne, p 83)*

2. (A) The trapezius muscle arises from the medial one-third of the superior nuchal line and the external occipital protuberance of the occipital bone, from ligamentum nuchae, from the spines of the 7th cervical and all thoracic vertebrae, and from the intervening supraspinal ligament. *(Woodburne, p 83)*

3. (C) The latissimus dorsi ends in a band-like tendon, 6 to 8 cm long, inserted in the floor of the intertubercular groove of the humerus. Its spinal course takes its tendon ventral to the tendon of the teres major muscle, a bursa intervening, and turns it so that the inferiorly arising muscle fibers lie more cranial in the tendon, and the dorsum of the muscle is represented ventrally. *(Woodburne, p 85)*

4. (C) The erector spinae extends the vertebral column and, acting on one side, bends the column toward that side. The muscle is innervated serially by branches of the dorsal rami of all spinal nerves. The erector spinae overlies the semispinalis and multifidus muscles of the transversospinal group. They occupy the vertebrocostal groove of the back and lie directly under the posterior layer of the thoracolumbar fascia. *(Woodburne, pp 326–327)*

5. (A) The iliocostalis begins at the crest of the ilium and inserts on the angles of the ribs. Its highest fascicles arise in lower ribs and insert in upper ribs and, at cervical levels, insert into transverse processes as high as the 4th cervical vertebrae. The longissimus, spinalis, semispinalis, and splenius muscles all have capitis portions. *(Woodburne, pp 326–327)*

6. (D) Vertebrae are composed of two parts—the anteriorly placed body and the posterior vertebral arch that encloses the vertebral foramen. The vertebral arch is formed of two pedicles and two laminae, from which arise four articular processes, two transverse processes, and one spinous process. *(Woodburne, p 329)*

7. (D) The thoracic vertebrae exhibit costal facets for articulation with the ribs. The spinous process of the thoracic vertebrae is long and sloped downward. The articular facets of the superior articular processes face backward, upward, and somewhat lateralward. The inferior articular facets of the inferior articular processes have facets that face forward, downward, and somewhat medialward. The facets of the thoracic vertebrae favor lateral bending and rotation of the column. *(Woodburne, p 330)*

8. (D) The articular surfaces of lumbar vertebrae facilitate flexion and extension and side-to-side bending. They do not permit rotation. They are capable of sliding superiorly and inferiorly. *(Woodburne, p 331)*

9. (C) The cervical vertebrae have spinous processes that are short and bifid. Each transverse process is perforated by a transverse foramen. They are the smallest of the vertebrae. The vertebral foramen is large and triangular and accommodates the largest portion of the spinal cord. The 1st, 2nd, and 7th cervical vertebrae are considered to be atypical. *(Woodburne, pp 331–333)*

10. (A) The 2nd cervical vertebra is known as the axis, and the 1st cervical vertebra is the atlas. The 1st and 2nd cervical vertebrae are modified from the basic plan, the changes being essentially the incorporation of a part of the body of the 1st vertebra into the body of the 2nd. This leaves only an anterior arch of bone in place of the body of the atlas (1st cervical). In the axis (2nd cervical), the bony addition forms the strong dens. *(Woodburne, p 332)*

11. **(B)** The laminae of the 5th sacral segment, and sometimes the 4th, fail to meet, and thus produce the sacral hiatus, an inferior entrance to the vertebral canal. *(Woodburne, p 334)*

12. **(E)** The majority of vertebral columns range between 72 and 75 cm in length, of which approximately one-fourth is accounted for the intervertebral disks. The adult vertebral column has four curvatures. Two primary curvatures exist in fetal life. The center of gravity of the body is located just anterior to the sacral promontory. *(Woodburne, pp 334–335)*

13. **(E)** The intervertebral disks vary in thickness and size in different regions of the column. In the cervical and lumbar regions, they are thicker in front than behind. The disks are of uniform thickness at thoracic levels. They are thickest in the lumbar region of the column. The disks are important shock absorbers. Ventrally and dorsally, their fibers are attached to the anterior longitudinal and posterior longitudinal ligaments. *(Woodburne, p 336)*

14. **(E)** The posterior longitudinal ligament is continuous with the tectorial membrane; it is attached to the occipital bone. It ends below in the sacral canal. It is located in the vertebral canal on the posterior borders of the vertebral bodies. *(Woodburne, p 336)*

15. **(D)** The ligamenta flava are yellow, elastic ligaments which connect the laminae of adjacent vertebrae. The portions of the two sides meet at the root of the spine, separated by intervals for the passage of veins that communicate between the internal vertebral venous and external vertebral venous plexuses. The ligamenta flava extend lateralward as far as the articular capsules. These strong, elastic ligaments assist in maintaining the upright posture. *(Woodburne, p 337)*

16. **(A)** The zygapophyseal (facet) joints are innervated by nerves that arise from medial branches of the dorsal rami of spinal nerves. As these nerves pass posteroinferiorly, they lie in grooves on the posterior surfaces of the medial parts of the transverse processes. *(Moore, pp 347–348)*

17. **(B)** Adjacent spinous processes are joined by weak interspinous ligaments and a strong cord-like supraspinous ligament. The ligamentum flavum joins the laminae of adjacent vertebral arches. The interspinous and supraspinous ligament of the cervical vertebrae are represented su-

periorly by the ligamentum nuchae. The tectorial membrane is the superior continuation of the posterior longitudinal ligament. *(Moore, pp 348–350)*

18. **(H)** The inferior oblique capitis arises from the lateral surface of the spinous process of the C2 vertebra and runs obliquely and anteriorly to insert on the inferior surface of the transverse process of the C1 vertebra. *(Moore, p 358)*

19. **(E)** The semispinalis capitis arises from the transverse processes of the T1 to T6 vertebrae and inserts into the medial half of the area between the superior and inferior nuchal lines on the occipital bone. *(Moore, p 355)*

20. **(E)** The semispinalis capitis forms the largest muscle mass in the posterior aspect of the neck. *(Moore, p 355)*

21. **(F)** The multifidus muscle covers the laminae of the S4 to C2 vertebrae. Its fibers pass superomedially from the vertebral arches to the spinous processes, spanning one to three vertebrae. *(Moore, p 355)*

22. **(G)** The rotators arise from the transverse process of one vertebra and insert into the base of the spinous process of the vertebra superior to it. *(Moore, p 355)*

23. **(B)** The lateral column of erector spinae arises from the common origin and inserts into the angles of the ribs. *(Moore, p 353)*

24. **(C)** The intermediate column of the erector spinae arises from the common origin and is attached to the transverse processes of the thoracic and cervical vertebrae and the mastoid process of the temporal bone of the skull. *(Moore, p 353)*

25. **(A)** The splenius capitis takes origin from the inferior half of the ligamentum nuchae and the spinous processes of the T1 to T6 vertebrae. *(Moore, p 353)*

26. **(D)** The atlas has no spinous process or body; it consists of anterior and posterior arches, each of which bears a tubercle and a lateral mass. *(Moore, pp 334–339)*

27. **(E)** The 2nd cervical vertebra, known as the axis, has two flat-bearing surfaces, the superior articular facets, upon which the atlas rotates. Its distinguishing feature is the blunt tooth-like dens. *(Moore, pp 334–339)*

28. **(B)** The 5th lumbar vertebra, the largest of all movable vertebra, is characterized by stout transverse processes. *(Moore, pp 334–339)*

29. **(C)** All 12 thoracic vertebrae articulate with ribs. Thus, they are characterized by articular facets for them. The spinous processes tend to be long and slender. *(Moore, pp 334–339)*

30. **(D)** The transverse ligament of the atlas is a strong band extending between the tubercles on the medial sides of the lateral masses of the atlas. It holds the dens of the axis against the anterior arch of the atlas, with a synovial joint between them. *(Moore, p 632)*

31. **(E)** The alar ligaments extend from the dens to the lateral margins of the foramen magnum. They check lateral rotation and side-to-side movements of the head and attach the skull to the axis. *(Moore, pp 349–350)*

32. **(A)** The tectorial membrane is the upward continuation of the posterior longitudinal ligament. It runs from the axis to the internal aspect of the occipital bone and covers the alar and transverse ligaments. *(Moore, pp 349–350)*

33. **(C)** The apical ligament is an adult derivative of the notochord in the embryo. It extends from the tip of the dens to the internal surface of the occipital bone. *(Moore, pp 349–350)*

34. **(D)** The extrinsic muscles of the back include the trapezius, latissimus dorsi, levator scapulae, and rhomboid muscles. They connect the upper limb to the axial skeleton and are related to movements of the upper limbs. *(Moore, pp 351–358)*

35. **(A)** The longissimus capitis inserts into the mastoid process of the temporal bone. *(Moore, pp 351–352)*

36. **(E)** The multifidus muscle extends the vertebral column and rotates it toward the opposite side. Each bundle of muscle ascends obliquely from its origin and inserts two to five vertebrae superiorly. *(Moore, pp 351–352)*

37. **(B)** The four suboccipital muscles include the rectus capitis posterior major, rectus capitis posterior minor, obliquus capitis inferior, and the obliquus capitis superior. *(Moore, p 342)*

38. **(B)** The spinalis muscle, the medial column of the erector spinae muscle, arises from spinous processes and inserts into spinous processes. It is an extensor of the vertebral column. *(Moore, p 353)*

39. **(E)** The muscles of the deep, or intrinsic, group—the true back muscles—are concerned with the maintenance of posture and movements of the vertebral column (flexion, extension, lateral bending, rotation, and circumduction). The intermediate layer of intrinsic muscles includes the erector spinae muscle, which contains large bundles known as the spinalis, longissimus, and iliocostalis. *(Moore, pp 353–355)*

Clinical Back
Questions

1. Which of the following terms correctly applies to the fusion of the 5th lumbar vertebra into the sacrum?

    (A) lumbarization
    (B) sacralization
    (C) lumbago
    (D) lordosis
    (E) scoliosis

2. Which of the following terms correctly applies to abnormal curvatures of the vertebral column?

    (A) sacralization
    (B) lumbarization
    (C) kyphosis
    (D) osteoporosis
    (E) osteomalacia

3. Lordosis is characterized by an increased curve of the vertebral column that is

    (A) convex posteriorly
    (B) convex anteriorly
    (C) convex to the side
    (D) concave laterally
    (E) concave anteriorly

4. The broad anterior longitudinal ligament tends to prevent

    (A) hyperextension of the vertebral column
    (B) coccydynia
    (C) scoliosis
    (D) osteoporosis
    (E) hemivertebra

5. A herniated or prolapsed disk usually occurs in which of the following directions?

    (A) anterior
    (B) posterior
    (C) posterolateral
    (D) anterolateral
    (E) inferiorly

6. Clinicians often refer to which of the following articulations as "facet joints"?

    (A) opposing articular processes of adjacent vertebral arches
    (B) ribs and transverse ventral processes
    (C) vertebrae and adjacent intervertebral disks
    (D) adjacent vertebral bodies
    (E) adjacent vertebral spinous processes

7. The broad, yellow, elastic bands that join the laminae of adjacent vertebral arches are known as the

    (A) interspinous ligaments
    (B) supraspinous ligaments
    (C) ligamentum nuchae
    (D) intertransverse ligaments
    (E) ligamenta flava

8. Which of the following statements correctly applies to the tectorial membrane?

    (A) it is the upward continuation of the posterior longitudinal ligament
    (B) it extends from the 1st thoracic vertebral body to the occipital bone
    (C) it is covered by the alar ligament
    (D) it covers the transverse ligament
    (E) it attaches to the dens

9. In severe neck flexion injuries, which of the following ligaments usually is torn?

   (A) anterior longitudinal
   (B) posterior longitudinal
   (C) apical
   (D) ligamentum nuchae
   (E) ligamentum flavum

10. The suboccipital triangle contains the

    (A) vertebral artery
    (B) lesser occipital nerve
    (C) spinal accessory nerve
    (D) occipital artery
    (E) posterior auricular artery

11. The spinal cord in adults usually ends opposite the intervertebral disk between which of the following vertebrae?

    (A) L4–L5
    (B) L1–L2
    (C) S2–S3
    (D) S4–S5
    (E) T10–T11

12. The spinal cord is suspended in the dura mater by the

    (A) filum terminale
    (B) cauda equina
    (C) conus medullaris
    (D) denticulate ligament
    (E) alar ligament

13. The principal site of absorption of cerebrospinal fluid into the venous system is through the

    (A) diploic veins
    (B) arachnoid villa
    (C) pterygoid plexus
    (D) vertebral venous plexus
    (E) cavernous sinus

14. Which of the following conditions are usually associated with a "whiplash injury"?

    (A) scoliosis
    (B) rachischisis
    (C) spina bifida
    (D) hyperextension injury of the neck
    (E) kyphosis

15. Protrusions of the nucleus pulposus usually occur in which direction?

    (A) posterolaterally
    (B) posteromedially
    (C) anteriorly
    (D) anterolaterally
    (E) anteromedially

16. All the following statements concerning the veins of the vertebral column are correct EXCEPT

    (A) they extend from the pelvis to the cranium
    (B) they contain valves
    (C) they communicate at all levels with the other major venous channels of the abdomen, the chest, and the neck
    (D) they are significant in the transfer of metastatic cancer
    (E) they are influenced by differences in venous pressure throughout the body

ANSWERS AND EXPLANATIONS

1. **(B)** In some people, the 5th lumbar vertebra is partly or completely incorporated into the sacrum (sacralization of the 5th lumbar vertebra). In others, the 1st sacral vertebra is separated from the sacrum (lumbarization of the 1st sacral vertebra). *(Moore, p 337)*

2. **(C)** Kyphosis is characterized by an abnormal curve that is convex posteriorly (dorsal curvature of the vertebral column) and that usually occurs in the thoracic region (humpback). *(Moore, p 327)*

3. **(B)** Lordosis is characterized by an increased curve of the vertebral column that is convex anteriorly (backward bending). *(Moore, p 327)*

4. **(A)** The anterior longitudinal ligament is a strong, broad, fibrous band that runs longitudinally along the anterior surfaces of the intervertebral disks and the bodies of the vertebrae. Its fibers are firmly fixed to the intervertebral disks and to the periosteum of the vertebral bodies. The broad anterior longitudinal ligament tends to prevent hyperextension of the vertebral column. *(Moore, p 347)*

5. **(C)** A herniated or prolapsed disk usually occurs in a posterolateral direction, where the anulus fibrosus is weakest and poorly supported by the posterior longitudinal ligament. The protruding part of the nucleus pulposus may compress an adjacent spinal nerve root, causing leg or low back pain. *(Moore, p 347)*

6. **(A)** True synovial joints of the plane variety, known as zygapophyseal joints, are formed by the opposing articular processes (zygapophyses) of adjacent vertebral arches. Because the contact surfaces of these articular processes are called articu-

lar facets, clinicians often refer to zygapophyseal joints as "facet joints." *(Moore, p 348)*

7. (E) The laminae of adjacent vertebral arches are joined by broad, yellow, elastic bands called ligamenta flava. Their fibers extend to the capsules of the zygapophyseal joints between the articular processes and contribute to the posterior boundary of the vertebral foramen. *(Moore, p 348)*

8. (A) The tectorial membrane is the upward continuation of the posterior longitudinal ligament. It runs from the body of the axis to the internal surface of the occipital bone and covers the alar ligaments and the transverse ligament. *(Moore, p 342)*

9. (B) In severe flexion injuries, the posterior longitudinal and interspinous ligaments may be torn, and the vertebral arches may be dislocated and/or fractured, along with crush fractures of the vertebral bodies. The anterior longitudinal ligament is usually not torn in flexion injuries. *(Moore, p 342)*

10. (A) The suboccipital triangle is important clinically because it contains the vertebral artery and the suboccipital nerve (dorsal ramus of the 1st cervical nerve). These structures lie in a groove on the superior surface of the posterior arch of the atlas. *(Moore, pp 358–359)*

11. (B) The spinal cord in adults often ends opposite the intervertebral disk between L1 and L2, but it may terminate as high as T12 or as low as L3. Thus, the spinal cord occupies only the upper two-thirds of the vertebral canal. *(Moore, p 359)*

12. (D) The spinal cord is suspended in the dura mater by a saw-toothed denticulate ligament on each side. This ribbon-like ligament, composed of pia mater, is attached along the lateral surface of the spinal cord, midway between the dorsal and ventral nerve roots. There are 21 tooth-like processes attached to the dura mater. *(Moore, p 366)*

13. (B) The principal site of absorption of cerebrospinal fluid into the venous blood is through the arachnoid villi projecting into the dural venous sinuses, particularly the superior sagittal sinus. Many arachnoid villi show hypertrophy in older persons and are called arachnoid granulations. *(Moore, p 670)*

14. (D) Although a hyperextension injury of the neck is popularly called a "whiplash injury," there is no well-defined clinical syndrome or fixed pathology associated with the injury. *(Moore, p 347)*

15. (A) Protrusions of the nucleus pulposus usually occur posterolaterally, where the anulus fibrosus is weak and poorly supported by the posterior longitudinal ligaments. *(Moore, p 347)*

16. (B) Batson pointed out that the veins of the vertebral column form a system of great blood-carrying capacity, extending, without valves, from the pelvis to the cranium and communicating at all levels with the other major venous channels of the abdomen, the chest, and the neck. It has been described as a significant route for the transfer of metastatic cancer cells to widely separated parts of the body under the influence of differences in venous pressure.

Developmental Back
Questions

DIRECTIONS (Questions 1 through 10): Each group of items in this section consists of lettered headings followed by a set of numbered words or phrases. For each numbered word or phrase, select the ONE lettered heading that is most closely associated with it. Each lettered heading may be selected once, more than once, or not at all.

Associate each of the following questions with one of the conditions listed below.

    (A) Klippel–Feil syndrome
    (B) spina bifida
    (C) achondroplasia

1. One of the best-known systemic abnormalities of the skeletal system

2. Patients have a reduced number of cervical vertebrae

3. Thoracic and lumbar vertebra are fused or abnormal in shape

4. One of the most serious vertebral defects

5. Imperfect fusion of the vertebral arches

6. Usually accompanied by abnormalities of the spinal cord

7. Nonunion of the vertebral arches

8. Regular number of vertebrae is increased

9. Regular number of vertebrae is decreased

10. Spinal cord may be exposed to the outside

1. **(C)** One of the best-known systemic abnormalities of the skeletal system is achondroplasia. *(Sadler, p 154)*

2. **(A)** Patients with Klippel–Feil syndrome have a reduced number of cervical vertebrae. *(Sadler, p 153)*

3. **(A)** Patients with Klippel–Feil syndrome have a reduced number of cervical vertebrae, while the remaining thoracic and lumbar vertebrae are fused or abnormal in shape. *(Sadler, p 153)*

4. **(B)** One of the most serious vertebral defects is the result of imperfect fusion or nonunion of the vertebral arches. Such an abnormality is known as cleft vertebra (spina bifida). *(Sadler, p 153)*

5. **(B)** The imperfect fusion of the vertebral arches is known as spina bifida. *(Sadler, p 153)*

6. **(B)** Spina bifida is usually accompanied by abnormalities of the spinal cord. *(Sadler, p 153)*

7. **(B)** The nonunion of the vertebral arches results in an abnormality known as cleft vertebrae (spina bifida). *(Sadler, p 153)*

8. **(A)** Klippel–Feil syndrome may be associated with an increase in the number of vertebrae. *(Sadler, p 153)*

9. **(A)** Klippel–Feil syndrome may be associated with a decrease in the number of vertebrae. *(Sadler, p 153)*

10. **(B)** Spina bifida is usually accompanied by abnormalities of the spinal cord, which herniates through the cleft and is thus exposed to the outside. *(Sadler, p 153)*

The Spinal Cord
Questions

1. All the following statements concerning the spinal cord are correct EXCEPT

    (A) it extends from the foramen magnum to the 2nd lumbar vertebra
    (B) it ranges from 42 to 45 cm in length
    (C) it occupies the superior two-thirds of the vertebral canal
    (D) the cervical enlargement extends from the C4 to T1 segment of the spinal cord
    (E) the spinal cord segments correspond with the vertebral levels

2. The cell bodies of axons making up the ventral roots are located in the

    (A) dorsal root ganglion
    (B) dorsal gray column
    (C) ventral gray column
    (D) ventral root
    (E) dorsal root

3. The dorsal root ganglia are located in the

    (A) vertebral furrow
    (B) coccyx
    (C) intervertebral foramina
    (D) intervertebral disks
    (E) sympathetic chain

4. The bundle of nerve rootlets in the subarachnoid space caudal to the termination of the spinal cord is known as the

    (A) lumbosacral plexus
    (B) femoral nerve
    (C) pelvic splanchnic nerve
    (D) sciatic nerve
    (E) cauda equina

5. All the following statements concerning the filum terminale are correct EXCEPT

    (A) it is a fibrous strand extending from the inferior end of the conus medullaris
    (B) it descends among the nerve rootlets comprising the cauda equina
    (C) it leaves the inferior end of the dural sac and passes through the sacral hiatus
    (D) it inserts into the sacrum
    (E) it contains neural tissue

6. All the following statements concerning the anterior spinal artery are correct EXCEPT

    (A) it is formed by the union of two small branches from the ventral arteries
    (B) it is located in the anterior median fissure
    (C) it runs the length of the spinal cord
    (D) it supplies the anterior two-thirds of the spinal cord
    (E) it is usually smallest in the L4 to S2 region of the cord

7. All the following structures are located in the epidural space EXCEPT

    (A) the posterior spinal arteries
    (B) fat
    (C) loose connective tissue
    (D) the anterior vertebral venous plexus
    (E) the posterior vertebral venous plexus

8. All the following statements concerning the denticulate ligament are correct EXCEPT

    (A) it attaches the spinal cord to the dural sac
    (B) it is composed of dura
    (C) its lateral edge is notched or serrated
    (D) its tooth-like processes are attached to the dura mater between the nerve roots
    (E) it attaches to the periosteum at the foramen magnum

9. Which of the following statements concerning the pia mater is correct?

    (A) it is the intermediate covering membrane of the spinal cord

    (B) it is composed of white fibrous and elastic tissue

    (C) it is composed of two layers of dense connective tissue

    (D) it is deep to the anterior spinal artery

    (E) it continues inferior to the conus medullaris as the filum terminale

10. The lumbar cistern contains the

    (A) posterior internal venous plexus

    (B) posterior spinal arteries

    (C) anterior external venous plexus

    (D) cauda equina

    (E) denticulate ligaments

ANSWERS AND EXPLANATIONS

1. **(E)** The spinal cord begins as a continuation of the medulla, the inferior part of the brain stem. It extends from the foramen magnum in the occipital bone to the level of the L2 vertebra. It ranges from 42 to 45 cm in length. The spinal cord occupies only the superior two-thirds of the vertebral canal. The cervical enlargement extends from the C4 to T1 segments of the spinal cord. The spinal cord segments do not correspond with the vertebral levels. *(Moore, p 359)*

2. **(C)** The cell bodies of axons making up the ventral roots are in the ventral gray column of the spinal cord, whereas the cell bodies of axons making up the dorsal roots are outside the spinal cord in the spinal ganglia (dorsal root ganglia). *(Moore, p 360)*

3. **(C)** The dorsal root ganglia are located in the intervertebral foramina, where they rest on the pedicles of the vertebral arches. Distal to the spinal ganglia, just outside the intervertebral foramina, the dorsal and ventral nerve roots unite to form a spinal nerve. *(Moore, p 360)*

4. **(E)** The lumbar and sacral spinal nerve rootlets are the longest. They must descend until they reach their intervertebral foramina of exit. This collection of rootlets reminded early anatomists of the hairs of a horse's tail, and, therefore, the bun-dle of nerve rootlets in the subarachnoid space caudal to the termination of the spinal cord is called the cauda equina. *(Moore, pp 360–362)*

5. **(E)** The conus medullaris has a slender fibrous strand at its inferior end called the filum terminale. It contains no neural tissue. It descends among the nerve rootlets comprising the cauda equina. It leaves the inferior end of the dural sac and passes through the sacral hiatus. Here it blends with the superior end of the anococcygeal ligament and ends with it by inserting into the dorsum of the coccyx. *(Moore, p 362)*

6. **(E)** The anterior spinal artery is formed by the union of two small branches from the vertebral arteries. It runs the length of the spinal cord in the anterior median fissure and supplies the anterior two-thirds of the spinal cord. It is usually smallest in the T4 to T8 region of the cord. *(Moore, p 362)*

7. **(A)** The extradural (epidural) space contains fat, loose connective tissue, and the anterior and posterior vertebral venous plexuses. The vessels of the spinal cord are located in the subarachnoid space. *(Moore, p 366)*

8. **(B)** The spinal cord is suspended in the dural sac by a saw-toothed denticulate ligament on each side. This ribbon-like ligament, composed of pia mater, is attached along the lateral surface of the spinal cord, midway between the dorsal and ventral nerve roots. The lateral edges of the denticulate ligament are notched or serrated. Their attachment is to the periosteum, starting at the foramen magnum; the last one is between T12 and L1 nerve roots. *(Moore, p 366)*

9. **(E)** Inferior to the conus medullaris, the pia continues as the filum terminale. It is the innermost covering membrane of the spinal cord. It is composed of two fused layers of loose connective tissue. It covers the roots of the spinal nerves and spinal blood vessels and ensheaths the anterior spinal artery. *(Moore, p 366)*

10. **(D)** The subarachnoid space within the dural sac extending from the L2 to S2 vertebrae is known as the lumbar cistern. In addition to CSF, the lumbar cistern contains the cauda equina and filum terminale. The spinal arteries are not in the subarachnoid space below L1 or L2, and the venous plexuses are not located in the subarachnoid space. *(Moore, p 367)*

Illustrations
Questions

THE CERVICAL VERTEBRAE
(Questions 1 through 11)

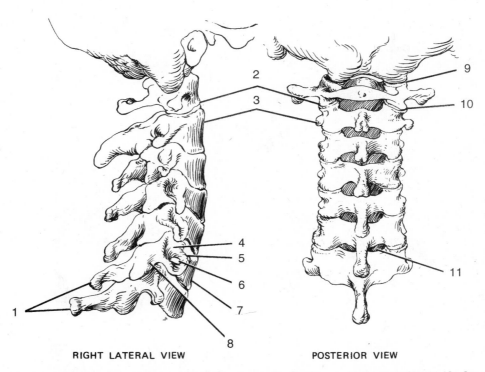

RIGHT LATERAL VIEW   POSTERIOR VIEW

Figure 5–1. The Cervical vertebrae. (Modified and reproduced, with permission, from Chusid JG: *Correlative Neuroanatomy & Functional Neurology,* 19th ed. Lange, 1985.)

Directions: With reference to the diagram, match the numbered structures with their corresponding lettered items.

(A) pedicle ✓
(B) spinous processes ✓
(C) axis ✓
(D) transverse process ○
(E) transverse foramen ✓
(F) vertebral canal ✓

(G) lamina ✓
(H) superior articular facet ✓
(I) inferior articular facet ✓
(J) atlas ✓
(K) body ✓

THE LUMBAR VERTEBRAE
(Questions 12 through 28)

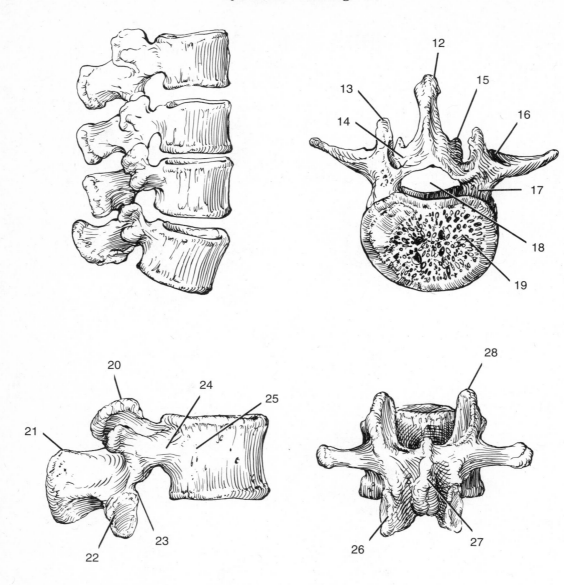

Figure 5–2. The lumbar vertebrae. (Modified and reproduced, with permission, from Chusid JG: *Correlative Neuroanatomy & Functional Neurology,* 19th ed. p. 102. Lange, 1985.)

Directions: With reference to the diagram, match the numbered structures with their corresponding lettered items.

(A) articular process

(B) transverse process

(C) spinous process

(D) inferior articular process

(E) vertebral foramen

(F) body

(G) pedicle

(H) lamina

(I) superior articular process

THE SACRUM AND COCCYX
(Questions 29 through 42)

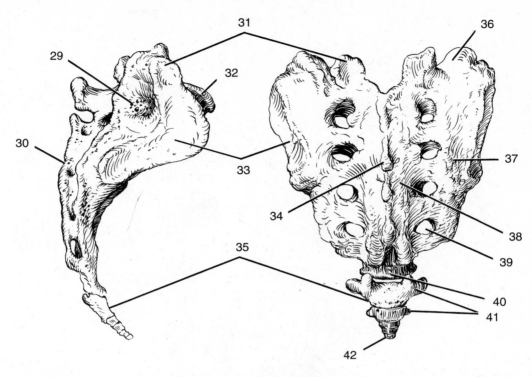

Figure 5–3. The sacrum and coccyx. (Modified and reproduced, with permission, from Chusid JG: *Correlative Neuroanatomy & Functional Neurology,* 19th ed. p. 103. Lange, 1985.)

Directions: With reference to the diagram, match the numbered structures with their corresponding lettered items.

(A) ala
(B) coccyx
(C) rudimentary transverse processes
(D) promontory of base
(E) apex of coccyx
(F) sacral tuberosity
(G) lateral sacral crest

(H) dorsal sacral foramen
(I) median sacral crest
(J) superior articular process
(K) apex of sacrum
(L) median sacral crest
(M) auricular surface
(N) spinous process

RIGHT LATERAL VIEW OF VERTEBRA IN THE THORACIC REGION, SHOWING ATTACHED LIGAMENTS AND INTERVERTEBRA DISKS
(Questions 43 through 49)

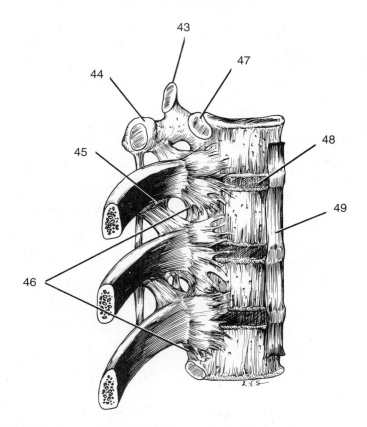

Figure 5–4. Right lateral view of vertebra in the thoracic region, showing attached ligaments and intervertebra disks. (Modified and reproduced, with permission, from Chusid JG: *Correlative Neuroanatomy & Functional Neurology,* 19th ed. p. 104. Lange, 1985.)

Directions: With reference to the diagram, match the numbered structures with their corresponding lettered items.

(A) posterior longitudinal ligament

(B) intervertebral disk

(C) superior articular process

(D) costal facet for articulation with head of rib

(E) anterior longitudinal ligament

(F) ligamenta flava

(G) transverse process

Answers

THE CERVICAL VERTEBRAE

1. (B)	7. (K)
2. (J)	8. (G)
3. (C)	9. (H)
4. (A)	10. (I)
5. (D)	11. (F)
6. (E)	

THE LUMBAR VERTEBRAE

12. (C)	21. (C)
13. (I)	22. (D)
14. (H)	23. (H)
15. (A)	24. (G)
16. (B)	25. (F)
17. (G)	26. (D)
18. (E)	27. (C)
19. (F)	28. (I)
20. (I)	

THE SACRUM AND COCCYX

29. (F)	36. (A)
30. (I)	37. (G)
31. (J)	38. (L)
32. (D)	39. (H)
33. (M)	40. (K)
34. (N)	41. (C)
35. (B)	42. (E)

RIGHT LATERAL VIEW OF VERTEBRA IN THE THORACIC REGION, SHOWING ATTACHED LIGAMENTS AND INTERVERTEBRA DISKS

43. (C)	47. (D)
44. (G)	48. (B)
45. (F)	49. (E)
46. (A)	

CHAPTER 6

Abdominal Region
Questions

DIRECTIONS (Questions 1 through 72): Each of the numbered items or incomplete statements in this section is followed by answers or by completions of the statement. Select the ONE lettered answer or completion that is BEST in each case.

1. All the following statements concerning the inferior epigastric artery are correct EXCEPT

   (A) it arises from the femoral artery
   (B) its origin is just medial to the deep inguinal ring
   (C) it is medial to the ductus deferens in the male at the deep inguinal ring
   (D) it pierces the transversalis fascia and enters the rectus sheath
   (E) it anastomoses with terminals of the superior epigastric

2. The gubernaculum testis remnant becomes the

   (A) epididymis
   (B) scrotal ligament
   (C) ductus deferens
   (D) tunica vaginalis testis
   (E) processus vaginalis

3. All the following structures are located in the spermatic cord EXCEPT the

   (A) ductus deferens
   (B) deferential artery
   (C) testicular artery
   (D) scrotal ligament
   (E) pampiniform plexus

4. The iliac crest is located at the transverse level of the

   (A) inguinal ligament
   (B) xiphosternal joint
   (C) 4th lumbar vertebra
   (D) anterior iliac spine
   (E) ischial tuberosity

5. The superficial inguinal ring is traversed by which of the following nerves?

   (A) iliohypogastric
   (B) subcostal
   (C) ilioinguinal
   (D) pudendal
   (E) obturator

6. The tunica dartos scroti contains

   (A) fat
   (B) striated muscle
   (C) the iliohypogastric nerve
   (D) the inferior epigastric artery
   (E) smooth muscle

7. The musculophrenic artery is a branch of which of the following arteries?

   (A) internal thoracic
   (B) inferior epigastric
   (C) superficial epigastric
   (D) superficial circumflex
   (E) deep external pudendal

8. The inferior epigastric artery arises from which of the following arteries?

   (A) internal thoracic
   (B) external iliac
   (C) femoral
   (D) obturator
   (E) musculophrenic

9. The superficial epigastric artery arises from which of the following arteries?

   (A) femoral
   (B) internal iliac
   (C) external iliac
   (D) inferior epigastric
   (E) superior epigastric

10. The superficial circumflex iliac artery arises from which of the following arteries?

    (A) external iliac
    (B) internal iliac
    (C) superior epigastric
    (D) inferior epigastric
    (E) femoral

11. The superficial external pudendal artery emerges through the

    (A) deep inguinal ring
    (B) saphenous opening
    (C) lumbar triangle
    (D) arcuate line
    (E) rectus sheath

12. The upper five slips of origin for the external abdominal oblique muscle interdigitate with which of the following muscles?

    (A) pectoralis major
    (B) rectus abdominis
    (C) latissimus dorsi
    (D) serratus anterior
    (E) subscapularis

13. Which of the following structures contributes to the formation of the lumbar triangle?

    (A) rectus sheath
    (B) crest of the ilium
    (C) ischial tuberosity
    (D) inguinal ligament
    (E) serratus posterior

14. Which of the following structures is not a specialization of the external abdominal oblique aponeurosis?

    (A) inguinal ligament
    (B) lacunar ligament
    (C) intercrural fibers
    (D) internal spermatic fascia
    (E) medial and lateral crura

15. The thickened, rolled-under portion of the external abdominal oblique aponeurosis, which is stretched between the anterior superior spine of the ilium and the pubic tubercle, is known as the

    (A) inguinal ligament
    (B) lacunar ligament
    (C) intercrural fibers
    (D) rectus sheath
    (E) linea alba

16. The lacunar ligament represents the more medial, rolled-under fibers of the

    (A) medial crura
    (B) reflected inguinal ligament
    (C) fundiform ligament
    (D) pectineal ligament
    (E) inguinal ligament

17. In the lower one-fourth of the abdomen, the internal abdominal oblique aponeurosis

    (A) splits to send one sheet anterior and one posterior to the rectus abdominis muscle
    (B) fails to split and passes to the median line entirely posterior to the rectus abdominis muscle
    (C) fails to split and passes to the median line entirely anterior to the rectus abdominis muscle
    (D) disappears
    (E) gives rise to the internal spermatic fascia

18. Among the coverings of the cord and testis, which of the following represents the internal abdominal oblique muscle layer?

    (A) tunica dartos
    (B) external spermatic fascia
    (C) cremaster muscle and fascia
    (D) internal spermatic fascia
    (E) subcutaneous layer

19. The cremaster muscle is innervated by which of the following nerves?

    (A) ilioinguinal
    (B) iliohypogastric
    (C) femoral
    (D) subcostal
    (E) genitofemoral

20. The aponeurosis of the transversus abdominis muscle contributes to the

    (A) inguinal ligament
    (B) lacunar ligament
    (C) falx inguinalis
    (D) external spermatic fascia
    (E) superficial inguinal ring

21. Which of the following statements correctly applies to the tendinous intersections?

    (A) they are firmly adherent to both layers of the rectus sheath
    (B) the lowest is at the level of the symphysis pubis

(C) the highest is near the xiphoid process

(D) the lowest is at the level of the arcuate line

(E) there are usually ten tendinous intersections

22. Which of the following statements correctly applies to the pyramidalis muscle?

(A) it is a large, well-developed muscle

(B) it is always present

(C) it is contained within the rectus sheath

(D) it is posterior to the rectus abdominis muscle

(E) it is innervated by the 10th thoracic nerve

23. The transversalis fascia contributes to the

(A) deep inguinal ring

(B) cremaster muscle and fascia

(C) inguinal ligament

(D) pectineal ligament

(E) external spermatic fascia

24. The innervation of the muscles of the abdominal wall is provided by which of the following cord segments?

(A) T3–S3

(B) T5–L2

(C) T1–S5

(D) T7–L4

(E) L1–S5

25. The 10th intercostal nerve enters the rectus sheath at the level of the

(A) xiphoid process

(B) umbilicus

(C) pyramidalis muscle

(D) pubic tubercle

(E) arcuate line

26. The four lumbar arteries arise from which of the following vessels?

(A) internal thoracic

(B) internal iliac

(C) femoral

(D) aorta

(E) external iliac

27. The iliolumbar artery is a branch of which of the following arteries?

(A) internal iliac

(B) external iliac

(C) internal thoracic

(D) femoral

(E) inferior epigastric

28. The esophagogastric junction is located at the level of which of the following vertebrae?

(A) 7th cervical

(B) 11th thoracic

(C) 2nd lumbar

(D) 5th lumbar

(E) 6th thoracic

29. The aortic hiatus of the diaphragm is located at the level of which vertebra?

(A) 4th cervical

(B) 6th cervical

(C) 5th thoracic

(D) 12th thoracic

(E) 4th lumbar

30. Which of the following arteries is a branch of the celiac trunk?

(A) gastroduodenal

(B) proper hepatic

(C) common hepatic

(D) right gastroepiploic

(E) cystic

31. The cystic artery arises from which of the following arteries?

(A) splenic

(B) left gastroepiploic

(C) right gastric

(D) right hepatic

(E) gastroduodenal

32. The left gastroepiploic artery arises from which of the following arteries?

(A) left hepatic

(B) gastroduodenal

(C) left gastric

(D) common hepatic

(E) splenic

33. Which of the following statements correctly applies to the spleen?

(A) it is located beneath the 6th, 7th, and 8th ribs

(B) it is retroperitoneal

(C) it develops in the ventral mesogastrium

(D) it normally descends below the costal margin

(E) it rests on the left flexure of the colon

34. Which of the following statements correctly applies to the first part of the duodenum?

    (A) it is surrounded by the hepatoduodenal ligament
    (B) it is related to the caudate lobe of the liver
    (C) the common bile duct passes ventrally
    (D) it is located at the level of the third lumbar vertebra
    (E) it has circular folds in its interior

35. The second portion of the duodenum is crossed by which of the following structures?

    (A) right renal artery
    (B) transverse colon
    (C) right ureter
    (D) portal vein
    (E) superior mesenteric vein

36. Which of the following arteries crosses the anterior aspect of the third part of the duodenum?

    (A) proper hepatic
    (B) left colic
    (C) superior mesenteric
    (D) inferior mesenteric
    (E) splenic

37. Which of the following statements correctly applies to the greater duodenal papilla?

    (A) it is the location for the terminal opening of the accessory pancreatic duct
    (B) it is located in the interior of the third part of the duodenum
    (C) it is continued below by the longitudinal fold of the duodenum
    (D) it is superior to the lesser duodenal papilla
    (E) it opens into the duodenojejunal flexure

38. The lower left portion of the head of the pancreas is inserted behind which of the following arteries?

    (A) left gastroepiploic
    (B) common hepatic
    (C) left colic
    (D) inferior mesenteric
    (E) superior mesenteric

39. The superior mesenteric and splenic veins unite to form the portal vein behind the

    (A) first part of the duodenum
    (B) transverse colon
    (C) spleen
    (D) neck of the pancreas
    (E) duodenojejunal junction

40. The tail of the pancreas enters the

    (A) epiploic foramen
    (B) lienorenal ligament
    (C) suspensory ligament of the duodenum
    (D) paracolic fossa
    (E) left coronary ligament

41. The pancreatica magna artery is a branch of which of the following arteries?

    (A) common hepatic
    (B) inferior mesenteric
    (C) superior mesenteric
    (D) left gastroepiploic
    (E) splenic

42. Which of the following structures represents the obliterated remains of the umbilical vein?

    (A) ligamentum teres hepatis
    (B) ligamentum venosum
    (C) ductus arteriosus
    (D) falciform ligament
    (E) porta hepatis

43. The hepatoduodenal ligament transmits the

    (A) hepatic vein
    (B) main pancreatic duct
    (C) portal vein
    (D) ligamentum venosum
    (E) superior mesenteric vein

44. The cystic artery usually arises from which of the following arteries?

    (A) splenic
    (B) gastroduodenal
    (C) right gastroepiploic
    (D) right hepatic
    (E) celiac trunk

45. The hepatic veins drain into which of the following veins?

    (A) portal
    (B) coronary
    (C) inferior vena cava
    (D) superior mesenteric
    (E) splenic

46. The portal vein ascends to the liver in the free margin of the

    (A) mesocolon
    (B) greater omentum
    (C) mesentery

(D) lesser omentum

(E) falciform ligament

47. All the following are supplied by the superior mesenteric artery EXCEPT the

(A) proximal part of the duodenum

(B) duodenojejunal junction

(C) jejunoileal junction

(D) distal end of the ileum

(E) descending portion of the duodenum

48. Which of the following statements correctly applies to the middle colic artery?

(A) it takes origin from the celiac trunk

(B) it supplies the cecum

(C) it anastomoses with the inferior pancreatico-duodenal artery

(D) it is a branch of the superior mesenteric artery

(E) it primarily supplies the left colic flexure

49. Epiploic appendages are located on the

(A) duodenum

(B) stomach

(C) ileum

(D) jejunum

(E) sigmoid

50. Which of the following statements correctly applies to the vermiform appendix?

(A) it is usually retroperitoneal

(B) it has a small mesentery

(C) it receives its blood supply from the inferior mesenteric artery

(D) it is usually located in a subhepatic position

(E) it receives its innervation from the pelvic splanchnic

51. The transverse mesocolon is attached posteriorly to the

(A) hepatoduodenal ligament

(B) spleen

(C) second portion of the duodenum

(D) lesser omentum

(E) gastrocolic ligament

52. The pampiniform plexis is located in the

(A) pancreas

(B) kidney

(C) spleen

(D) inguinal canal

(E) liver

53. The psoas major muscle inserts onto the

(A) greater trochanter

(B) anterior superior iliac spine

(C) crest of the ilium

(D) lesser trochanter

(E) ischial spine

54. Which of the following layers of fasciae is associated with the diaphragm?

(A) alar

(B) superficial

(C) transversalis

(D) buccopharyngeal

(E) innominate

55. The right suprarenal vein drains into which of the following veins?

(A) right renal

(B) inferior mesenteric

(C) superior mesenteric

(D) portal

(E) inferior vena cava

56. Which of the following statements correctly applies to the suprarenal gland?

(A) the cortex is essential to life

(B) the medulla is essential to life

(C) the medulla is concerned with carbohydrate metabolism

(D) the medulla is concerned with the body fluid and electrolyte balance

(E) the medulla receives only a postganglionic innervation

57. Which of the following structures is located in the renal column?

(A) interlobular arteries

(B) collecting tubule

(C) arcuate arteries

(D) interlobar arteries

(E) minor calyx vein

58. Which of the following structures is important in the selective reabsorption of water and the return of dissolved materials back into the circulation?

(A) glomerular capsule

(B) renal papilla

(C) straight and convoluted tubules

(D) glomerulus

(E) major calyx

59. The pelvic splanchnic nerves provide parasympathetic fibers to all the following structures EXCEPT the

   (A) bladder
   (B) right colic flexure
   (C) descending colon
   (D) sigmoid colon
   (E) distal one-third of the transverse colon

60. Which of the following statements correctly applies to the sigmoid colon?

   (A) it begins at the brim of the pelvis
   (B) it has no mesocolon
   (C) it continues as the rectum at the level of the 5th sacral segment
   (D) it receives its blood supply from the left colic artery
   (E) it has no teniae coli

61. Which of the following statements correctly applies to the small intestine?

   (A) the upper three-fifths is considered jejunum
   (B) the lower three-fifths contains aggregated lymph nodules
   (C) none of it is retroperitoneal
   (D) the parasympathetic innervation is provided by the pelvic splanchnic nerves
   (E) the blood supply is provided by both the superior and inferior mesenteric arteries

62. Which of the following statements correctly applies to the gallbladder?

   (A) the submucosal layer is well developed
   (B) the mucous membrane is thrown into circular folds
   (C) its epithelium concentrates the contents of the gallbladder
   (D) it produces bile
   (E) it lies to the left of the falciform ligament

63. Which of the following statements correctly applies to the falciform ligament?

   (A) it represents the inferior limit of the common mesentery
   (B) it encloses the ligamentum teres of the liver
   (C) it extends from the umbilicus to the liver
   (D) it contains the common bile duct
   (E) it does not extend over the diaphragmatic surface of the liver

64. The anterior surface of the liver lies against all the following structures EXCEPT the

   (A) diaphragm
   (B) costal margin
   (C) xiphoid process
   (D) abdominal wall
   (E) spleen

65. Which of the following structures are situated between the celiac trunk and the superior mesenteric artery?

   (A) duodenum and pancreas
   (B) spleen and stomach
   (C) transverse colon and ileum
   (D) stomach and cecum
   (E) pancreas and jejunum

66. Which of the following statements correctly applies to the pancreas?

   (A) it extends from the right kidney to the spleen
   (B) it is inferior to the stomach
   (C) it is crossed by the transverse mesocolon
   (D) it overlies the 4th lumbar vertebra
   (E) its uncinate process extends behind the inferior mesenteric vessels

67. Which of the following statements correctly applies to the fourth portion of the duodenum?

   (A) it is located at the level of the 1st lumbar vertebra
   (B) it is entirely retroperitoneal
   (C) the root of the mesentery begins at the duodenojejunal flexure
   (D) it is in direct continuity with the pylorus of the stomach
   (E) it overlies the hilum of the right kidney

68. All the following statements correctly apply to the duodenum EXCEPT

   (A) it is the shortest portion of the small intestine
   (B) it is usually the breadth of twelve fingers
   (C) it is the fixed portion of the small intestine
   (D) it is suspended by a mesentery
   (E) it is continuous with the completely peritonealized stomach and jejunum

69. Which of the following statements correctly applies to the innervation of the stomach?

    (A) the parasympathetic innervation enhances muscular movement
    (B) the sympathetic innervation exerts the greater influence on the secretion of water
    (C) the sympathetic innervation exerts the greater influence on the secretion of hydrochloric acid
    (D) the parasympathetic innervation has the major influence in the secretion of enzymes
    (E) afferents principally accompany the parasympathetic system

70. Which of the following structures forms the inferior boundary of the epiploic foramen?

    (A) inferior vena cava
    (B) hepatoduodenal ligament
    (C) caudate lobe of the liver
    (D) lesser omentum
    (E) first part of the duodenum

71. The lesser omentum includes which of the following ligaments?

    (A) phrenicocolic
    (B) coronary
    (C) hepatogastric
    (D) gastrocolic
    (E) gastrolienal

72. The lesser peritoneal sac is closed off from the greater peritoneal sac except for the communication through the

    (A) aortic hiatus
    (B) esophageal hiatus
    (C) caval foramen
    (D) deep inguinal ring
    (E) epiploic foramen

DIRECTIONS (Questions 73 through 102): Each group of items in this section consists of lettered headings followed by a set of numbered words or phrases. For each numbered word or phrase, select the ONE lettered heading that is most closely associated with it. Each lettered heading may be selected once, more than once, or not at all.

Questions 73 through 76

For each nerve listed below, choose the spinal cord segments associated with it.

    (A) L1
    (B) T5–T9
    (C) L2–L4
    (D) T1–T5
    (E) S2–S4

73. Greater splanchnic

74. Iliohypogastric

75. Pelvic splanchnic

76. Obturator

Questions 77 through 80

For each structure listed below, choose the term that identifies it.

    (A) haustra
    (B) longitudinal folds
    (C) circular folds
    (D) spiral fold
    (E) coronary ligament

77. Gallbladder

78. Liver

79. Transverse colon

80. Jejunum

Questions 81 through 84

For each structure listed below, choose the source of its origin.

(A) external abdominal oblique aponeurosis
(B) internal abdominal oblique aponeurosis
(C) transverse abdominis muscle
(D) transversalis fascia
(E) extraperitoneal fat

81. Cremaster muscle and fascia

82. Inguinal ligament

83. Superficial inguinal ring

84. Deep inguinal ring

Questions 85 through 88

For each artery listed below, choose the artery from which it arises.

(A) superior mesenteric artery
(B) celiac trunk
(C) inferior mesenteric artery
(D) external iliac artery
(E) femoral artery

85. Inferior epigastric artery

86. Superior rectal artery

87. Superficial circumflex iliac artery

88. Splenic artery

Questions 89 through 92

For each vein listed below, choose the vein that it empties into.

(A) splenic vein
(B) portal vein
(C) superior mesenteric vein
(D) inferior vena cava
(E) internal iliac vein

89. Hepatic vein

90. Left gastric vein

91. Right colic vein

92. Pancreatic magna vein

DIRECTIONS (Questions 93 through 100): Each of the numbered items or incomplete statements in this section is followed by answers or by completions of the statement. Select the ONE lettered answer or completion that is BEST in each case.

93. The dorsal pancreatic artery usually arises from which of the following arteries?

(A) splenic
(B) celiac
(C) superior mesenteric
(D) left renal
(E) gastroduodenal

94. All the following structures may be observed on the visceral surface of the liver EXCEPT the

(A) porta hepatis
(B) gallbladder
(C) fissure for the ligamentum teres
(D) fissure for the ligamentum venosum
(E) bare area

95. All the following statements correctly apply to the common bile duct EXCEPT

(A) it descends in the free border of the lesser omentum
(B) it usually lies to the right of the hepatic artery
(C) it usually lies anterior to the portal vein
(D) it descends behind the first portion of the duodenum
(E) it is retroperitoneal

96. All the following arteries anastomose to form the marginal artery EXCEPT the

(A) ileocolic
(B) right colic
(C) middle colic
(D) left colic
(E) splenic

97. All the following statements correctly applies to the superior mesenteric vein EXCEPT

(A) it lies anterior and to the right of the superior mesenteric artery
(B) it crosses the third part of the duodenum
(C) it crosses the uncinate process of the pancreas
(D) it joins the splenic vein behind the neck of the pancreas to form the portal vein
(E) it drains the rectum

98. All the following statements correctly applies to the portal vein EXCEPT

    (A) it is formed behind the neck of the pancreas by the union of the superior mesenteric vein and the splenic vein
    (B) it ascends behind the first part of the duodenum
    (C) it ascends in the free margin of the hepatoduodenal ligament
    (D) it lies behind the common bile duct and the proper hepatic artery
    (E) it empties directly into the inferior vena cava

99. Which of the following structures is located at the level of the 8th thoracic vertebra?

    (A) caval foramen
    (B) celiac trunk
    (C) esophageal hiatus
    (D) aortic hiatus
    (E) suprasternal notch

100. The sternocostal hiatus allows the passage of the

    (A) aorta
    (B) esophagus
    (C) vagus nerve
    (D) phrenic nerve
    (E) lymphatic channels

DIRECTIONS (Questions 101 through 122): Each group of items in this section consists of lettered headings followed by a set of numbered words or phrases. For each numbered word or phrase, select the ONE lettered heading that is most closely associated with it. Each lettered heading may be selected once, more than once, or not at all.

Questions 101 through 104

For each structure listed below, select the vertebral level at which it is located.

    (A) 2nd lumbar
    (B) 10th thoracic
    (C) 8th thoracic
    (D) 4th lumbar
    (E) 12th thoracic

101. Crest of the ilium

102. Vena caval foramen

103. Esophageal hiatus

104. Renal arteries

Questions 105 through 108

The collateral circulation of the portal vein involves the veins listed below. Choose the tributaries into which these veins drain.

    (A) testicular vein
    (B) superior epigastric vein
    (C) femoral vein
    (D) internal iliac vein
    (E) azygos vein

105. Esophageal tributaries of the left gastric

106. Superior rectal

107. Paraumbilical

108. Retroperitoneal

Questions 109 through 112

For each characteristic listed below, choose the segment of the intestinal tract with which it is associated.

    (A) stomach
    (B) duodenum
    (C) jejunum
    (D) ascending colon
    (E) ileum

109. Teniae coli

110. Sacculations

111. Epiploic appendages

112. Transverse folds

Questions 113 through 116

    (A) common bile duct
    (B) portal vein
    (C) both
    (D) neither

113. Located in the porta hepatis

114. Located in the hepatoduodenal ligament

115. Empties into the liver

116. Empties into the first part of the duodenum

Questions 117 through 120

    (A) main pancreatic duct

    (B) accessory pancreatic duct

    (C) both

    (D) neither

117. Develops from the proximal part of the duct of the dorsal primordium

118. Empties into the second portion of the duodenum

119. Joins the common bile duct

120. Develops from the distal part of the duct of the dorsal primordium and the proximal part of the duct of the ventral primordium

Questions 121 and 122

    (A) neurons in the myenteric plexus

    (B) neurons in the submucosal plexus

    (C) both

    (D) neither

121. Postganglionic parasympathetic neurons

122. Send pain afferents to the central nervous system

ANSWERS AND EXPLANATIONS

1. (A) The inferior epigastric artery arises from the external iliac immediately above the inguinal ligament. Its origin is just medial to the deep inguinal ring and, consequently, the ductus deferens in the male (or round ligament of the uterus in the female) passes behind and then lateral to the artery to enter the inguinal canal. Nearing the arcuate line, the inferior epigastric artery pierces the transversalis fascia and enters the rectus sheath between the muscle and the posterior layer of the sheath. The inferior epigastric artery anastomoses with terminal branches of the superior epigastric. *(Woodburne, p 420)*

2. (B) The gubernaculum testis becomes much reduced in the adult, its remnant constituting the scrotal ligament which extends from the inferior pole of the testis and the tail of the epididymis to the skin of the bottom of the scrotum. *(Woodburne, p 422)*

3. (D) The scrotal ligament extends from the inferior pole of the testis and the tail of the epididymis to the skin of the bottom of the scrotum. The spermatic cord includes the ductus deferens, the deferential artery and vein, the testicular artery, the pampiniform plexus of veins, the lymphatics, and the autonomic nerves of the testis. *(Woodburne, p 423)*

4. (C) The prominent iliac crest forms the upper limit of the region of the hip; the curve of the crest ends ventrally in the anterior superior spine of the ilium, dorsally in the posterior superior iliac spine. The highest point of the iliac crest is at the transverse level of the body of the 4th lumbar vertebra. *(Woodburne, p 407)*

5. (C) The ilioinguinal nerve traverses the inguinal canal to the superficial inguinal ring, where it emerges on the lateral aspect of the spermatic cord. *(Woodburne, p 409)*

6. (E) The tunica dartos scroti is directly continuous with the subcutaneous tissue of the abdominal wall. It is without fat and contains smooth muscle intermingled with its areolar tissue. This muscle is the cause of the wrinkling of the skin of the scrotum. *(Woodburne, p 409)*

7. (A) The musculophrenic branch of the internal thoracic artery supplies twigs to the skin of the abdomen along the costal arch. *(Woodburne, p 409)*

8. (B) The inferior epigastric artery enters the rectus sheath posterior to the rectus sheath from below after arising from the external iliac artery. *(Woodburne, p 409)*

9. (A) The superficial epigastric artery arises from the anterior aspect of the femoral artery about 1 cm below the inguinal ligament. Piercing the femoral sheath and cribriform fascia, the artery turns superiorly over the inguinal ligament and runs toward the umbilicus. *(Woodburne, p 409)*

10. (E) The superficial circumflex iliac artery arises from the femoral artery about 1 cm below the inguinal ligament. It pierces the fascia lata lateral to the saphenous opening and runs laterally across the upper thigh below and parallel to the inguinal ligament. *(Woodburne, p 410)*

11. (B) The superficial external pudendal artery emerges through the saphenous opening and then passes medially and upward across the spermatic cord in the male (or the round ligament of the uterus in the female) to be distributed to the skin of the suprapubic region of the abdomen and to the penis and scrotum (or the labium majus in the female). *(Woodburne, p 410)*

12. (D) The upper five slips of origin for the external abdominal oblique muscle interdigitate with those of the serratus anterior muscle; the lower three digitations with the costal attachments of the latissimus dorsi muscle. *(Woodburne, p 411)*

13. (B) The posterior margin of the external abdominal oblique is free and forms, with the converging border of the latissimus dorsi muscle and the iliac crest below, the lumbar triangle. *(Woodburne, p 411)*

14. **(D)** Additional specializations of the external abdominal oblique aponeurosis are the inguinal ligament, the lacunar ligament, the reflected inguinal ligament, the medial and lateral crura of the superficial inguinal ring, the intercrural fibers, and the external spermatic fascia. *(Woodburne, pp 411–412)*

15. **(A)** The external abdominal oblique aponeurosis has, at its inferior extremity, a thickened, rolled-under border that is stretched between the anterior superior spine of the ilium and the pubic tubercle. This is the inguinal ligament. *(Woodburne, p 412)*

16. **(E)** The lacunar ligament represents the more medial, rolled-under fibers of the inguinal ligament which, flattening down into a horizontal shelf, attach to the pecten of the pubis for about 2 cm. *(Woodburne, pp 412–413)*

17. **(C)** Above the umbilicus, the posterior layer of the internal oblique aponeurosis fuses with the aponeurosis of the transversus abdominis muscle; the anterior layer fuses with that of the external abdominal oblique muscle. Thus, an equal split of the abdominal aponeurosis forms the sheath of the rectus abdominis muscle. In the lower one-fourth of the abdomen, the internal abdominal oblique aponeurosis fails to split and passes to the median line entirely anterior to the rectus abdominis. *(Woodburne, p 414)*

18. **(C)** The cremaster muscle and fascia are the representatives of the internal abdominal oblique muscle layer among the coverings of the cord and testis. They form a layer that immediately underlies the external spermatic fascia. *(Woodburne, p 414)*

19. **(E)** The cremaster muscle is innervated by the genital branch of the genitofemoral nerve. This nerve, a derivative of the lumbar plexus, joins the spermatic cord from within the abdomen at the deep inguinal ring, traverses the inguinal canal, and lies under the cremaster muscle. *(Woodburne, p 414)*

20. **(C)** Like the internal abdominal oblique, the lowest fibers of the transversus abdominis arch downward to the pubis. They insert into the superior border of the pubis and into the medial 2 cm of the pecten. Together with the lowermost fibers of the internal abdominal oblique muscle, which end in the superior border of the pubis, they constitute the falx inguinalis. *(Woodburne, p 415)*

21. **(C)** In the anterior surface of the rectus abdominis, there are three tendinous intersections. They are firmly adherent to the anterior layer of the rectus sheath. The lowest is at the level of the umbilicus; the highest is near the xiphoid process; and the third is halfway between these levels. *(Woodburne, p 416)*

22. **(C)** The pyramidalis muscle is an insignificant muscle, frequently absent and contained in the rectus sheath, where it lies anterior to the inferior portion of the rectus abdominis muscle. It is supplied by a branch of the 12th thoracic nerve. *(Woodburne, p 417)*

23. **(A)** The principal outpouching of the transversalis fascia is the internal spermatic fascia, which invests the ductus deferens and the testicular vessels as they leave the abdominal cavity. The mouth of this outpouching constitutes the deep inguinal ring, located about 1.5 cm above the middle of the inguinal ligament. *(Woodburne, p 418)*

24. **(D)** The innervation of the muscles of the abdominal wall is by ventral rami of spinal nerves T7–L4. This is the same segmental sequence that provides the cutaneous nerves in the region. *(Woodburne, pp 418–419)*

25. **(B)** The 10th intercostal nerve enters the sheath just below the tendinous intersection at the level of the umbilicus. The higher nerves (T7–T9) are above, and the lower nerves distribute, in sequence, below this level. *(Woodburne, p 419)*

26. **(D)** The lumbar arteries are in series with the posterior intercostal and subcostal vessels. Four in number, they arise from the back of the abdominal aorta at the levels of the bodies of the upper four lumbar vertebrae. *(Woodburne, p 419)*

27. **(A)** The iliolumbar artery is a branch of the internal iliac artery, usually of its posterior trunk. *(Woodburne, p 421)*

28. **(B)** The esophagogastric junction is on the horizontal plane of the tip of the xiphoid process and to the left of the 11th thoracic vertebral body. *(Woodburne, p 440)*

29. **(D)** The aorta begins its abdominal distribution by passing through the aortic hiatus of the diaphragm in front of the lower border of the 12th thoracic vertebra. *(Woodburne, pp 440–441)*

30. **(C)** The celiac trunk arises from the abdominal aorta just below the aortic hiatus and at the level of the upper portion of the 1st lumbar vertebra. It gives rise to the left gastric, common hepatic, and splenic arteries. *(Woodburne, pp 440–441)*

31. **(D)** The right hepatic artery passes to the right, usually behind the common hepatic duct, to gain the right end of the liver hilum. Here it breaks up into several branches, which enter the right lobe of the liver with radicles of the portal vein and hepatic duct. As it passes between the hepatic duct and the cystic duct, it gives rise to the small cystic artery, which follows the cystic duct to the gallbladder. *(Woodburne, pp 443–444)*

32. **(E)** The left gastroepiploic artery arises from the splenic artery or an inferior terminal branch and passes toward the greater curvature of the stomach through the gastrolienal ligament. *(Woodburne, p 444)*

33. **(E)** The 9th, 10th, and 11th ribs are in relation to the spleen. It develops in the dorsal mesogastrium. It is entirely surrounded by peritoneum and normally does not descend below the costal margin but rests on the left flexure of the colon and the phrenicocolic ligament. *(Woodburne, p 447)*

34. **(A)** The first part of the duodenum is surrounded by the hepatoduodenal ligament. It is related to the quadrate lobe of the liver and the common bile duct passes behind the first part of the duodenum. The first part of the duodenum passes posteriorly along the right side of the body of the 1st lumbar vertebra. *(Woodburne, pp 448–449)*

35. **(B)** The middle one-third of the second portion of the duodenum is crossed ventrally by the transverse colon. *(Woodburne, p 410)*

36. **(C)** The superior mesenteric artery arises above and crosses the anterior aspect of the third part of the duodenum, whereas the inferior mesenteric artery arises from the aorta directly below the duodenum. *(Woodburne, p 449)*

37. **(C)** The greater duodenal papilla, on which are the terminal openings of the common bile duct and the pancreatic duct, is found at the junction of the middle and lower thirds of the second part of the duodenum. The papilla is continued below by the tapered longitudinal fold of the duodenum. The lesser duodenal papilla marks the termination of the accessory pancreatic duct. *(Woodburne, p 450)*

38. **(E)** The lower left portion of the head of the pancreas is inserted behind the superior mesenteric vessels, forming the uncinate process. *(Woodburne, p 450)*

39. **(D)** Behind the neck of the pancreas, the superior mesenteric and splenic veins unite to form the portal vein. The anterior surface of the neck is covered by peritoneum and lies in the floor of the omental bursa. *(Woodburne, p 450)*

40. **(B)** The tail of the pancreas is usually blunted and turned upward. It enters the lienorenal ligament and frequently makes contact with the spleen; inferiorly, it is in relation with the left flexure of the colon. *(Woodburne, p 450)*

41. **(E)** The pancreatica magna artery is the largest of the series of superior pancreatic branches of the splenic artery. It enters the pancreas in the region of the junction of the middle and left thirds of the gland. *(Woodburne, p 455)*

42. **(A)** Extending from the inferior border to the porta, there is a deep fissure for the ligamentum teres; the ligamentum teres, the obliterated remains of the umbilical vein, passes through this to end in the left branch of the portal vein. *(Woodburne, pp 456–457)*

43. **(C)** The hepatoduodenal ligament transmits the hepatic artery, the portal vein, and the common bile duct. *(Woodburne, p 457)*

44. **(D)** The cystic artery usually arises from a normal right hepatic artery as that vessel crosses the cystohepatic angle. As its most frequent variation, the cystic artery may arise as a branch of either a right hepatic or a common hepatic artery from the superior mesenteric artery. *(Woodburne, p 425)*

45. **(C)** The hepatic veins drain into the inferior vena cava. They are entirely intrahepatic. *(Woodburne, p 460)*

46. **(D)** The portal vein, formed behind the neck of the pancreas by the junction of the superior mesenteric and splenic veins, ascends to the liver in the free margin of the lesser omentum posterior to the common bile duct and the proper hepatic artery. *(Woodburne, pp 464–465)*

47. **(A)** The superior mesenteric artery supplies all of the small intestine except the proximal part of the duodenum; it also supplies the cecum, the ascending colon, and most of the transverse colon, the embryonic midgut. *(Woodburne, p 469)*

48. **(D)** The middle colic artery takes origin from the front of the superior mesenteric artery immediately below the neck of the pancreas. It divides into right and left branches. The right branch anastomoses with the right colic artery and the left branch with the left colic branch of the inferior mesenteric artery. *(Woodburne, p 470)*

49. **(E)** Three surface features serve to distinguish the small intestine from the large. Longitudinal musculature of the large intestine forms three bands called teniae coli. These bands are shorter

than the colon and therefore force the wall to bulge between the teniae, forming sacculations, or haustra coli. The third characteristic of the large intestine is the occurrence along its length of epiploic appendages, which are fat-filled tabs of peritoneum that hang down from the serous coat of the large intestine. *(Woodburne, pp 472–473)*

50. (B) The vermiform appendix has a complete peritoneal investment and a small mesentery, the mesoappendix. It receives its blood supply from the ileocolic artery and is innervated by the vagus and thoracic splanchnic nerves. It is usually located in the pelvis. *(Woodburne, p 475)*

51. (C) The transverse colon is attached posteriorly by the transverse mesocolon on a line that crosses the second part of the duodenum and passes across the pancreas except for its distal extremity. *(Woodburne, pp 475–476)*

52. (D) The testicular veins arise from the testis and the epididymis. They form the pampiniform plexus which, consisting of 8 to 10 anastomosing veins, ascends along the ductus deferens. The plexus, as a constituent of the spermatic cord, traverses the inguinal canal and ends near the deep inguinal ring by forming two accompanying veins of the testicular artery. *(Woodburne, p 503)*

53. (D) The psoas major muscle ends in the iliopsoas tendon, which inserts on the lesser trochanter of the femur. This tendon also receives most of the fibers of the iliac muscle. *(Woodburne, pp 504–505)*

54. (C) The diaphragm consists of a central tendon and muscle covered on both surfaces by a membranous layer of fascia. For the thoracoabdominal diaphragm, the inferior fascia is provided by the upper portion of the parietal abdominopelvic fascia, the transversalis fascia. Its superior fascia is the parietal thoracic fascia (endothoracic fascia), which lines the interior of the thoracic cavity. *(Woodburne, pp 489–490)*

55. (E) The right suprarenal vein empties directly into the posterior surface of the inferior vena cava. On the left side (after union with the inferior phrenic vein), it is a tributary of the renal. *(Woodburne, p 488)*

56. (A) The cortex is essential to life. It secretes hormones that influence the fluid and electrolyte balance in the body. It is also concerned with carbohydrate metabolism. The medulla receives only a preganglionic innervation and produces epinephrine and norepinephrine. *(Woodburne, p 487)*

57. (D) Traversing each renal column is a principal branch of a renal artery, the interlobar artery; its name is a reflection of the lobar character of a single medullary pyramid and the cortical tissue on all sides of it. *(Woodburne, pp 482–483)*

58. (C) The double capillary network in relation to the tubular nephron forms the essential mechanism of the kidney, for the glomerulus and the glomerular capsule provide for filtration of the blood plasma, and the second capillary plexus around the tubules provides for selective reabsorption of water and the return of dissolved materials to the circulation. *(Woodburne, pp 482–483)*

59. (B) The preganglionic parasympathetic fibers of the pelvic splanchnic nerves distribute to the viscera of the pelvis and the perineum as components of this plexus. However, their supply of the left colic flexure, the descending colon, and the sigmoid colon is by independent routes. *(Woodburne, p 479)*

60. (A) The sigmoid colon is characterized by its S-shaped loop and by the presence of a mesocolon. It begins at the brim of the pelvis on the left side and ends at the median line opposite the 3rd segment of the sacrum. *(Woodburne, p 476)*

61. (B) The upper two-fifths (8 feet) is considered jejunum; the lower three-fifths (12 feet) is ileum. Aggregated lymph nodules occur in patches along the antimesenteric border of the ileum. *(Woodburne, p 448)*

62. (C) The gallbladder serves as a reservoir for bile, and its epithelium concentrates it by extracting water. The gallbladder has only serous, fibromuscular, and mucosal layers. The mucous membrane has a honeycomb appearance due to the elevation of folds in low criss-crossing ridges. *(Woodburne, pp 461–462)*

63. (C) The falciform ligament represents the inferior limit of the ventral mesogastrium and encloses the ligamentum teres of the liver in its free border. This double layer extends from the umbilicus upward to the liver. Here its layers pass over both the diaphragmatic and visceral surfaces of the liver. *(Woodburne, p 457)*

64. (E) The anterior surface of the liver lies against the diaphragm, the costal margin, the xiphoid process, and the abdominal wall. *(Woodburne, p 456)*

65. (A) The duodenum and the pancreas are situated between the celiac trunk and the superior mesenteric artery and receive major blood vessels from both. *(Woodburne, p 453)*

66. **(C)** The pancreas lies transversely across the posterior abdominal wall from the duodenum to the spleen and is behind the stomach. The head overlies the 2nd and 3rd lumbar vertebrae, and the uncinate process inserts behind the superior mesenteric vessels. It is crossed by the transverse mesocolon. *(Woodburne, p 450)*

67. **(C)** The end of the duodenum is covered by peritoneum and is movable, but most of the fourth segment is retroperitoneal. The root of the mesentery begins at the duodenojejunal flexure. This portion of the duodenum is stabilized by a fibromuscular band, the suspensory ligament of the duodenum. *(Woodburne, p 450)*

68. **(D)** The duodenum is the fixed and retroperitoneal portion of the small intestine. It receives its name from the fact that its length is equal to the breadth of 12 fingers. At its extremities, the duodenum is continuous with the completely peritonealized stomach and jejunum. *(Woodburne, pp 448– 449)*

69. **(A)** The parasympathetic innervation enhances muscular movements, exerting the greater influence on the secretion of water and hydrochloric acid. The sympathetic innervation is important in vasomotor control and has the major influence in the secretion of enzymes. Afferent impulses principally accompany the sympathetic system. *(Woodburne, p 446)*

70. **(E)** The caudate lobe of the liver forms the superior boundary of the epiploic foramen. The posterior boundary is formed by the inferior vena cava. The hepatoduodenal ligament and its contents form the ventral boundary. The inferior boundary is the first part of the duodenum. *(Woodburne, p 446)*

71. **(C)** The lesser omentum, the double layer remaining in the interval between the stomach and the liver, encloses the common bile duct (hepatic diverticulum) and is a continuous sheet that includes both the hepatogastric and the hepatoduodenal ligaments. *(Woodburne, p 457)*

72. **(E)** The adult bursa omentalis (lesser peritoneal sac) is a peritoneal space behind the stomach that is closed off from the major peritoneal cavity (greater peritoneal sac) except for the communication through the epiploic foramen. *(Woodburne, p 433)*

73. **(B)** The greater thoracic splanchnic nerve (T5–T9 or 10) terminates in the abdomen in the lateral border of the celiac ganglion. The lesser thoracic splanchnic nerve (T10,11) terminates in

the aorticorenal ganglion. The least thoracic splanchnic nerve (last thoracic ganglion), when present, ends in the renal plexus. *(Woodburne, p 494)*

74. **(A)** The iliohypogastric arises from the 1st lumbar nerve, together with a frequent contribution from the 12th thoracic nerve. *(Woodburne, p 507)*

75. **(E)** The pelvic splanchnic nerves have their cells of origin in the 2nd, 3rd, and 4th segments of the sacral spinal cord and arise from the corresponding sacral spinal nerves. *(Woodburne, p 496)*

76. **(C)** The obturator nerve is the principal preaxial nerve of the lumbar plexus. It arises from the anterior branches of lumbar nerves 2, 3, and 4 and descends along the medial border of the psoas muscle. *(Woodburne, p 506)*

77. **(D)** The neck of the gallbladder is directed toward the porta hepatis, makes an S-shaped curve, and is continuous with the cystic duct. Crescentic folds of mucous membrane in its interior are spirally arranged and constitute the spiral fold. *(Woodburne, p 461)*

78. **(E)** The layers of the falciform ligament pass over both the diaphragmatic and visceral surfaces of the liver. The layers of the diaphragmatic surface spread to the right and left anterior layers of the coronary ligament until they reach the sharp reversals of peritoneal reflection to the diaphragm known as the right and left triangular ligaments. *(Woodburne, p 457)*

79. **(A)** The longitudinal bands of muscle of the large intestine are about one-sixth shorter than the colon, so that the wall is forced to bulge between the teniae. The colon, therefore, presents three rows of sacculations, or haustra coli, alternating between the teniae. *(Woodburne, p 473)*

80. **(C)** The wall of the intestine, like that of the stomach, is composed of four coats: mucosal, submucosal, muscular, and serous. The mucous membrane exhibits circular folds and intestinal villi. The circular folds are well developed in the jejunum but become very small or absent in the ileum. *(Woodburne, pp 448–449)*

81. **(B)** Among the coverings of the spermatic cord and testis, the cremaster muscle and fascia are the representatives of the internal abdominal oblique muscle layer. *(Woodburne, pp 423–424)*

82. **(A)** The external oblique aponeurosis has, at its inferior extremity, a thickened, rolled-under border that is stretched between the anterior superior

spine of the ilium and the pubic tubercle. This is the inguinal ligament. *(Woodburne, pp 412–413)*

83. **(A)** The superficial inguinal ring lies at the end of a triangular cleft in the external oblique aponeurosis and is located just above and lateral to the pubic tubercle. The long triangular cleft represents a weakness in the aponeurosis. *(Woodburne, p 413)*

84. **(D)** The principal outpouching of the transversalis fascia is the internal spermatic fascia, which invests the ductus deferens and the testicular vessels as they leave the abdominal cavity. The mouth of this outpouching constitutes the deep inguinal ring. *(Woodburne, pp 417–418)*

85. **(D)** The inferior epigastric artery enters the rectus sheath from below after arising from the external iliac artery. *(Woodburne, p 369)*

86. **(C)** The superior rectal artery is the continuation of the inferior mesenteric artery. The artery arises from the aorta at approximately the level of the 3rd or 4th lumbar vertebra. *(Woodburne, p 420)*

87. **(E)** The superficial circumflex iliac artery arises from the femoral artery about 1 cm below the inguinal ligament. *(Woodburne, p 419)*

88. **(B)** The splenic artery is the largest branch of the celiac trunk. It arises from the left side of the trunk distal to the left gastric artery. The splenic artery runs a highly tortuous course, partially embedded in the superior border of the pancreas. *(Woodburne, p 444)*

89. **(D)** The hepatic veins have no valves and usually empty individually into the inferior vena cava. *(Woodburne, p 460)*

90. **(B)** The left gastric vein ends in the portal vein. Its circular course along the lesser curvature and inferiorly on the body wall is expressed in the old name "coronary vein." *(Woodburne, pp 444–445)*

91. **(C)** The right colic vein enters the right side of the superior mesenteric vein. *(Woodburne, p 471)*

92. **(A)** The caudal pancreatic and pancreatica magna veins empty into the splenic vein on the back of the pancreas. *(Woodburne, p 455)*

93. **(A)** The dorsal pancreatic artery arises most commonly from the proximal portion of the splenic artery or as a 4th branch of the celiac trunk. It may arise as a branch of the superior mesenteric artery or even the hepatic artery. *(Woodburne, p 454)*

94. **(E)** The bare area is on the dorsal or diaphragmatic surface of the liver. The visceral surface of the liver lodges the gallbladder and is deeply indented posteriorly by the inferior vena cava. The porta hepatis is located at about the middle of the visceral surface. The deep fissure for the ligamentum teres extends from the inferior border to the porta hepatis. The deep fissure for the ligamentum venosum extends from the porta hepatis to the posterior surface. *(Woodburne, p 456)*

95. **(E)** The common bile duct descends in the free border of the lesser omentum to the duodenum. It lies to the right of the hepatic artery and anterior to the portal vein. The duct descends behind the first portion of the duodenum and then crosses the posterior surface of the head of the pancreas. It is not retroperitoneal; it is located within the hepatoduodenal ligament. *(Woodburne, p 449)*

96. **(E)** The anastomotic channels along the large intestine are frequently so large as to constitute a marginal artery that follows the arch of the colon. The right branch of the middle colic anastomose with the right colic, and the left branch anastomose with the left colic branch of the inferior mesenteric. The splenic artery is a branch of the celiac trunk and does not contribute to the marginal artery. *(Woodburne, p 477)*

97. **(E)** The superior mesenteric vein accompanies the superior mesenteric artery and lies anterior and to its right in the root of the mesentery. Like the artery, the vein crosses the third part of the duodenum and the uncinate process of the pancreas. It terminates behind the neck of the pancreas by joining the splenic vein to form the portal vein. It drains most of the small intestine and a portion of the large intestine. *(Woodburne, pp 470–471)*

98. **(E)** The portal vein is formed behind the neck of the pancreas by the union of the superior mesenteric vein and the splenic vein. The portal vein ascends behind the first part of the duodenum and, in the free margin of the hepatoduodenal ligament, behind the common bile duct and the proper hepatic duct. It drains into the liver. *(Woodburne, p 479)*

99. **(A)** The aortic hiatus occurs at the lower border of the 12th thoracic vertebra or at the level of the disk below it. The esophageal hiatus occurs at the level of the 10th thoracic vertebra. The vena cava foramen lies at the level of the 8th thoracic vertebra. The celiac trunk arises from the front of the abdominal aorta just below the aortic hiatus at the level of the upper portion of the 1st lumbar vertebra. *(Woodburne, pp 490–491)*

100. **(E)** The sternocostal interval between the adjacent sternal and costal muscular fasciculi, allows passage of lymphatic channels from the convex surface of the liver to the phrenic nodes. *(Woodburne, pp 490–491)*

101. **(D)** The highest point of the iliac crest is at the transverse level of the body of the 4th lumbar vertebra. *(Woodburne, p 367)*

102. **(C)** The vena caval foramen is an opening in the central tendon. It is the highest of the three openings and lies at the level of the 8th thoracic vertebra or the disk below it. *(Woodburne, p 451)*

103. **(B)** The elliptical esophageal hiatus lies in the muscular part of the diaphragm at the level of the 10th thoracic vertebra. It is formed by the divergence and subsequent decussation of the bundles of the right crus. *(Woodburne, p 451)*

104. **(A)** The renal arteries arise, one on each side of the aorta, at the level of the upper border of the 2nd lumbar vertebra. Their origin is about 1 cm below that of the superior mesenteric artery. *(Woodburne, p 446)*

105. **(E)** The esophageal tributaries of the left gastric vein communicate with esophageal veins that empty into the azygos vein of the chest. *(Woodburne, p 440)*

106. **(D)** The rectal plexus of the anal canal and the lower rectum allow communication between tributaries of the superior rectal, middle rectal, and inferior rectal veins. The middle rectal and inferior rectal veins transmit their blood to the inferior vena cava. *(Woodburne, p 440)*

107. **(B)** The paraumbilical veins anastomose with small veins of the anterior abdominal wall which, as radicales of the superior epigastric, inferior epigastric, thoracoepigastric, and segmental vessels, connect with the superior or the inferior vena cava. *(Woodburne, p 440)*

108. **(A)** The retroperitoneal veins draining the colon (ileocolic, right colic, middle colic, and left colic veins) have anastomotic connections with testicular (or ovarian) veins and especially with small veins of the pararenal fat. *(Woodburne, p 440)*

109. **(D)** Three surface features serve to distinguish isolated loops of the small or the large intestine presenting through an abdominal opening: (1) teniae coli; (2) sacculations, or haustra coli; and (3) epiploic appendages. *(Woodburne, p 434)*

110. **(D)** The colon presents three rows of sacculations, or haustra coli, alternating between the teniae. *(Woodburne, p 434)*

111. **(D)** The third characteristic of the colon is the occurrence along its length of epiploic appendages. These are fat-filled tabs, or pendants, of peritoneum that project from the serous coat of the large intestine except on the rectum. *(Woodburne, p 434)*

112. **(C)** Little fat exists in the mesentery of the upper jejunum, and "windows" of translucency between the blood vessels of the mesentery are numerous. *(Woodburne, p 429)*

113. **(C)** The porta of the liver is the region of branching and entrance of the hepatic artery and the portal vein and of exit of the hepatic bile ducts. *(Woodburne, p 417)*

114. **(C)** The hepatoduodenal ligament transmits the hepatic artery, the portal vein, and the common bile duct. *(Woodburne, p 419)*

115. **(B)** The hepatic artery conducts arterial blood for the nourishment of the liver tissues, whereas the portal vein carries to the liver blood from the gastrointestinal tract containing certain of the products of digestion. *(Woodburne, p 419)*

116. **(D)** The common bile duct is the excretory duct of the liver and empties into the second portion of the duodenum. It is formed near the porta hepatis by the junction of the common hepatic duct from the liver and the cystic duct from the gallbladder. *(Woodburne, p 419)*

117. **(B)** The ducts of the two primordia fuse in the upper part of the head of the gland, thus the pancreatic duct of the adult is formed from the distal part of the duct of the dorsal primordium and the proximal part of the duct of the ventral primordium. The remaining proximal part of the duct of the dorsal primordium becomes the accessory pancreatic duct in the adult. *(Woodburne, pp 413–414)*

118. **(C)** The greater duodenal papilla marks the termination of the main pancreatic duct and the common bile duct. Typically, the accessory pancreatic duct empties at the lesser duodenal papilla, about 2 cm proximal to the greater papilla, in the anteromedial duodenal wall. Both empty into the second portion of the duodenum. *(Woodburne, p 413)*

119. **(A)** The greater duodenal papilla marks the termination of the main

120. **(A)** The pancreatic duct of the adult is formed from the distal part of the duct of the dorsal primordium and the proximal part of the duct of the ventral primordium. *(Woodburne, pp 413–414)*

121. **(C)** The cell bodies within these plexuses are those of the postganglionic neurons in the two-neuron parasympathetic innervation of the intestinal tract. *(Woodburne, p 399)*

122. **(C)** The parasympathetic nerves increase motility in the tract and are important in keeping the chyme moving along. *(Woodburne, p 399)*

Clinical Abdominal Region
Questions

Questions 1 through 5

    (A) hydrocele
    (B) cryptorchidism
    (C) persistent "canal of nuck"
    (D) tunica vaginalis testis

1. Persistence of the vaginal process in the female

2. Fluid accumulation within the tunica vaginalis testis

3. Ectopic testis

4. Peritoneum covering the anterior and lateral aspect of the testis

5. Undescended testis

Questions 6 through 10

    (A) Meckel's diverticulum
    (B) volvulus
    (C) diverticulosis

6. Herniation of the lining mucous membrane through the circular layer of muscle between the teniae coli

7. Twisting of the sigmoid colon on its mesentery, causing an obstruction

8. Occasional feature of the ileum

9. Represents the remains of the vitelline duct of early fetal life

10. Rarely has a fistulous opening at the umbilicus

11. Hydrocele is a fluid accumulation within the

    (A) round ligament
    (B) gubernaculum testis
    (C) scrotal ligament
    (D) tunica vaginalis testis
    (E) vas deferens

12. Herniation of abdominal contents into an unobliterated vaginal process and within the coverings of the spermatic cord results in which of the following herniae?

    (A) umbilical
    (B) indirect inguinal
    (C) direct inguinal
    (D) lumbar
    (E) femoral

13. The inferior epigastric artery is lateral to the herniating mass in which of the following herniae?

    (A) direct inguinal
    (B) indirect inguinal
    (C) femoral
    (D) umbilical
    (E) lumbar

14. Meckel's diverticulum is an occasional feature of the

    (A) duodenum
    (B) cecum
    (C) ileum
    (D) jejunum
    (E) liver

15. Femoral herniae descend into the thigh behind which of the following ligaments?

   (A) iliopectineal
   (B) lacunar
   (C) reflected inguinal
   (D) falx inguinalis
   (E) inguinal

16. A fusion fascia has surgical importance because of the absence of

   (A) blood vessels
   (B) lymph nodes
   (C) ligaments
   (D) lymphatic channels
   (E) white cells

ANSWERS AND EXPLANATIONS

1. **(C)** Persistence of the vaginal process in the female (persistent "canal of nuck") leads to cysts and herniae of congenital origin. *(Woodburne, p 422)*

2. **(A)** Hydrocele is a fluid accumulation within the tunica vaginalis testis due to secretion of abnormal amounts of serous fluid by the serous membrane. *(Woodburne, p 422)*

3. **(B)** Abnormalities in testis descent may occur, as into the thigh or the perineum. Such testes are said to be ectopic in position. *(Woodburne, p 422)*

4. **(D)** The peritoneum covering the anterior and lateral aspects of the testis, a closed serous sac, is known as the tunica vaginalis. *(Woodburne, p 422)*

5. **(B)** Occasionally, the testis fails to descend or fails to make a complete descent. *(Woodburne, p 422)*

6. **(C)** Diverticulosis is a herniation of the lining mucous membrane through the circular layer of muscle between teniae coli. *(Woodburne, p 476)*

7. **(B)** A twisting of the sigmoid colon on its mesentery, causing obstruction, is known as volvulus. *(Woodburne, p 476)*

8. **(A)** Meckel's diverticulum is an occasional feature of the ileum. It is a finger-like pouch which springs from the free border of the intestine. *(Woodburne, p 468)*

9. **(A)** Meckel's diverticulum is the remains of the vitelline duct of early fetal life. *(Woodburne, p 468)*

10. **(A)** Meckel's diverticulum rarely has a fistulous opening at the umbilicus. *(Woodburne, p 468)*

11. **(D)** Hydrocele is a fluid accumulation within the tunica vaginalis testis due to secretion of abnormal amounts of serous fluid by the serous membrane. *(Woodburne, p 422)*

12. **(B)** Herniation of abdominal contents into an unobliterated vaginal process and within the coverings of the spermatic cord results in an indirect inguinal hernia. *(Woodburne, pp 424–425)*

13. **(A)** Another type of inguinal hernia, the direct inguinal hernia, occurs less commonly (one-third as frequently as indirect herniae in males). The direct inguinal hernia bulges at the superficial inguinal ring and almost never descends into the scrotum. The inferior epigastric artery is lateral to the herniating mass in the direct type. *(Woodburne, pp 424–425)*

14. **(C)** The Meckel's diverticulum is an occasional feature of the ileum. It occurs in about 1% of individuals, somewhere in the last meter of the ileum. It represents the remains of the vitelline duct. *(Woodburne, p 468)*

15. **(E)** Femoral herniae descend into the thigh behind the inguinal ligament, using a tubular compartment of the femoral sheath, the femoral canal. *(Woodburne, p 426)*

16. **(A)** A fusion fascia has surgical importance: because it is a peritoneal remnant along which or across which no blood vessels, nerves, or other accessory structures pass, it can be invaded in the adult body without fear of encountering any important vessels or nerves. *(Woodburne, p 433)*

Developmental Abdominal Region Questions

DIRECTIONS (Questions 1 through 11): Each of the numbered items or incomplete statements in this section is followed by answers or by completions of the statement. Select the ONE lettered answer or completion that is BEST in each case.

1. The scrotal ligament develops from the

    (A) processus vaginalis
    (B) tunica vaginalis testis
    (C) inguinal canal
    (D) gubernaculum testis
    (E) genital ridge

2. Which of the following structures is not located in the spermatic cord?

    (A) ductus deferens
    (B) deferential artery
    (C) testicular artery
    (D) pampiniform plexus of veins
    (E) urethra

3. The following structures traverse the inguinal canal EXCEPT the *wrote*

    (A) inferior epigastric artery
    (B) ilioinguinal nerve
    (C) genital branch of the genitofemoral nerve
    (D) cremasteric artery
    (E) internal spermatic fascia

4. The tunica vaginalis testis is a remnant of which of the following?

    (A) urachus
    (B) processus vaginalis
    (C) scrotal ligament
    (D) gubernaculum testis
    (E) round ligament

5. Which of the following is a derivative of the dorsal common mesentery?

    (A) transverse mesocolon
    (B) lienorenal ligament *splenorenal*
    (C) falciform ligament
    (D) hepatogastric ligament
    (E) gastrocolic ligament

6. Which of the following is a derivative of the dorsal mesogastrium?

    (A) hepatogastric ligament
    (B) hepatocolic ligament
    (C) phrenicocolic ligament
    (D) sigmoid mesocolon
    (E) coronary ligament

7. Which of the following is a derivative of the ventral mesogastrium?

    (A) mesoappendix
    (B) gastrolienal ligament *(gastrosplenic)*
    (C) lienorenal ligament *(splenorenal)*
    (D) hepatoduodenal ligament
    (E) sigmoid mesocolon

8. The primordia of the pancreas, liver, and gallbladder appear as outgrowths of the gut tube during which of the following weeks of development?

    (A) 2nd
    (B) 4th
    (C) 8th
    (D) 16th
    (E) 21st

9. Which of the following statements correctly applies to the rotation of the gastrointestinal tube?

   (A) rotation is clockwise when viewed from the ventral side

   (B) rotation occurs during the 2nd week of development

   (C) rotation takes place around an axis represented by the superior mesenteric artery

   (D) rotation is usually complete by the 4th week of development

   (E) rotation only involves the small intestine

10. Which of the following structures develops in two parts from a dorsal and ventral primordium?

   (A) liver
   (B) spleen
   (C) gallbladder
   (D) pancreas
   (E) cecum

11. Which of the following ducts formed from the distal part of the duct of the dorsal primordium and the proximal part of the duct of the ventral primordium?

   (A) cystic
   (B) hepatic
   (C) common hepatic
   (D) accessory pancreatic
   (E) main pancreatic

ANSWERS AND EXPLANATIONS

1. **(D)** The gubernaculum testis becomes much reduced in the adult, its remnant constituting the scrotal ligament that extends from the inferior pole of the testis and the tail of the epididymis to the skin of the bottom of the scrotum. *(Woodburne, p 422)*

2. **(E)** The spermatic cord contains the ductus deferens, the deferential artery and vein, the testicular artery, the pampiniform plexus of veins, the lymphatics, and the autonomic nerves of the testis. *(Woodburne, p 422)*

3. **(A)** Traversing the inguinal canal are the ilioinguinal nerve, the genital branch of the gen-

itofemoral nerve, and the cremasteric artery. The components of the spermatic cord are invested by the internal spermatic fascia all the way through the canal. *(Woodburne, pp 422–423)*

4. **(B)** The tunica vaginalis testis is the invaginated serous sac that partially covers the testis and represents the lower closed-off portion of the processus vaginalis of the peritoneum. The visceral layer is closely applied to the testis, the epididymis, and the lower part of the spermatic cord. *(Woodburne, p 385)*

5. **(A)** The derivatives of the dorsal common mesentery include the mesentery, transverse mesocolon, sigmoid mesocolon, and mesoappendix. *(Woodburne, p 388)*

6. **(C)** The derivatives of the dorsal mesogastrium include the greater omentum, the lienorenal ligament, and the phrenicocolic ligament. *(Woodburne, p 388)*

7. **(D)** The derivatives of the ventral mesogastrium include the hepatogastric, hepatoduodenal, hepatocolic, falciform, coronary, right triangular, and left triangular ligaments. *(Woodburne, p 388)*

8. **(B)** The primordia of the pancreas, liver, and gallbladder appear as outgrowths of the gut tube just caudal to the stomach during the 4th week of development. *(Woodburne, p 388)*

9. **(C)** Viewed from the ventral side, the rotation is counterclockwise and brings up cephalically and to the right the caudal part of the loop, representing the cecum and the large intestine, and turns the originally cephalic limb of the loop (small intestine) downward and to the left. The rotation of the loop takes place around an axis represented by the superior mesenteric artery. *(Woodburne, pp 388–389)*

10. **(D)** The pancreas develops in two parts, from a dorsal and a ventral primordium. *(Woodburne, p 452)*

11. **(E)** The ducts of the two primordia fuse in the upper part of the head of the gland. Thus, the pancreatic duct of the adult is formed from the distal part of the duct of the dorsal primordium and the proximal part of the duct of the ventral primordium. *(Woodburne, p 452)*

Nervous Abdominal Region Questions

DIRECTIONS (Questions 1 through 10): Each group of items in this section consists of lettered headings followed by a set of numbered words or phrases. For each numbered word or phrase, select the ONE lettered heading that is most closely associated with it. Each lettered heading may be selected once, more than once, or not at all.

(A) vagus nerve
(B) pelvic splanchnic nerves
(C) phrenic nerve
(D) thoracic splanchnic nerves
(E) superior hypogastric plexus

1. Motor to the diaphragm

2. Innervation of the suprarenal glands

3. Parasympathetic innervation of the descending colon

4. Parasympathetic innervation to the gallbladder

5. Parasympathetic innervation to the pancreas

6. Sympathetic innervation to the jejunum

7. Sympathetic to the descending colon

8. Sympathetic innervation to the sigmoid

9. Sympathetic innervation to the kidney

10. Parasympathetic innervation to the vermiform appendix

DIRECTIONS (Questions 11 and 12): Each of the numbered items or incomplete statements in this section is followed by answers or by completions of the statement. Select the ONE lettered answer or completion that is BEST in each case.

11. Which of the following statements correctly applies to the innervation of the stomach?

    (A) the sacral plexus provides the parasympathetic fibers
    (B) the anterior vagal trunk carries preganglionic visceral efferents only
    (C) the stomach has no sympathetic innervation
    (D) the vagal trunks contain preganglionic visceral efferent and general visceral afferent fibers
    (E) the postganglionic parasympathetic cell bodies are located in the celiac plexus

12. Both the vagal parasympathetic innervation and the thoracic splanchnic sympathetic innervation of the gastrointestinal tract terminate at the

    (A) duodenojejunal junction
    (B) junction of the middle and left thirds of the transverse colon
    (C) jejunoileal junction
    (D) ileocecal junction
    (E) distal one-third of the sigmoid colon

ANSWERS AND EXPLANATIONS

1. **(C)** The entire motor supply to the diaphragm is from the phrenic nerves, which arise from the ventral rami of segments C3 to C5 of the spinal cord. The phrenic nerves also supply sensory fibers (pain and proprioception) to most of the diaphragm. *(Moore, p 228)*

2. **(D)** The suprarenal glands have a rich nerve supply from the adjacent celiac plexus and the greater thoracic splanchnic nerves. *(Moore, p 224)*

3. **(B)** The parasympathetic innervation for the descending colon is derived from the pelvic splanchnic nerves. *(Moore, p 207)*

4. **(A)** The vagus nerve provides parasympathetic innervation to the gallbladder. The celiac plexus provides the sympathetic innervation. *(Moore, p 202)*

5. **(A)** The parasympathetic innervation of the pancreas is provided by the vagus nerve. The pain fibers are carried by the splanchnic nerves. *(Moore, p 189)*

6. **(D)** The sympathetic innervation to the jejunum and ileum is derived from the thoracic splanchnic nerves. *(Moore, p 181)*

7. **(E)** The sympathetic innervation to the descending colon is provided by the superior hypogastric plexus. *(Moore, p 221)*

8. **(E)** The sympathetic innervation to the sigmoid colon is provided by the superior hypogastric plexus. The parasympathetic supply is derived from the pelvic splanchnic nerves. *(Moore, p 209)*

9. **(D)** The sympathetic innervation of the kidney is provided by the lesser and least thoracic splanchnic nerves. *(Moore, p 221)*

10. **(A)** The parasympathetic innervation to the vermiform appendix is provided by the vagus nerve. The celiac and superior mesenteric plexus contain both sympathetic and parasympathetic fibers. *(Moore, p 205)*

11. **(D)** The anterior and posterior vagal trunks pass through the esophageal hiatus of the diaphragm anterior and posterior to the terminal esophagus, and both lie toward its right side. They contain preganglionic visceral efferent and general visceral afferent fibers. *(Woodburne, p 407)*

12. **(B)** Both the vagal parasympathetic innervation and the thoracic splanchnic sympathetic innervation of the gastrointestinal tract terminate with the end of the distribution of the superior mesenteric artery at about the junction of the middle and left thirds of the transverse colon. *(Woodburne, pp 471–472)*

Illustrations
Questions

STOMACH
(Questions 1 through 8)

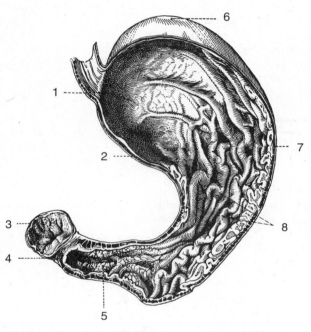

Figure 6–1. Stomach (internal aspect). (Modified and reproduced, with permission, from Montgomery RL: *Basic Anatomy,* Urban & Schwarzenberg, p. 259, 1980.)

Directions: With reference to the diagram, match the numbered structures with their corresponding lettered items.

(A) pyloric sphincter

(B) fundus

(C) greater curvature

(D) lesser curvature

(E) cardiac opening

(F) rugae

(G) duodenum

(H) pylorus

LIVER AND GALLBLADDER
(Questions 9 through 31)

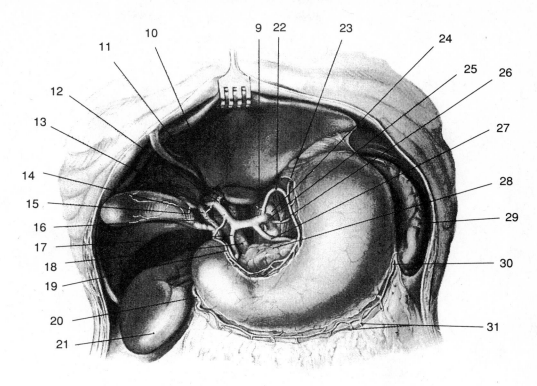

Figure 6–2. Liver and gallbladder. (Modified and reproduced, with permission, from Montgomery RL: *Basic Anatomy,* Urban & Schwarzenberg, p. 268, 1980.)

Directions: With reference to the diagram, match the numbered structures with their corresponding lettered items.

(A) right hepatic artery

(B) gastroduodenal artery

(C) esophageal artery

(D) splenic artery

(E) portal vein

(F) common hepatic duct

(G) pancreas

(H) inferior phrenic artery

(I) epiploic arteries

(J) left hepatic artery

(K) proper hepatic artery

(L) inferior phrenic artery

(M) left lobe of liver

(N) left gastroepiploic artery

(O) right gastric artery

(P) inferior vena cava

(Q) spleen

(R) celiac trunk

(S) cystic artery

(T) abdominal aorta

(U) kidney

(V) right gastroepiploic artery

(W) left gastric artery

LIVER AND GALLBLADDER
(Questions 32 through 50)

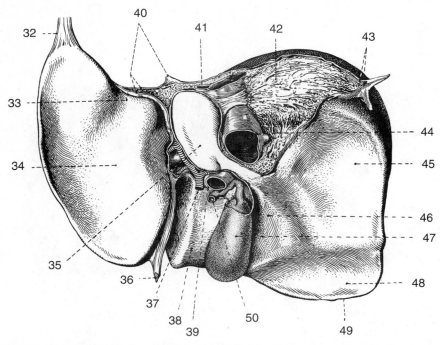

Figure 6–3. Liver and gallbladder (inferiodorsal view). (Modified and reproduced, with permission, from Montgomery RL: *Basic Anatomy,* Urban & Schwarzenberg, p. 268, 1980.)

Directions: With reference to the diagram, match the numbered structures with their corresponding lettered items.

(A) quadrate lobe
(B) hepatic vein
(C) esophageal impression
(D) inferior vena cava
(E) portal vein
(F) duodenal impression
(G) appendix fibrosa hepatis
(H) common bile duct
(I) inferior margin
(J) gastric impression

(K) colic impression
(L) right renal impression
(M) bare area
(N) left triangular ligament
(O) caudate lobe
(P) hepatic artery
(Q) gallbladder
(R) right triangular ligament
(S) round ligament of liver

GALLBLADDER
(Questions 51 through 57)

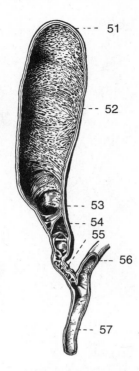

Figure 6–4. Gallbladder (sagittal view) (Modified and reproduced, with permission, from Montgomery RL: *Basic Anatomy,* Urban & Schwarzenberg, p. 271, 1980.)

Directions: With reference to the diagram, match the numbered structures with their corresponding lettered items.

(A) body of gallbladder

(B) cystic duct

(C) common bile duct

(D) spiral folds

(E) hepatic duct

(F) fundus of gallbladder

(G) neck of gallbladder

COMMON BILE DUCT
(Questions 58 through 64)

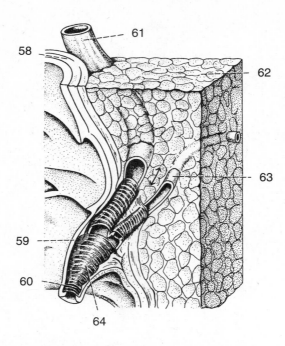

Figure 6–5. Common bile duct. (Modified and reproduced, with permission, from Montgomery RL: *Basic Anatomy,* Urban & Schwarzenberg, p. 271, 1980.)

Directions: With reference to the diagram, match the numbered structures with their corresponding lettered items.

(A) sphincter ampullae

(B) pancreas

(C) major duodenal papillae

(D) duodenum

(E) mucosa

(F) major pancreatic duct

(G) common bile duct

PANCREATIC DUCTS
(Questions 65 through 75)

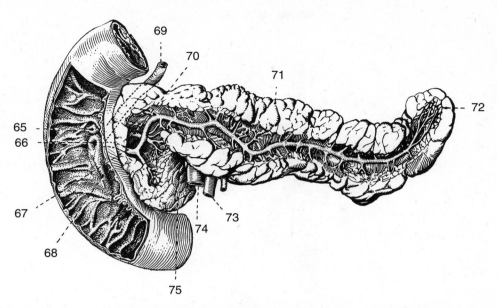

Figure 6–6. Pancreatic ducts. (Modified and reproduced, with permission, from Montgomery RL: *Basic Anatomy,* Urban & Schwarzenberg, p. 273, 1980.)

Directions: With reference to the diagram, match the numbered structures with their corresponding lettered items.

(A) longitudinal duodenal fold
(B) accessory pancreatic duct
(C) tail of pancreas
(D) major duodenal papillae
(E) superior mesenteric vein
(F) uncinate process

(G) common bile duct
(H) body of pancreas
(I) minor duodenal papillae
(J) superior mesenteric artery
(K) main pancreatic duct

VARIATIONS IN THE LENGTH OF THE CYSTIC DUCT AND ITS LEVEL
AND MODE OF ENTRY INTO THE JUNCTION OF THE COMMON HEPATIC
AND THE COMMON BILE DUCTS
Questions 76 through 85)

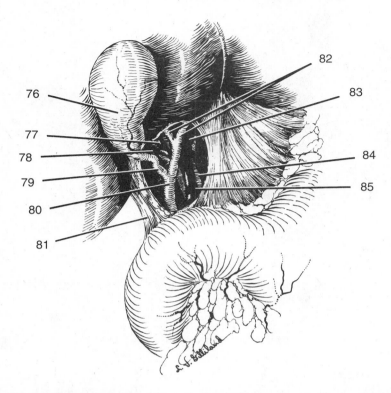

Figure 6–7 Variations in the length of the cystic duct and its level and mode of entry into the junction of the common hepatic and the common bile ducts. (Modified and reproduced, with permission, from Way LW [editor]: *Current Surgical Diagnosis & Treatment,* 7th ed. Lange, 1985.)

Directions: With reference to the diagram, match the numbered structures with their corresponding lettered items.

(A) proper hepatic artery

(B) cystic artery

(C) left and right hepatic ducts

(D) gallbladder

(E) free edge of hepatoduodenal ligament

(F) left hepatic artery

(G) portal vein

(H) right hepatic artery

(I) cystic duct

(J) common bile duct

PANCREAS
(Questions 86 through 106)

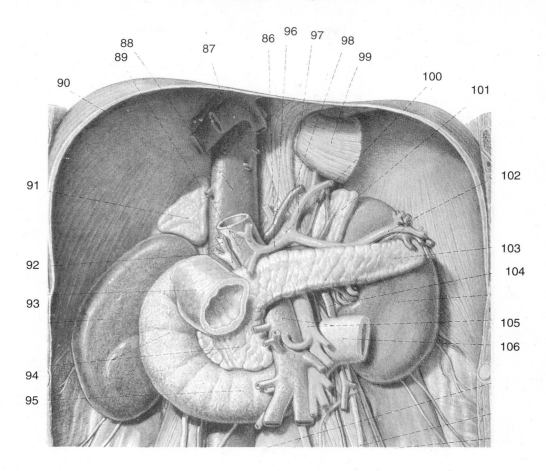

Figure 6–8. Pancreas. (Modified and reproduced, with permission, from Montgomery RL: *Basic Anatomy,* Urban & Schwarzenberg, p. 280, 1980.)

Directions: With reference to the diagram, match the numbered structures with their corresponding lettered items.

(A) common bile duct, portal vein, and hepatic artery

(B) second portion of duodenum and head of pancreas

(C) aortic hiatus

(D) inferior mesenteric vein

(E) common hepatic artery

(F) esophageal hiatus

(G) tail of pancreas

(H) left gastric artery and vein

(I) hepatic veins

(J) diaphragm

(K) inferior vena cava

(L) third portion of duodenum

(M) first portion of duodenum

(N) cardiac portion of stomach

(O) suprarenal gland

(P) celiac trunk

(Q) hepatic duct and cystic duct

(R) superior mesenteric artery and vein

(S) jejunum

(T) splenic artery and vein

DEVELOPMENT OF EXTRAHEPATIC BILIARY TRACT
IN THE EMBRYO
(Questions 107 through 125)

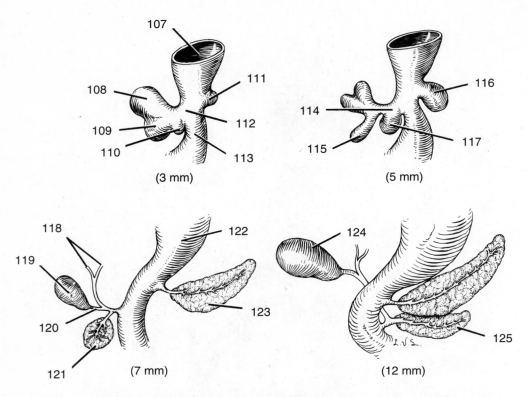

Figure 6–9. Development of extrahepatic biliary tract in the embryo from the 3-mm to the 12-mm stage. (Modified and reproduced, with permission, from Way LW [editor]: *Current Surgical Diagnosis & Treatment,* 6th ed. Lange, p. 410, 1983.)

Directions: With reference to the diagram, match the numbered structures with their corresponding lettered items.

(A) cranial bud

(B) hepatic ducts

(C) gallbladder

(D) dorsal pancreas

(E) dorsal bud of pancreas

(F) caudal bud

(G) common bile duct

(H) stomach

(I) ventral pancreas

(J) ventral bud of pancreas

(K) cystic duct

(L) hindgut

(M) foregut

(N) midgut

(O) ventral pancreas and common bile duct have rotated dorsal to the duodenum

COMMUNICATION OF PORTAL SYSTEM
WITH SYSTEMIC VENOUS SYSTEM
(Questions 126 through 144)

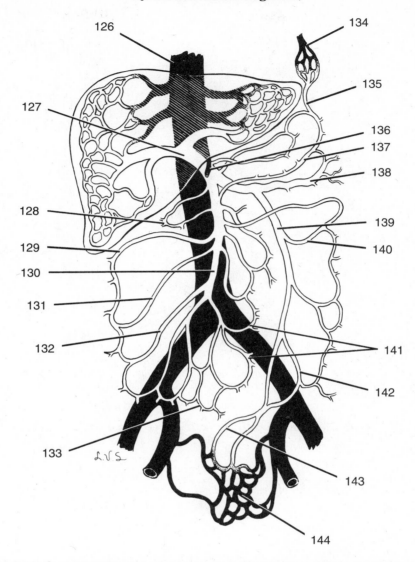

Figure 6–10. Communication of portal system with systemic venous system. (Modified and reproduced, with permission, from Way LW [editor]: *Current Surgical Diagnosis & Treatment,* 6th ed. Lange, p. 405, 1983.)

Directions: With reference to the diagram, match the numbered structures with their corresponding lettered items.

(A) inferior mesenteric vein

(B) jejunal veins

(C) sigmoid vein

(D) portal vein

(E) right colic vein

(F) ileocolic vein

(G) superior rectal vein

(H) right gastroepiploic vein

(I) left colic vein

(J) esophageal vein

(K) inferior vena cava

(L) inferior and middle rectal veins

(M) superior mesenteric vein

(N) middle colic vein

(O) ascending branch of gastric vein

(P) ileal vein

(Q) paraumbilical vein

(R) left gastroepiploic vein

(S) splenic vein

THE VISCERAL SURFACE OF THE LIVER
(Questions 145 through 164)

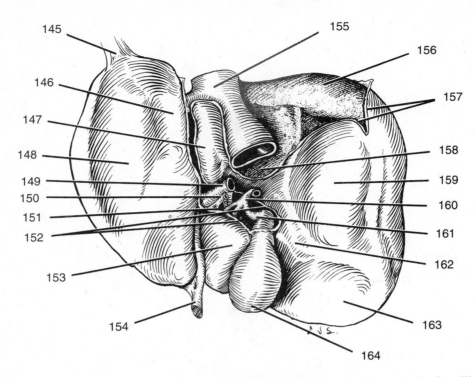

Figure 6–11. The visceral surface of the liver. (Modified and reproduced, with permission, from Way LW [editor]: *Current Surgical Diagnosis & Treatment,* 6th ed. Lange, p. 399, 1983.)

Directions: With reference to the diagram, match the numbered structures with their corresponding lettered items.

(A) suprarenal impression

(B) round ligament

(C) inferior vena cava

(D) appendix fibrosa

(E) quadrate lobe

(F) caudate lobe

(G) colic impression

(H) portal vein

(I) coronary ligament

(J) cystic duct

(K) bare area of the liver

(L) esophageal impression

(M) renal impression

(N) common hepatic duct

(O) duodenal impression

(P) gastric impression

(Q) gallbladder

(R) hepatic artery

(S) porta hepatis

(T) edge of lesser omentum

GREATER OMENTUM AND ITS ABDOMINAL RELATIONSHIPS
(Questions 165 through 179)

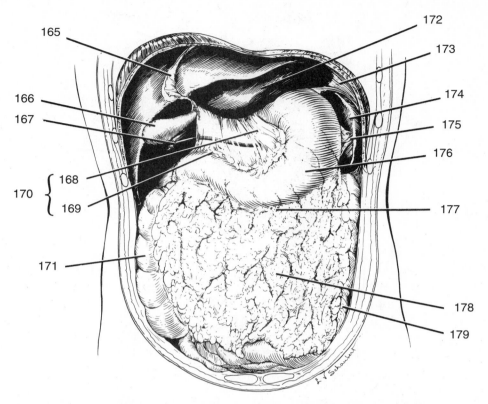

Figure 6–12. Greater omentum and its abdominal relationships. (Modified and reproduced, with permission, from Way LW [editor]: *Current Surgical Diagnosis & Treatment,* 6th ed. Lange, p. 393, 1983.)

Directions: With reference to the diagram, match the numbered structures with their corresponding lettered items.

(A) gastrocolic ligament
(B) falciform ligament
(C) ascending colon
(D) left lobe of liver
(E) stomach
(F) gallbladder
(G) lesser omentum
(H) gastrohepatic ligament

(I) spleen
(J) splenorenal ligament
(K) probe in epiploic foramen
(L) hepatoduodenal ligament
(M) gastrosplenic ligament
(N) greater omentum
(O) descending colon

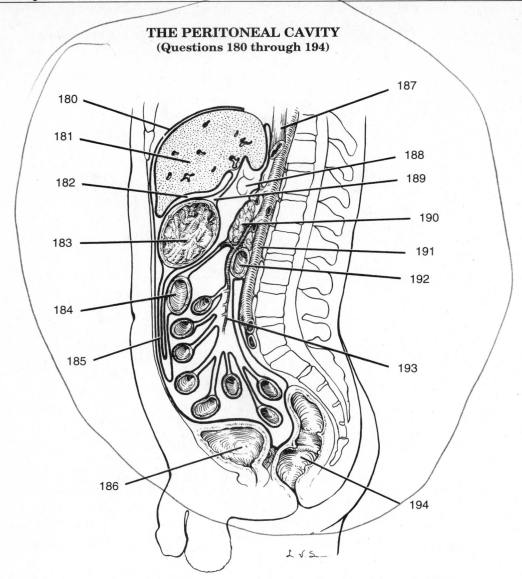

Figure 6–13. The peritoneal cavity, showing 4 layers of the greater omentum and abdominal relationships. (Modified and reproduced, with permission, from Way LW [editor]: *Current Surgical Diagnosis & Treatment,* 6th ed. Lange, p. 392, 1983.)

Directions: With reference to the diagram, match the numbered structures with their corresponding lettered items.

(A) superior mesenteric artery

(B) urinary bladder

(C) greater omentum

(D) pancreas

(E) aorta

(F) esophagus

(G) lesser peritoneal cavity

(H) duodenum

(I) liver

(J) anteroinferior subphrenic space

(K) anterosuperior subphrenic space

(L) stomach

(M) transverse colon

(N) rectum

(O) gastrohepatic ligament (lesser omentum)

ARTERIAL SUPPLY OF THE RECTOSIGMOID
AND RECTUM
(Questions 195 through 207)

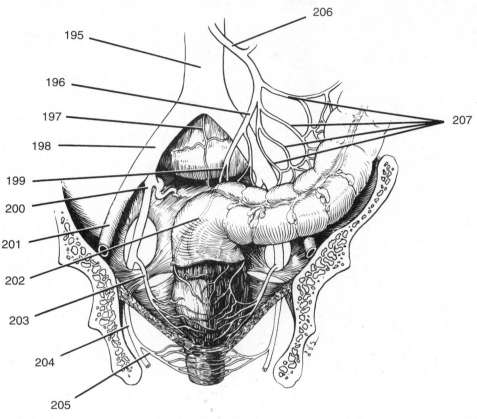

Figure 6–14. Arterial supply of the rectosigmoid and rectum (anterior view). (Modified and reproduced, with permission, from Way LW [editor]: *Current Surgical Diagnosis & Treatment,* 6th ed. Lange, p. 383, 1983.)

Directions: With reference to the diagram, match the numbered structures with their corresponding lettered items.

(A) aorta

(B) sigmoid arteries

(C) superior rectal artery

(D) inferior mesenteric artery

(E) middle sacral artery

(F) common iliac artery

(G) inferior rectal artery

(H) middle rectal artery

(I) internal pudendal artery

(J) rectosigmoid arteries

(K) internal iliac artery

(L) external iliac artery

(M) superior rectal artery

ANATOMY OF THE RECTOSIGMOID
RECTUM AND ANUS
(Questions 208 through 224)

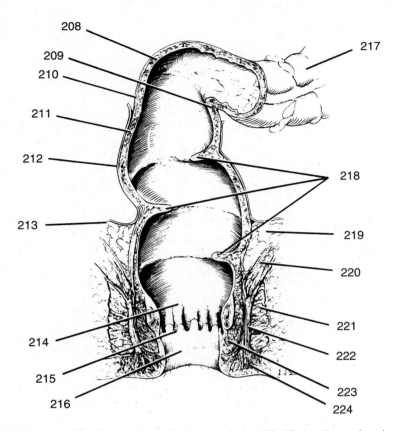

Figure 6–15. Anatomy of the rectosigmoid rectum and anus. (Modified and reproduced, with permission, from Way LW [editor]: *Current Surgical Diagnosis & Treatment,* 7th ed. Lange, p. 379, 1985.)

Directions: With reference to the diagram, match the numbered structures with their corresponding lettered items.

(A) transverse rectal folds (Houston)

(B) mucosa

(C) sigmoid colon

(D) rectosigmoid junction

(E) supralevator space

(F) longitudinal muscle

(G) levator ani muscle

(H) circular muscle

(I) deep external sphincter

(J) serosa

(K) longitudinal muscle fibers

(L) peritoneum

(M) internal sphincter

(N) rectal column

(O) external sphincter

(P) pectinate line

(Q) intersphincteric line (white line of Hilton)

ARTERIES AND VEINS OF THE COLON
(Questions 225 through 247)

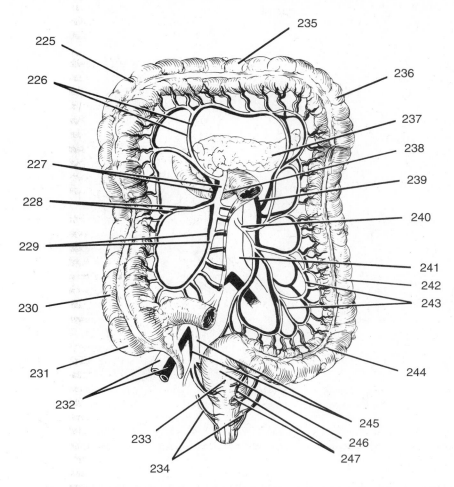

Figure 6–16. Arteries and veins of the colon. (Modified and reproduced, with permission, from Way LW [editor]: *Current Surgical Diagnosis & Treatment,* 7th ed. Lange, p. 367, 1985.)

Directions: With reference to the diagram, match the numbered structures with their corresponding lettered items.

(A) hepatic flexure

(B) splenic flexure

(C) middle colic artery and vein

(D) transverse colon

(E) superior mesenteric artery and vein

(F) pancreas

(G) inferior rectal arteries and veins

(H) middle rectal artery and vein

(I) rectosigmoid

(J) rectum

(K) sigmoid

(L) external iliac artery and vein

(M) cecum

(N) ascending colon

(O) sigmoidal vessels

(P) descending colon

(Q) aorta

(R) right colic artery and vein

(S) transverse duodenum

(T) inferior mesenteric vein

(U) ileocolic artery and vein

(V) inferior mesenteric artery

(W) internal iliac artery and vein

THE COLON
(Questions 248 through 259)

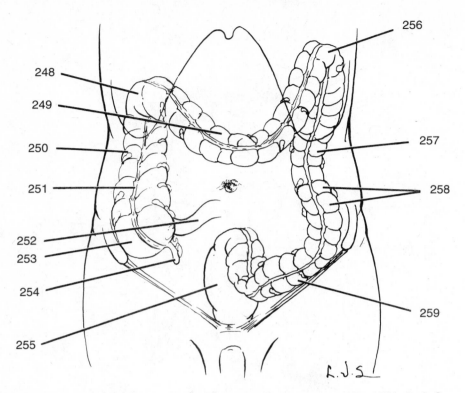

Figure 6–17. The colon. (Modified and reproduced, with permission, from Way LW [editor]: *Current Surgical Diagnosis & Treatment,* 6th ed. Lange, p. 353, 1983.)

Directions: With reference to the diagram, match the numbered structures with their corresponding lettered items.

(A) hepatic flexure

(B) descending colon

(C) transverse colon

(D) splenic flexure

(E) teniae coli

(F) rectum

(G) haustra

(H) ileum

(I) ascending colon

(J) sigmoid colon

(K) cecum

(L) appendix

ARTERIAL SUPPLY TO THE SMALL BOWEL
(Questions 260 through 268)

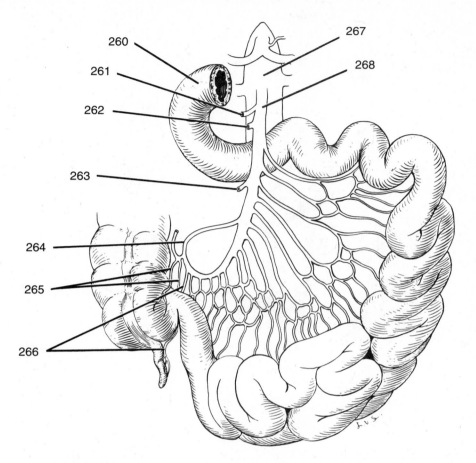

Figure 6–18. Arterial supply to the small bowel. (Modified and reproduced, with permission, from Way LW [editor]: *Current Surgical Diagnosis & Treatment,* 6th ed. Lange, p. 353, 1983.)

Directions: With reference to the diagram, match the numbered structures with their corresponding lettered items.

(A) aorta

(B) middle colic artery

(C) duodenum

(D) right colic artery

(E) inferior pancreaticoduodenal artery

(F) appendicular artery

(G) superior mesenteric artery

(H) ileocolic artery

(I) anterior and posterior cecal arteries

ARTERIAL SUPPLY AND VENOUS RETURN
TO THE DESCENDING AND TRANSVERSE DUODENUM,
PANCREAS, AND SPLEEN
(Questions 269 through 289)

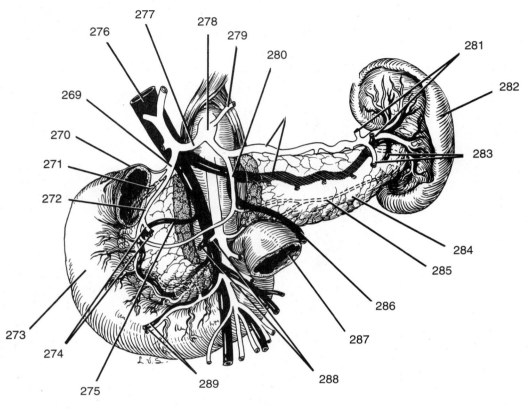

Figure 6–19. Arterial supply and venous return to the descending and transverse duodenum, pancreas, and spleen. (Modified and reproduced, with permission, from Way LW [editor]: *Current Surgical Diagnosis & Treatment,* 6th ed. Lange, p. 346, 1983.)

Directions: With reference to the diagram, match the numbered structures with their corresponding lettered items.

(A) celiac artery

(B) superior pancreatic artery

(C) portal vein

(D) gastroduodenal artery

(E) short gastric arteries and veins

(F) middle colic artery and vein

(G) superior duodenal artery

(H) left gastroepiploic artery and vein

(I) right colic artery and vein

(J) transverse pancreatic artery

(K) posterosuperior pancreaticoduodenal artery

(L) left gastric artery

(M) duodenum

(N) jejunum

(O) pancreas

(P) inferior mesenteric vein

(Q) gastroduodenal vein

(R) common hepatic artery

(S) spleen

(T) anterosuperior pancreaticoduodenal artery

(U) right gastroepiploic artery and vein

THE PERITONEAL REFLECTIONS AND THE LOCATION
OF THE LESSER PERITONEAL CAVITY
(Questions 290 through 300)

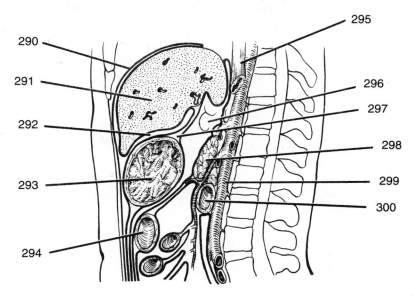

Figure 6–20. The peritoneal reflections and the location of the lesser peritoneal cavity. (Modified and reproduced, with permission, from Way LW [editor]: *Current Surgical Diagnosis & Treatment*, 6th ed. Lange, p. 342, 1983.)

Directions: With reference to the diagram, match the numbered structures with their corresponding lettered items.

(A) lesser peritoneal cavity

(B) anterior inferior subphrenic space

(C) transverse colon

(D) anterior superior subphrenic space

(E) pancreas

(F) duodenum

(G) aorta

(H) esophagus

(I) stomach

(J) liver

(K) gastrohepatic ligament (lesser omentum)

DUODENAL RELATIONSHIPS
(Questions 301 through 312)

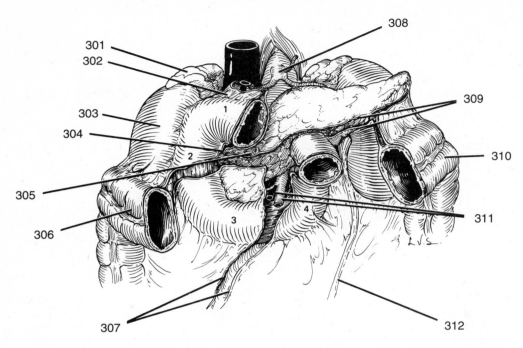

Figure 6–21. Duodenal relationships. 1 = superior segment; 2 = descending segment; 3 = transverse segment; 4 = ascending segment. (Modified and reproduced, with permission, from Way LW [editor]: *Current Surgical Diagnosis & Treatment,* 6th ed. Lange, p. 341, 1983.)

Directions: With reference to the diagram, match the numbered structures with their corresponding lettered items.

(A) attachment of greater omentum

(B) attachment of transverse mesocolon

(C) celiac arteries and branches

(D) superior mesenteric vessels

(E) root of mesentery of the small bowel

(F) right suprarenal gland

(G) pancreas

(H) hepatic flexure of colon

(I) splenic flexure of colon

(J) left ureter

(K) right kidney

(L) right free border of lesser omentum (hepato-duodenal ligament)

VENOUS DRAINAGE OF THE STOMACH
(Questions 313 through 323)

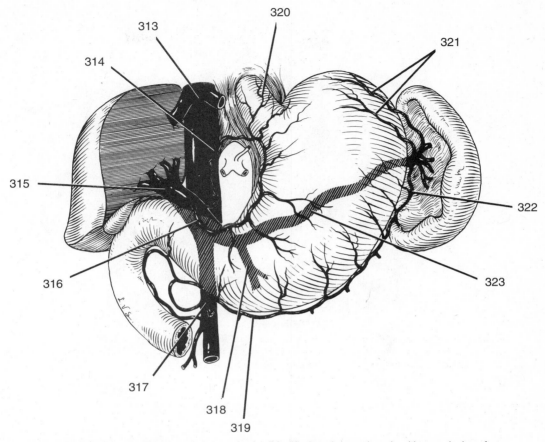

Figure 6–22. Venous drainage of the stomach. (Modified and reproduced, with permission, from Way LW [editor]: *Current Surgical Diagnosis & Treatment,* 6th ed. Lange, p. 336, 1983.)

Directions: With reference to the diagram, match the numbered structures with their corresponding lettered items.

(A) inferior vena cava

(B) right gastroepiploic vein

(C) left gastroepiploic vein

(D) ascending esophageal veins

(E) superior mesenteric vein

(F) inferior mesenteric vein

(G) short gastric veins

(H) left gastric vein

(I) portal vein

(J) right gastric vein

(K) splenic vein

ARTERIES OF THE STOMACH
(Questions 324 through 342)

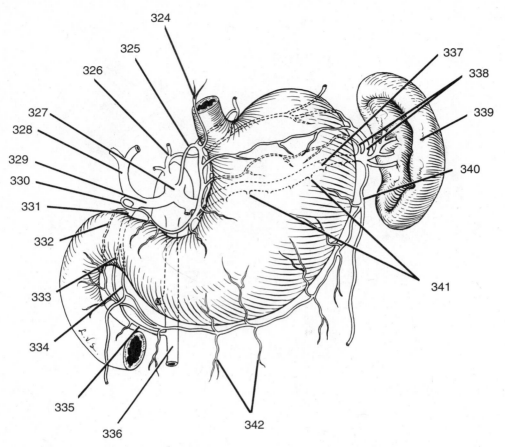

Figure 6–23. Arteries of the stomach. (Modified and reproduced, with permission, from Way LW [editor]: *Current Surgical Diagnosis & Treatment,* 6th ed. Lange, p. 334, 1983.)

Directions: With reference to the diagram, match the numbered structures with their corresponding lettered items.

(A) splenic artery

(B) ascending branch of left gastric artery

(C) inferior phrenic artery

(D) left gastroepiploic artery

(E) inferior pancreaticoduodenal artery

(F) celiac artery

(G) gastroduodenal artery

(H) superior mesenteric artery

(I) right gastroepiploic artery

(J) pancreatic branches

(K) left gastric artery

(L) short gastric artery

(M) common hepatic artery

(N) spleen

(O) proper hepatic artery

(P) right gastric artery

(Q) epiploic arteries (omental branches)

(R) posterior superior pancreaticoduodenal artery

(S) anterior superior pancreaticoduodenal artery

GASTRIC RELATIONSHIPS
(Questions 343 through 355)

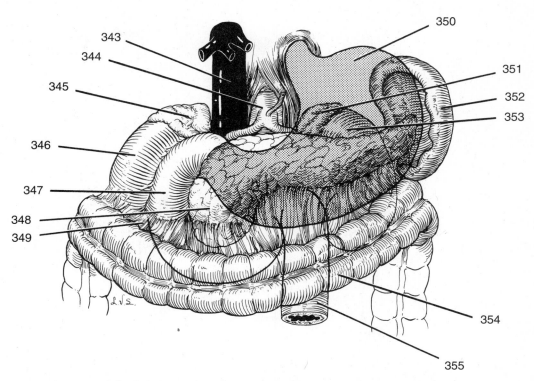

Figure 6–24. Gastric relationships. The stomach is made transparent to show its posterior relationship to the pancreas, spleen, and transverse mesocolon. (Modified and reproduced, with permission, from Lindner HH: *Clinical Anatomy,* Appleton & Lange, p. 330, 1989.)

Directions: With reference to the diagram, match the numbered structures with their corresponding lettered items.

(A) inferior vena cava

(B) stomach

(C) aorta

(D) left suprarenal (adrenal) gland

(E) right kidney

(F) spleen

(G) left kidney

(H) transverse colon

(I) right suprarenal (adrenal) gland

(J) duodenum

(K) jejunum

(L) pancreas

(M) transverse mesocolon

ABDOMINAL VISCERA IN SITU
(Questions 356 through 366)

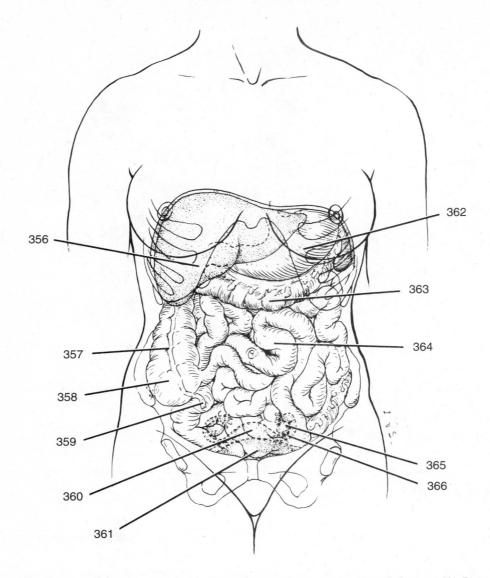

Figure 6–25. Abdominal viscera in situ. (Reproduced, with permission, from deCherney AH, Pernoll ML [editors]: *Current Obstetric & Gynecologic Diagnosis & Treatment,* 8th ed. Appleton & Lange, 1994.)

Directions: With reference to the diagram, match the numbered structures with their corresponding let-

(A) liver
(B) transverse colon
(C) ascending colon
(D) stomach
(E) ovary
(F) appendix

(G) small intestine
(H) uterine tube
(I) cecum
(J) uterus
(K) bladder

EARLY (SEVENTH WEEK) EMBRYONIC DEVELOPMENT OF THE STOMACH
(Questions 367 through 380)

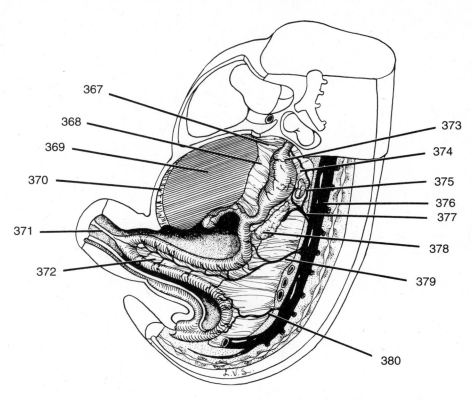

Figure 6–26. Early (seventh week) embryonic development of the stomach. (Modified and reproduced, with permission, from Lindner HH: *Clinical Anatomy,* Appleton & Lange, p. 326, 1989.)

Directions: With reference to the diagram, match the numbered structures with their corresponding lettered items.

(A) stomach

(B) ventral mesogastrium

(C) liver

(D) dorsal mesogastrium

(E) hepatogastric ligament

(F) superior mesenteric artery

(G) herniated midgut loop

(H) inferior mesenteric artery

 (I) falciform ligament

 (J) spleen

(K) aorta

 (L) vitellointestinal duct

(M) celiac artery

(N) pancreas

AUTONOMIC PLEXUSES
OF THE RETROPERITONEUM
(Questions 381 through 389)

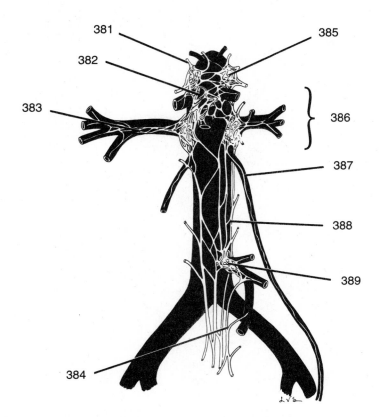

Figure 6–27. Autonomic plexuses of the retroperitoneum. (Modified and reproduced, with permission, from Lindner HH: *Clinical Anatomy,* Appleton & Lange, p. 325, 1989.)

Directions: With reference to the diagram, match the numbered structures with their corresponding lettered items.

(A) celiac ganglion

(B) inferior mesenteric plexus

(C) superior mesenteric plexus

(D) abdominal aortic plexus

(E) superior hypogastric plexus

(F) right renal plexus

(G) greater splanchnic nerve

(H) celiac plexus

(I) spermatic or ovarian plexus

THE LUMBAR SYMPATHETIC CHAIN AND ITS RELATIONSHIP TO THE BRANCHES OF THE LUMBAR PLEXUS
(Questions 390 through 397)

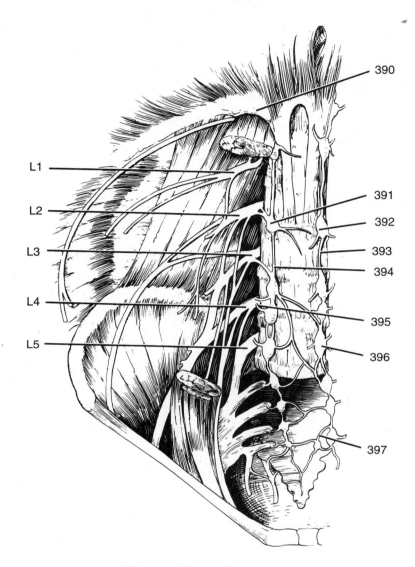

Figure 6–28. The lumbar sympathetic chain and its relationship to the branches of the lumbar plexus. (Modified and reproduced, with permission, from Lindner HH: *Clinical Anatomy,* Appleton & Lange, p. 324, 1989.)

Directions: With reference to the diagram, match the numbered structures with their corresponding lettered items.

(A) right second lumbar ganglion

(B) gray rami communication to lumbar nerve

(C) left second lumbar ganglion

(D) medial lumbocostal arch

(E) left lumbar sympathetic trunk

(F) right lumbar sympathetic trunk

(G) pelvic portion of sympathetic trunk

(H) fifth lumbar ganglion

THE LUMBAR PLEXUS
(Questions 398 through 406)

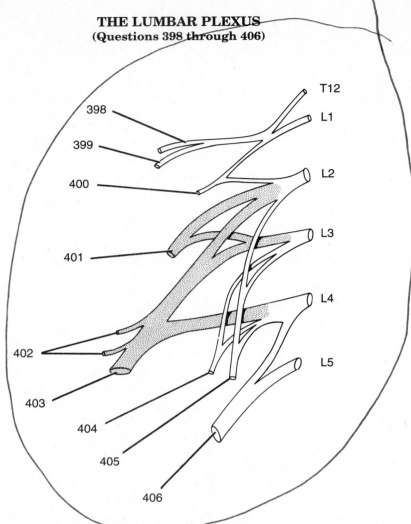

Figure 6–29. The lumbar plexus. (Modified and reproduced, with permission, from Lindner HH: *Clinical Anatomy,* Appleton & Lange, p. 322, 1989.)

Directions: With reference to the diagram, match the numbered structures with their corresponding lettered items.

(A) obturator nerve

(B) iliohypogastric nerve

(C) ilioinguinal nerve

(D) branches to psoas and iliacus muscles

(E) femoral nerve

(F) genitofemoral nerve

(G) lateral cutaneous nerve of thigh

(H) accessory obturator nerve

(I) lumbosacral trunk

Answers

STOMACH

1.	(E)	5.	(H)
2.	(D)	6.	(B)
3.	(G)	7.	(C)
4.	(A)	8.	(F)

LIVER AND GALLBLADDER

9.	(H)	21.	(U)
10.	(M)	22.	(W)
11.	(P)	23.	(C)
12.	(J)	24.	(T)
13.	(A)	25.	(R)
14.	(F)	26.	(L)
15.	(S)	27.	(D)
16.	(K)	28.	(G)
17.	(B)	29.	(Q)
18.	(E)	30.	(N)
19.	(O)	31.	(I)
20.	(V)		

LIVER AND GALLBLADDER

32.	(G)	42.	(M)
33.	(C)	43.	(R)
34.	(J)	44.	(D)
35.	(O)	45.	(L)
36.	(S)	46.	(F)
37.	(P)	47.	(Q)
38.	(A)	48.	(K)
39.	(E)	49.	(I)
40.	(N)	50.	(H)
41.	(B)		

GALLBLADDER

51.	(F)	55.	(B)
52.	(A)	56.	(E)
53.	(G)	57.	(C)
54.	(D)		

COMMON BILE DUCTS

58.	(D)	62.	(B)
59.	(E)	63.	(F)
60.	(A)	64.	(C)
61.	(G)		

PANCREATIC DUCTS

65.	(I)	71.	(H)
66.	(D)	72.	(C)
67.	(K)	73.	(J)
68.	(A)	74.	(E)
69.	(G)	75.	(F)
70.	(B)		

VARIATIONS IN THE LENGTH OF THE CYSTIC DUCT AND ITS LEVEL AND MODE OF ENTRY INTO THE JUNCTION OF THE COMMON HEPATIC AND THE COMMON BILE DUCTS

76.	(D)	81.	(E)
77.	(H)	82.	(C)
78.	(B)	83.	(F)
79.	(I)	84.	(G)
80.	(J)	85.	(A)

PANCREAS

86.	(E)	97.	(F)
87.	(I)	98.	(H)
88.	(K)	99.	(N)
89.	(A)	100.	(P)
90.	(J)	101.	(O)
91.	(O)	102.	(T)
92.	(Q)	103.	(G)
93.	(M)	104.	(D)
94.	(B)	105.	(R)
95.	(L)	106.	(S)
96.	(C)		

DEVELOPMENT OF EXTRAHEPATIC BILIARY TRACT IN THE EMBRYO

107.	(M)	117.	(J)
108.	(A)	118.	(B)
109.	(F)	119.	(C)
110.	(J)	120.	(K)
111.	(E)	121.	(I)
112.	(N)	122.	(H)
113.	(L)	123.	(D)
114.	(G)	124.	(C)
115.	(C)	125.	(O)
116.	(E)		

COMMUNICATION OF PORTAL SYSTEM WITH VENOUS SYSTEM

126.	(K)	136.	(Q)
127.	(D)	137.	(R)
128.	(H)	138.	(S)
129.	(N)	139.	(A)
130.	(M)	140.	(I)
131.	(E)	141.	(B)
132.	(F)	142.	(C)
133.	(P)	143.	(G)
134.	(J)	144.	(L)
135.	(O)		

THE VISCERAL SURFACE OF THE LIVER

145.	(D)	155.	(C)
146.	(L)	156.	(K)
147.	(F)	157.	(I)
148.	(P)	158.	(A)
149.	(H)	159.	(M)
150.	(R)	160.	(N)
151.	(S)	161.	(J)
152.	(T)	162.	(O)
153.	(E)	163.	(G)
154.	(B)	164.	(Q)

GREATER OMENTUM AND ITS ABDOMINAL RELATIONSHIPS

165.	(B)	173.	(J)
166.	(F)	174.	(I)
167.	(K)	175.	(M)
168.	(H)	176.	(E)
169.	(L)	177.	(A)
170.	(G)	178.	(N)
171.	(C)	179.	(O)
172.	(D)		

PERITONEAL CAVITY

180.	(K)	188.	(G)
181.	(I)	189.	(O)
182.	(J)	190.	(D)
183.	(L)	191.	(E)
184.	(M)	192.	(H)
185.	(C)	193.	(A)
186.	(B)	194.	(N)
187.	(F)		

ARTERIAL SUPPLY OF THE RECTOSIGMOID AND RECTUM

195.	(A)	202.	(M)
196.	(C)	203.	(H)
197.	(E)	204.	(I)
198.	(F)	205.	(G)
199.	(J)	206.	(D)
200.	(K)	207.	(B)
201.	(L)		

ANATOMY OF THE RECTOSIGMOID RECTUM AND ANUS

208.	(B)	217.	(C)
209.	(D)	218.	(A)
210.	(F)	219.	(E)
211.	(H)	220.	(G)
212.	(J)	221.	(I)
213.	(L)	222.	(K)
214.	(N)	223.	(M)
215.	(P)	224.	(O)
216.	(Q)		

ARTERIES AND VEINS OF THE COLON

225.	(A)	237.	(F)
226.	(C)	238.	(S)
227.	(E)	239.	(T)
228.	(R)	240.	(V)
229.	(U)	241.	(Q)
230.	(N)	242.	(P)
231.	(M)	243.	(O)
232.	(L)	244.	(K)
233.	(J)	245.	(W)
234.	(G)	246.	(I)
235.	(D)	247.	(H)
236.	(B)		

THE COLON

248.	(A)	254.	(L)
249.	(C)	255.	(F)
250.	(I)	256.	(D)
251.	(E)	257.	(B)
252.	(H)	258.	(G)
253.	(K)	259.	(J)

ARTERIAL SUPPLY TO THE SMALL BOWEL

260.	(C)	265.	(I)
261.	(E)	266.	(F)
262.	(B)	267.	(A)
263.	(D)	268.	(G)
264.	(H)		

ARTERIAL SUPPLY AND VENOUS RETURN TO THE DESCENDING AND TRANSVERSE DUODENUM, PANCREAS, AND SPLEEN

269.	(D)	280.	(B)
270.	(G)	281.	(E)
271.	(K)	282.	(S)
272.	(T)	283.	(H)
273.	(M)	284.	(O)
274.	(U)	285.	(J)
275.	(D)	286.	(P)
276.	(C)	287.	(N)
277.	(R)	288.	(F)
278.	(A)	289.	(I)
279.	(L)		

THE PERITONEAL REFLECTIONS AND THE LOCATION OF THE LESSER PERITONEAL CAVITY

290.	(D)	296.	(A)
291.	(J)	297.	(K)
292.	(B)	298.	(E)
293.	(I)	299.	(G)
294.	(C)	300.	(F)
295.	(H)		

DUODENAL RELATIONSHIPS

301.	(F)	307.	(E)
302.	(L)	308.	(C)
303.	(K)	309.	(B)
304.	(A)	310.	(I)
305.	(G)	311.	(D)
306.	(H)	312.	(J)

VENOUS DRAINAGE OF THE STOMACH

313.	(A)	319.	(B)
314.	(H)	320.	(D)
315.	(I)	321.	(G)
316.	(J)	322.	(C)
317.	(E)	323.	(K)
318.	(F)		

ARTERIES OF THE STOMACH

324.	(B)	334.	(I)
325.	(K)	335.	(E)
326.	(C)	336.	(H)
327.	(F)	337.	(A)
328.	(O)	338.	(L)
329.	(M)	339.	(N)
330.	(P)	340.	(D)
331.	(G)	341.	(J)
332.	(R)	342.	(Q)
333.	(S)		

GASTRIC RELATIONSHIPS

343.	(A)	350.	(B)
344.	(C)	351.	(D)
345.	(I)	352.	(F)
346.	(E)	353.	(G)
347.	(J)	354.	(H)
348.	(L)	355.	(K)
349.	(M)		

ABDOMINAL VISCERA IN SITU

356.	(A)	362.	(D)
357.	(C)	363.	(B)
358.	(I)	364.	(G)
359.	(F)	365.	(E)
360.	(J)	366.	(H)
361.	(K)		

EARLY (SEVENTH WEEK) EMBRYONIC DEVELOPMENT OF THE STOMACH

367.	(B)	374.	(D)
368.	(E)	375.	(J)
369.	(C)	376.	(K)
370.	(I)	377.	(M)
371.	(L)	378.	(N)
372.	(G)	379.	(F)
373.	(A)	380.	(H)

AUTONOMIC PLEXUSES OF THE RETROPERITONEUM

381.	(G)	386.	(H)
382.	(C)	387.	(I)
383.	(F)	388.	(D)
384.	(B)	389.	(B)
385.	(A)		

THE LUMBAR SYMPATHETIC CHAIN AND ITS RELATIONSHIP TO THE BRANCHES OF THE LUMBAR PLEXUS

390.	(D)	394.	(F)
391.	(A)	395.	(B)
392.	(C)	396.	(H)
393.	(E)	397.	(G)

THE LUMBAR PLEXUS

398.	(B)	403.	(E)
399.	(C)	404.	(H)
400.	(F)	405.	(A)
401.	(G)	406.	(I)
402.	(D)		

CHAPTER 7

The Upper and Lower Limbs
Questions

DIRECTIONS (Questions 1 through 75): Each of the numbered items or incomplete statements in this section is followed by answers or by completions of the statement. Select the ONE lettered answer or completion that is BEST in each case.

1. The base of the scapular spine lies opposite which of the following vertebrae?

    (A) vertebra prominens
    (B) 3rd thoracic vertebral spine
    (C) 7th thoracic vertebral spine
    (D) 1st thoracic vertebral spine
    (E) 6th cervical vertebral spine

2. The inferior angle of the scapula is located under the skin and marks the level of the

    (A) crest of the ilium
    (B) vertebra prominens
    (C) 7th thoracic vertebral spine
    (D) 1st lumbar vertebra
    (E) 9th rib

3. Which of the following muscles insert at the medial border of the scapula at the root of the scapular spine?

    (A) levator scapulae
    (B) trapezius
    (C) supraspinatus
    (D) rhomboideus minor
    (E) semispinalis

4. The deltoid muscle is innervated by which of the following nerves?

    (A) dorsal scapular
    (B) axillary
    (C) accessory
    (D) thoracodorsal
    (E) subscapular

5. Which of the following structures pass through the scapular notch below the superior transverse scapular ligament?

    (A) suprascapular nerve
    (B) axillary nerve
    (C) dorsal scapular nerve
    (D) dorsal scapular artery
    (E) superior lateral brachial cutaneous nerve

6. The pectoralis minor muscle is invested by the

    (A) pectoral fascia
    (B) axillary fascia
    (C) costocoracoid membrane
    (D) suspensory ligament of the axilla
    (E) clavipectoral fascia

7. The axillary artery extends from the outer border of the 1st rib to the lower border of which of the following muscles?

    (A) latissimus dorsi
    (B) pectoralis major
    (C) coracobrachialis
    (D) teres major
    (E) subscapularis

8. All of the following statements concerning the thoracoacromial artery are correct EXCEPT

    (A) it arises from the second part of the axillary artery
    (B) it pierces the costocoracoid membrane
    (C) it divides into 4 branches deep to the clavicular head of pectoralis major
    (D) it arises beneath the upper border of the pectoralis minor
    (E) it arises at the lower border of the subscapularis muscle

9. The thoracodorsal artery is the principal supply to which of the following muscles?

   (A) latissimus dorsi
   (B) teres major
   (C) pectoralis minor
   (D) subscapularis
   (E) supraspinatus

10. The branches of the third part of the axillary artery include the

   (A) lateral thoracic
   (B) superior thoracic
   (C) thoracoacromial
   (D) dorsal scapular
   (E) posterior circumflex humeral

11. The cephalic vein perforates the costocoracoid membrane to terminate in which of the following veins?

   (A) internal jugular
   (B) axillary
   (C) brachial
   (D) azygos
   (E) external jugular

12. The long thoracic nerve supplies which of the following muscles?

   (A) pectoralis major
   (B) infraspinatus
   (C) serratus anterior
   (D) trapezius
   (E) supraspinatus

13. All of the following statements concerning the axillary nerve are correct EXCEPT

   (A) it enters the triangular space
   (B) it arises from the posterior cord of the brachial plexus
   (C) it accompanies the posterior circumflex humeral artery
   (D) it innervates the deltoid
   (E) it innervates the teres minor

14. The pectoralis minor muscle arises from which of the following structures?

   (A) sternum
   (B) clavicle
   (C) outer surface of the 3rd, 4th, and 5th ribs
   (D) medial border of the coracoid process
   (E) xiphoid process

15. Which of the following muscles take origin from the coracoid process?

   (A) short head of the biceps
   (B) triceps
   (C) long head of the biceps
   (D) teres minor
   (E) subclavius

16. All of the following structures may be located in the cubital fossa EXCEPT the

   (A) tendon of the biceps brachii muscle
   (B) bicipital aponeurosis
   (C) ulnar nerve
   (D) median cubital vein
   (E) brachial artery

17. Which of the following carpal bones is regarded as a sesamoid bone in the tendon of the flexor carpi ulnaris muscle?

   (A) lunate
   (B) triquetrum
   (C) scaphoid
   (D) pisiform
   (E) capitate

18. All of the following statements concerning the capitate bone are correct EXCEPT

   (A) it articulates with the trapezoid on the ulnar side
   (B) it articulates with the 2nd, 3rd, and 4th metacarpals distally
   (C) it articulates with the scaphoid and lunate proximally
   (D) it occupies the center of the wrist
   (E) it is the largest of the carpal bones

19. The distinguishing characteristic of the third metacarpal is

   (A) it is shorter and stouter than the others
   (B) it is the longest
   (C) it has a styloid process
   (D) it has a deep groove for articulation
   (E) it articulates with the hamate bone

20. Which of the following structures is located within the hypothenar compartment?

   (A) abductor pollicis brevis
   (B) adductor pollicis
   (C) motor branch of the median nerve
   (D) flexor digiti minimi brevis
   (E) lumbrical muscles

21. Which of the following structures enters the palm of the hand through the gap separating the two heads of the adductor pollicis muscle?

    (A) radial artery
    (B) ulnar nerve
    (C) median nerve
    (D) radial nerve
    (E) ulnar artery

22. Which of the following joints represents the only point of bony connection between the trunk and the upper limb?

    (A) sternoclavicular
    (B) acromioclavicular
    (C) scapulohumeral
    (D) costocervical
    (E) sternocostal

23. Which of the following ligaments restrains backward movement of the scapula?

    (A) trapezoid
    (B) coracohumeral
    (C) conoid
    (D) superior glenohumeral
    (E) superior transverse scapular

24. Which of the following joints has the greatest freedom of movement of all the joints in the body?

    (A) acromioclavicular
    (B) scapulohumeral
    (C) sacroiliac
    (D) talocalcaneonavicular
    (E) costovertebral

25. All of the following muscles are medial rotators of the upper limb EXCEPT the

    (A) subscapularis
    (B) teres major
    (C) infraspinatus
    (D) latissimus dorsi
    (E) pectoralis major

26. All of the following muscles extend the upper limb EXCEPT the

    (A) latissimus dorsi
    (B) teres major
    (C) deltoid (posterior fibers)
    (D) triceps (long head)
    (E) coracobrachialis

27. The long head of the biceps brachii arises from the

    (A) acromion
    (B) olecranon process
    (C) radial tuberosity
    (D) coracoid process
    (E) supraglenoid tubercle

28. Which of the following carpal bones is located in the distal row, radial side?

    (A) lunate
    (B) triquetrum
    (C) trapezium
    (D) trapezoid
    (E) pisiform

29. The flexor retinaculum is crossed anteriorly by the

    (A) radial nerve
    (B) median nerve
    (C) palmaris longus tendon
    (D) tendons of the long flexors of the fingers
    (E) tendon of the extensor pollicis longus

30. Which of the following muscles abduct the digits from the midline of the middle digit?

    (A) lumbricals
    (B) dorsal interossei
    (C) thenar muscles
    (D) hypothenar muscles
    (E) palmaris brevis

31. The forearm can be defined correctly as the

    (A) upper extremity
    (B) brachium
    (C) antebrachium
    (D) upper limb
    (E) shoulder girdle

32. All of the following statements relating to the vascular system of the upper limb are correct EXCEPT

    (A) the basilic is a deep vein
    (B) the arteries are regularly accompanied by one or two deep veins
    (C) the subclavian artery is the arterial stem to the limb
    (D) the named arteries are all deep ones
    (E) the cephalic vein runs up the radial side of the limb

33. A correct description of the lymphatics of the upper limb includes

    (A) superficial lymphatics begin with brachial vessels

    (B) deep lymphatics are more numerous than are superficial lymphatics

    (C) superficial lymphatics usually remain on the palmar side of the limb

    (D) lymphatics usually do not accompany deep blood vessels

    (E) lymphatics end in axillary lymph nodes

34. In the development of nerve-muscle relations, which of the following statements is correct?

    (A) the nerve supply of the latissimus dorsi originates at lumbar levels

    (B) nerves retain original connection to their muscle mass

    (C) most muscles of the upper limb receive their nerve supply from a single spinal nerve

    (D) nerves do not parallel muscles in their development

    (E) fibers of upper limb muscles are innervated by dorsal branches of spinal nerves

35. Which of the following is a correct statement regarding distribution of nerves within muscle?

    (A) no fixed pattern of distribution has been noted

    (B) distribution is not influenced by the shape of the muscle

    (C) in skeletal muscle, each individual muscle fiber receives a nerve fiber

    (D) nerve fibers to skeletal muscle are known as adrenergic fibers

    (E) all nerve fibers entering a voluntary muscle are motor to muscle fibers

36. All of the following statements are true in relation to development of the upper limb EXCEPT the

    (A) limb projects early at approximately a right angle to the body

    (B) anatomical position is with the forearm supinated and palm facing forward

    (C) limb, later in growth, adducts to almost parallel the trunk

    (D) little finger develops on the preaxial border

    (E) developing musculature of the limb divides into ventral and dorsal parts

37. Correct patterns of cutaneous nerve supply of the upper limb include

    (A) the 3rd and 4th cervical nerves supply a limited area of skin over the pectoral region and shoulder

    (B) the 3rd thoracic nerve usually sends a branch to the skin of the medial and upper parts of the arm

    (C) the cervical plexus supplies most of the skin of the arm

    (D) antebrachial cutaneous nerves supply the region of the humerus

    (E) branches of the brachial plexus supply only the arm and forearm

38. Characteristics of muscles of the upper limb include

    (A) anterior muscles are extensors

    (B) the anterior group of forearm muscles arises chiefly on the radial side of the arm

    (C) the anterior group of forearm muscles extends the wrist and fingers

    (D) the anterior group of forearm muscles pronates the forearm

    (E) the posterior group of forearm muscles flexes the wrist and fingers

39. Which of the following is an accurate description of nerve supply to upper limb muscles?

    (A) the radial nerve supplies the supinator muscle of the forearm

    (B) the musculocutaneous nerve supplies the extensor muscles of the arm

    (C) the median nerve supplies flexor muscles of the arm

    (D) the axillary nerve supplies pectoral muscles

    (E) the ulnar nerve supplies the coracobrachialis muscle

40. Arterial blood supply to the upper limb is correctly described by which of the following statements?

    (A) the axillary artery is a branch of the arch of the aorta

    (B) the brachial artery is a direct branch of the subclavian artery

    (C) the radial artery is a direct branch of the axillary artery

    (D) the humeral circumflex arteries are branches of the brachial artery

    (E) the ulnar artery is a direct division of the brachial artery

41. The pectoral girdle consists of the

    (A) humerus and scapula
    (B) sternum and humerus
    (C) sternum and scapula
    (D) clavicle and scapula
    (E) clavicle and sternum

42. The clavicle has attachment to the scapula

    (A) through the scapuloclavicular ligament
    (B) at the sternoclavicular joint
    (C) through the coracoacromial ligament
    (D) through the coracohumeral ligament
    (E) through the conoid and trapezoid ligaments

43. All of the following characterize the structure of the scapula EXCEPT

    (A) a thickened medial border adjacent to the coracoid
    (B) a subscapular fossa on its costal surface
    (C) a spine continuing into the acromion
    (D) three angles and three borders
    (E) the glenoid cavity at its lateral angle

44. The humerus presents

    (A) an olecranon fossa on its anterior surface
    (B) a radial fossa on its medial distal end
    (C) a capitulum on its distal lateral condyle
    (D) a deltoid tuberosity adjoining its head
    (E) a greater tubercle at its midregion

45. The pectoralis major muscle inserts on the

    (A) lesser tubercle of the humerus
    (B) lateral third of the clavicle
    (C) coracoid process of the scapula
    (D) crest of the greater tubercle of the humerus
    (E) head of the humerus

46. The chief action of the pectoralis major is

    (A) abduction and lateral rotation of the humerus
    (B) elevation and upward rotation of the scapula
    (C) elevation of the sternum
    (D) adduction and medial rotation of the humerus
    (E) elevation of the clavicle

47. The pectoralis minor muscle usually has its insertion on the

    (A) coracoid process of the scapula
    (B) anterior manubrium
    (C) medial third of the clavicle
    (D) acromion of the scapula
    (E) greater tubercle of the humerus

48. Innervation of the triceps brachii involves which of the following nerves?

    (A) long thoracic
    (B) lower subscapular
    (C) musculocutaneous
    (D) axillary
    (E) radial

49. Which of the following statements correctly describes the axillary artery?

    (A) it originates from the arch of the aorta
    (B) it gives origin to the thoracoacromion artery
    (C) it has the lateral thoracic artery as its first branch
    (D) it divides into radial and ulnar arteries
    (E) it provides no blood supply to the humerus

50. The central structure of the axilla is stated to be the

    (A) subscapular artery
    (B) brachial plexus
    (C) axillary artery
    (D) lateral thoracic artery
    (E) axillary nerve

51. Which of the following statements correctly describes the lateral cord of the brachial plexus?

    (A) it represents lateral divisions of the plexus
    (B) typically it has five branches
    (C) it contains nerve fibers from C8 and T1
    (D) it gives rise to the ulnar nerve
    (E) it gives rise to the musculocutaneous nerve

52. The posterior cord of the brachial plexus is described correctly by all the following statements EXCEPT

    (A) it is formed by union of all the posterior divisions of the plexus
    (B) it gives off the upper subscapular nerve
    (C) it gives off the median nerve
    (D) it gives off the axillary nerve
    (E) it has the radial nerve as a terminal branch

53. The long thoracic nerve innervates which of the following muscles?

    (A) triceps brachii
    (B) serratus anterior
    (C) pectoralis minor
    (D) latissimus dorsi
    (E) deltoid

54. Attachments of the trapezius muscle may correctly be described as

   (A) an origin on spinous processes of all lumbar vertebrae
   (B) an origin from the spine of the scapula
   (C) an origin from the vertebral border of the scapula
   (D) an origin from the occipital bone
   (E) an insertion on the thoracic spinous processes of all thoracic vertebrae

55. Which of the following nerves provides motor innervation for the latissimus dorsi muscle?

   (A) accessory
   (B) dorsal scapular
   (C) thoracodorsal
   (D) transverse cervical
   (E) axillary

56. The axillary nerve innervates which of the following muscles?

   (A) supraspinatus
   (B) infraspinatus
   (C) deltoid
   (D) teres major
   (E) trapezius

57. Primary lateral rotators of the arm are described as including the

   (A) infraspinatus and teres minor
   (B) subscapularis and teres major
   (C) supraspinatus and anterior deltoid
   (D) triceps brachii and latissimus dorsi
   (E) serratus anterior and rhomboidus major

58. The deltoid is assisted in its primary action of abduction of the arm by the

   (A) teres major
   (B) latissimus dorsi
   (C) levator scapulae
   (D) supraspinatus
   (E) serratus anterior

59. An important artery to the shoulder that arises in the neck is the

   (A) thoracoacromial
   (B) subscapular
   (C) scapular circumflex
   (D) posterior humeral circumflex
   (E) thyrocervical trunk

60. All of the following muscles comprise the musculotendinous cuff of the shoulder joint EXCEPT the

   (A) subscapularis
   (B) supraspinatus
   (C) infraspinatus
   (D) deltoid
   (E) teres minor

61. When the arm is abducted, the strength of the shoulder joint is largely dependent on the

   (A) depth of the glenoid fossa
   (B) heavy joint capsule
   (C) transverse humeral ligament
   (D) musculotendinous cuff
   (E) glenohumeral ligaments

62. The biceps muscle is the only member of the anterior group of arm muscles that

   (A) originates on the supraglenoid tubercle of the scapula
   (B) originates on the coracoid process of the scapula
   (C) inserts on the ulnar tuberosity
   (D) is innervated by the musculocutaneous nerve
   (E) partly arises from the body of the humerus

63. A correct description of innervation of the upper limb includes which of the following?

   (A) musculocutaneous nerve, a derivative of the medial cord of the brachial plexus
   (B) median nerve, innervating no muscles in the arm
   (C) ulnar nerve, a derivative of the lateral cord of the brachial plexus
   (D) radial nerve, innervating the coracobrachialis muscle
   (E) lateral antebrachial cutaneous nerve, terminating above the elbow

64. The anatomical snuffbox is described correctly by which of the following?

   (A) being located medial to the extensor pollicis longus
   (B) having the abductor pollicis longus as part of its posterior boundary
   (C) having the extensor pollicis longus as its anterior boundary
   (D) being located between the tendons of the extensor pollicis brevis and the extensor indicis
   (E) being a depression at the base of the first metacarpal, distal to the end of the radius

65. A structure found at the distal end of the ulna is the

(A) olecranon
(B) trochlear notch
(C) styloid process
(D) ulnar tuberosity
(E) coronoid process

66. All of the following muscles attach to the radius EXCEPT the

(A) biceps
(B) supinator
(C) brachioradialis
(D) brachialis
(E) pronator quadratus

67. Which of the following bones is found in the proximal row of carpals?

(A) lunate
(B) trapezium
(C) trapezoid
(D) capitate
(E) hamate

68. Which of the following statements is true concerning the radial nerve?

(A) it carries only motor fibers
(B) it supplies the flexor carpi ulnaris muscle
(C) it is accompanied by the profunda brachii artery
(D) it innervates the biceps muscle
(E) it is a terminal branch of the medial cord of the brachial plexus

69. Which of the following muscles originates on the humerus, the radius, and the ulna?

(A) flexor digitorum superficialis
(B) flexor carpi radialis
(C) palmaris longus
(D) flexor pollicis longus
(E) flexor digitorum profundus

70. The radial artery is described correctly as

(A) arising as the medial terminal branch of the brachial artery
(B) giving rise to the common interosseous artery
(C) giving rise to the superficial palmar artery
(D) providing the major components of the superficial palmar arch
(E) giving rise to all four common digital arteries

71. Which of the following statements correctly describes the median nerve?

(A) it gives rise to the posterior interosseous nerve
(B) it passes superficial to the flexor retinaculum
(C) it innervates all flexor muscles on the anterior forearm
(D) it gives a muscular branch to the thenar muscles
(E) it innervates all the lumbrical muscles

72. In a typical innervation pattern of the hand, which of the following muscles is supplied by branches of the median nerve?

(A) abductor pollicis brevis
(B) abductor pollicis longus
(C) adductor pollicis
(D) palmaris brevis
(E) 2nd and 3rd interossei

73. Which of the following statements correctly describes the arteries of the palm?

(A) the ulnar artery is the source of the superficial palmar arch
(B) palmar metacarpal arteries arise from the superficial palmar arch
(C) the princeps pollicis artery arises from the ulnar artery
(D) deep palmar arch branches do not connect with common digital arteries
(E) proper digital arteries run only on the radial side of the fingers

74. A muscle that is both a strong flexor at the elbow and a supinator of the forearm is the

(A) brachialis
(B) supinator
(C) biceps brachii
(D) brachioradialis
(E) flexor carpi radialis

75. Anomalous innervation of the hand muscles has been found in all the following forms EXCEPT

(A) the opponens pollicis being supplied by both median and ulnar nerves
(B) the short flexor of the thumb being supplied by only the ulnar nerve
(C) the median nerve sending a branch into the first dorsal interosseous
(D) deep penetration of the ulnar nerve into the thenar mass
(E) the median nerve sending a direct branch across the palm to the hypothenar muscles

Questions 76 through 79

(A) radial nerve
(B) median nerve
(C) ulnar nerve
(D) musculocutaneous nerve
(E) axillary nerve

76. Supplies the deltoid

77. Supplies the coracobrachialis

78. Supplies the interossei

79. Supplies the abductor pollicis brevis

Questions 80 and 81

(A) palmar metacarpal artery
(B) princeps pollicis artery
(C) ulnar artery
(D) radial artery
(E) common digital artery

80. Arterial origin of the superficial palmar arch

81. Arterial origin of the deep palmar arch

82. All of the following statements are true of wrist joint structure EXCEPT

(A) the radius articulates with the scaphoid, lunate, and triquetrum
(B) the articular disk at the distal ulna articulates with the proximal row of carpals
(C) articular nerves are derived from the anterior interosseous nerve
(D) an articular disk is present between the radius and ulna
(E) the radiocarpal joint is a ball-and-socket type of synovial joint

83. The ulnar artery has all of the following characteristics EXCEPT it

(A) is the larger terminal branch of the brachial artery
(B) gives off the anterior ulnar recurrent branch
(C) gives off the common interosseous artery
(D) has palpable pulsations anterior to the head of the ulna
(E) leaves the forearm by passing deep to the flexor retinaculum

84. Fibrous joints include

(A) syndesmosis
(B) synchondroses
(C) trochoidal
(D) ginglymus
(E) symphysis

85. Which of the following synovial joints provides greatest freedom of movement?

(A) saddle joint
(B) ball-and-socket joint
(C) condyloid articulation
(D) ginglymus joint
(E) trochoidal joint

ANSWERS AND EXPLANATIONS

1. **(B)** The lateral border of the acromion can be followed backward into the scapular spine, the root of which lies opposite the 3rd thoracic vertebral spine. *(Woodburne, p 80)*

2. **(C)** The inferior angle of the scapula can be located under the skin and marks the level of the 7th thoracic vertebral spine. *(Woodburne, p 80)*

3. **(D)** The rhomboideus minor is a slender slip parallel to and poorly separated from the rhomboideus major. It is inserted on the medial border on the scapula at the root of the scapular spine. *(Woodburne, p 86)*

4. **(B)** The axillary nerve from the posterior cord of the brachial plexus supplies the deltoid. The axillary nerve also supplies the teres minor muscle by a lower branch. *(Woodburne, p 88)*

5. **(A)** The suprascapular nerve from the superior trunk of the brachial plexus enters the supraspinatus fossa through the scapular notch. Passing under the superior transverse scapular ligament, it is deep to the muscle and supplies it from the underside. *(Woodburne, p 88)*

6. **(E)** The pectoral fascia is attached above to the clavicle and medially to the sternum and encloses the pectoralis major muscle. The deeper clavipectoral fascia invests the subclavius and pectoralis minor muscles. The costocoracoid membrane is in the interval between the subclavius and the pectoralis minor. The suspensory ligament of the axilla forms lateral to the axillary border of the pectoralis minor muscle. *(Woodburne, p 108)*

7. **(D)** The axillary artery is defined by the limits of the axilla; it extends from the outer border of the first rib to the lower border of the teres major muscle, where its name is changed to brachial. *(Woodburne, p 109)*

8. **(E)** The thoracoacromial artery arises from the second part of the axillary artery beneath the upper border of the pectoralis minor muscle. It pierces the costocoracoid membrane and then divides into four branches deep to the clavicular head of pectoralis major. The subscapular artery arises at the lower border of the subscapularis muscle. *(Woodburne, pp 109–110)*

9. **(A)** The thoracodorsal artery is the principal supply to the latissimus dorsi muscle, entering it on its deep axillary surface, accompanied by the thoracodorsal nerve. *(Woodburne, p 111)*

10. **(E)** The branches of the third part of the axillary artery include the subscapular, the anterior circumflex humeral, and the posterior circumflex humeral. *(Woodburne, p 110)*

11. **(B)** The cephalic vein perforates the costocoracoid membrane at the upper border of the tendon of the pectoralis minor muscle to terminate in the axillary vein. *(Woodburne, p 112)*

12. **(C)** The long thoracic nerve supplies the serratus anterior muscle. Its three roots arise from the back of the ventral rami of the 5th, 6th, and 7th cervical nerves. *(Woodburne, p 113)*

13. **(A)** The lateral divergence of the teres minor and teres major muscles produces a long, horizontally oriented triangle, which is bisected vertically by the long head of the triceps muscle. The humerus forms the fourth side of the quadrangular space laterally. The axillary nerve and the posterior circumflex artery pass through the quadrangular space. The circumflex scapular vessels pass through the triangular space.

14. **(C)** The pectoralis minor muscle arises from the outer surfaces of the 3rd, 4th, and 5th ribs near their costal cartilages, with a slip from the 2nd rib being a frequent addition. The muscle converges to

an insertion on the medial border and upper surface of the coracoid process. *(Woodburne, p 105)*

15. **(A)** The short head of the biceps arises by a thick, flattened tendon from the tip of the coracoid process, in common with the coracobrachialis. The round tendon of the long head arises from the supraglenoid tubercle of the scapula. *(Woodburne, p 119)*

16. **(C)** The cubital fossa is a triangular space at the bend of the elbow. It is bounded by a line connecting the epicondyles of the humerus, and its sides are formed by the covering borders of the brachioradialis muscle laterally and the pronator teres muscle medially. The following structures may be located in this space: the tendon of the biceps, the brachial artery, the bicipital aponeurosis, the median nerve, the radial nerve, and the median cubital vein. *(Woodburne, pp 126–127)*

17. **(D)** The pisiform bone is a small, pea-shaped bone with a single articular facet. It projects palmarward from the triquetral bone at the ulnar side of the wrist and is regarded as a sesamoid bone in the tendon of the flexor carpi ulnaris muscle. *(Woodburne, p 147)*

18. **(A)** The capitate is the largest of the carpal bones and occupies the center of the wrist. It articulates with seven bones: the scaphoid and lunate proximally; the 2nd, 3rd, and 4th metacarpals distally; the trapezoid radially; and the hamate to the ulnar side. *(Woodburne, p 148)*

19. **(C)** The distinguishing characteristic of the 3rd metacarpal is its styloid process. The 1st metacarpal bone is shorter and stouter than the others. The 2nd metacarpal bone is the longest and has a grooved base for articulation with the wedge of the trapezoid bone. The 4th and 5th metacarpals articulate proximally with the hamate bone. *(Woodburne, pp 148–149)*

20. **(D)** The flexor digiti minimi brevis, abductor digiti minimi, and opponens digiti minimi are located in the hypothenar compartment. The motor branch of the median nerve is located in the thenar compartment, along with the abductor pollicis brevis, flexor pollicis brevis, and opponens pollicis. The lumbrical muscles are located in the central compartment. *(Woodburne, pp 153–155)*

21. **(A)** The adductor pollicis muscle has two heads of origin separated by a gap, through which the radial artery enters the palm of the hand. *(Woodburne, p 158)*

22. **(A)** The sternoclavicular joint represents the only point of bony connection between the trunk

and the upper limb. The scapula articulates with the clavicle at the acromioclavicular joint, but it is joined to the trunk by muscles only. *(Woodburne, p 162)*

23. **(C)** The conoid ligament restrains backward movement of the scapula. The trapezoid ligament prevents excessive forward movement of the scapula and is especially important in resisting displacing forces that would cause the acromion to be carried down and under the clavicle. *(Woodburne, p 164)*

24. **(B)** The scapulohumeral joint is a ball-and-socket joint. It has the greatest freedom of movement of all the joints of the body, a freedom which is inevitably accompanied by a considerable loss in stability. *(Woodburne, p 165)*

25. **(C)** Medial rotators of the upper limb include the subscapularis, teres major, latissimus dorsi, pectoralis major, and the anterior fibers of the deltoid muscle. The infraspinatus is a lateral rotator of the upper limb. *(Woodburne, p 167)*

26. **(E)** Extensors of the upper limb include the latissimus dorsi, teres major, deltoid (posterior fibers), triceps (long head), and subscapularis muscles. The coracobrachialis muscle is a flexor of the upper limb. *(Woodburne, p 166)*

27. **(E)** The long head of the biceps brachii arises from the supraglenoid tubercle of the scapula. It inserts on the radial tuberosity and the bicipital aponeurosis. The short head of the biceps brachii arises from the tip of the coracoid process. *(Hollinshead, p 209)*

28. **(C)** The distal row of carpal bones, radial-to-ulnar side, is the trapezium, trapezoid, capitate, and hamate bones. The proximal row of carpal bones, radial-to-ulnar side, is the scaphoid, lunate, triquetral, and pisiform. *(Hollinshead, p 225)*

29. **(C)** The palmaris longus tendon passes anterior to the flexor retinaculum, as do the ulnar nerve and vessels. The median nerve and tendons of the long flexors of the fingers and of the thumb pass posterior to the flexor retinaculum in the carpal canal. *(Hollinshead, p 248)*

30. **(B)** The dorsal interossei are abductors of the digits from the midline of the middle digit. The palmaris brevis tightens the skin of the hypothenar eminence. The lumbricals are primarily extensors of the interphalangeal joints; secondarily, they flex the metacarpophalangeal joints. *(Hollinshead, pp 263,267,271)*

31. **(C)** The chief named parts of the upper limb are the acromion, or tip of the shoulder; the axilla, or armpit; the brachium, or arm; the cubitus, or elbow; the antebrachium, or forearm; the manus, or hand; the carpus, or wrist; and the digits, or fingers, and the thumb. In anatomical descriptions, the antebrachium, or forearm refers to the region of the radius and ulna and related structures. *(Hollinshead, p 148)*

32. **(A)** The superficial veins of the upper limb begin as networks on the digits and drain mostly onto the dorsum of the hand. They unite to form two chief channels: the cephalic vein, from the radial side, and the basilic vein, from the ulnar side. The named arteries of the limb are all deep ones, and they are accompanied regularly by one or two deep veins. The subclavian artery is the arterial stem to the limb. *(Hollinshead, p 161)*

33. **(E)** Both superficial and deep lymphatics of the upper limb end in axillary lymph nodes. Superficial lymphatics begin as a dense capillary plexus in the skin of the digits. Deep lymphatics are much less numerous than superficial lymphatics. Lymphatic vessels from the palmar surface tend to run onto the dorsum; thus, infections of the palm may be evidenced by swelling on the dorsum of the hand. The deep lymphatics follow the deep arteries and veins. *(Hollinshead, pp 161–164)*

34. **(B)** Muscle masses migrate, but nerves retain their original connection to their muscle mass. The latissimus dorsi, for example, spreads as far caudally as the pelvis but actually is derived from mesenchyme originating at the lower cervical region, and its nerve contains fibers from lower cervical nerves. Most muscles of the limbs receive their nerve supply from two or more spinal nerves. Since the relationship between nerves and muscle is so close and so nearly constant, nerves tend to parallel muscle in their development. Muscle fibers of the limb muscles are supplied by ventral (motor) branches of spinal nerves. *(Hollinshead, pp 102–103)*

35. **(C)** In skeletal muscle, every individual muscle fiber receives a nerve fiber. The distribution of a nerve within a muscle typically follows a fixed pattern—the nerve branches and rebranches in the connective tissue of the muscle, and the branches follow such courses as to bring them into contact with all the fibers within the muscle. The pattern of nerve distribution depends in part on the shape of the muscle; in a long muscle, major nerve branches run longitudinally, and in a short muscle, they run transversely. Nerve fibers to skeletal muscle release acetylcholine at the neuromuscular junction, an essential part of the mechanism for muscle contraction. These nerve fibers, therefore, are known as cholinergic, not adrenergic, fibers.

Not all nerve fibers entering a voluntary muscle are motor fibers destined for muscle fibers; sympathetic fibers innervate blood vessels, and afferent fibers conduct sensory impulses toward the spinal cord. (Hollinshead, pp 105–107)

36. **(D)** In the original position of the developing limb, the palm faces forward, with the thumb on the cranial, or preaxial, border and the little finger on the caudal, or postaxial, border. The limb first projects out at approximately a right angle but later adducts to become almost parallel to the trunk. The anatomical position, therefore, is described as the palm facing forward, with the ulnar side medial and the radial side lateral. The developing musculature of the limb divides into ventral and dorsal parts. This division is accompanied by a corresponding division of the nerves growing into the muscle. (Hollinshead, p 147)

37. **(A)** The 3rd and 4th cervical nerves supply a limited area of skin over the pectoral region and shoulder. The 2nd, not the 3rd, thoracic nerve usually sends a branch to the skin of the medial and upper parts of the arm. Most of the skin of the upper limb is supplied by branches of the brachial plexus, not the cervical plexus. Antebrachial cutaneous nerves supply skin of the forearm, not the arm (humeral region). (Hollinshead, p 151)

38. **(D)** The anterior muscles of the arm originally are ventral ones and are flexors. The anterior muscles of the forearm arise chiefly on the ulnar side of the arm or forearm and flex the wrist and fingers; they also pronate the forearm. The posterior group of forearm muscles arises chiefly on the radial side of the arm and on the back of the forearm and extends the wrist and digits; it also supinates the forearm. (Hollinshead, pp 156–157)

39. **(A)** With minor exceptions, all the major nerves of the upper limb are derived from the brachial plexus. The brachial plexus is divisible into anterior and posterior parts. Anterior nerves are the musculocutaneous, the median, and the ulnar; posterior nerves are the axillary and the radial. The radial nerve supplies the supinator muscle. The musculocutaneous nerve supplies anterior (flexor) muscles of the arm. The median and ulnar nerves run through the arm without supplying any muscles there. The axillary nerve supplies two posterior muscles of the shoulder (deltoid and teres minor). The ulnar nerve, as previously stated, is derived from anterior portions of the brachial plexus. (Hollinshead, pp 156–157)

40. **(E)** The subclavian artery derives its blood directly or indirectly from the arch of the aorta. As it enters the axilla, its name changes to the axillary artery, continuing into the arm as the brachial artery. The brachial artery ends in front of the elbow by dividing into the radial and ulnar arteries. The anterior and posterior humeral circumflex arteries are branches of the axillary artery. (Hollinshead, p 161)

41. **(D)** The anteriorly situated clavicle and the posteriorly situated scapula constitute the shoulder girdle. Neither the sternum nor the humerus is considered part of the shoulder girdle. (Hollinshead, p 165)

42. **(E)** The clavicle has attachment to the coracoid process of the scapula through the coracoclavicular ligament, composed of the conoid and trapezoid ligaments. There is no scapuloclavicular ligament. The clavicle articulates with the sternum only at the sternoclavicular joint. The coracoacromial ligament is situated between the coracoid process and acromion of the scapula. The coracohumeral ligament is not attached to the clavicle. (Hollinshead, pp 167–168)

43. **(A)** The scapula is a rather thin, triangular, flat bone strengthened by the scapular spine and a thickened lateral, not medial, border. The coracoid process is located superiorly near the lateral angle. The subscapular fossa is located on the costal surface of the bone and the spine on the dorsal surface, continuing laterally into the acromion. The scapula has three borders (medial, lateral, and superior) and three angles (inferior, lateral, and superior) where these borders meet. The lateral angle is expanded to form the glenoid cavity, which articulates with the head of the humerus. (Hollinshead, p 169)

44. **(C)** The humerus has at its expanded distal end the condyle, consisting of the capitulum on the lateral anterior inferior surface and the trochlea, the pulleylike medial surface. The olecranon fossa is located on the lower posterior surface for reception of the olecranon of the ulna. The radial fossa for reception of the head of the radius is located proximal to the capitulum. The deltoid tuberosity is located on the anterolateral surface of the humerus midway its length, not adjoining the head, and the greater tubercle adjoins the head. (Hollinshead, pp 172–173)

45. **(D)** The pectoralis major muscle inserts on the crest of the greater tubercle of the humerus (lateral lip of the intertubercular groove). It originates from the medial third of the clavicle, from the lateral part of the entire length of the anterior surface of the manubrium and body of the sternum, and from the cartilages of about the first six ribs. It has no attachment to the head of the humerus. (Hollinshead, pp 177–178)

46. **(D)** The chief action of the pectoralis major is adduction and medial rotation of the humerus. It as-

sists the anterior deltoid in flexion of the arm. The lower fibers can help to extend the limb until it is by the side. It is not in a position to abduct the humerus, does not attach to the scapula, and cannot elevate the clavicle. *(Hollinshead, p 180)*

47. (A) The pectoralis minor usually takes origin from three ribs—the 2nd or 3rd to the 5th or 6th. It inserts into the medial side of the coracoid process of the scapula. It does not attach to the greater tubercle of the humerus. *(Hollinshead, p 179)*

48. (E) The radial nerve supplies the triceps muscle. The long thoracic innervates the serratus anterior muscle; the lower subscapular innervates the subscapularis and the teres major; the musculocutaneous nerve innervates the anterior muscles of the arm; and the axillary nerve innervates the deltoid and teres minor muscles. *(Hollinshead, p 181)*

49. (B) The axillary artery gives off the two chief arteries of the pectoral region: the thoracoacromial and the lateral thoracic. The axillary artery is the continuation of the subclavian as the vessel crosses the 1st rib. The axillary artery becomes the brachial artery as it leaves the axilla at the lower border of the teres major muscle. The axillary artery usually is described as giving off 6 branches, the first being the supreme thoracic artery and the last the anterior and posterior humeral circumflex arteries to the upper end of the humerus. *(Hollinshead, pp 188–189)*

50. (C) The axilla houses the great vessels and nerves of the limb, which are closely grouped together and enclosed in a layer of fascia, the axillary sheath. Most of the nerve trunks appearing in the axilla are the lower part of the brachial plexus and its major branches and rather closely surround the axillary artery. This artery is, therefore, thought of as the central structure of the axilla. The cords of the brachial plexus are named lateral, medial, and posterior according to their position relative to the axillary artery. *(Hollinshead, pp 183–185)*

51. (E) The lateral cord of the brachial plexus typically has only three branches, the musculocutaneous nerve being one of these. The lateral and medial cords represent anterior divisions of the brachial plexus, not lateral divisions. The lateral cord contains fibers from C5, C6, and C7, and perhaps from C4 if these fibers join the plexus. The ulnar nerve continues into the arm from the medial cord of the plexus. *(Hollinshead, p 185)*

52. (C) The posterior cord of the brachial plexus does not give off the median nerve; this nerve is formed from branches of the lateral and medial cords. The posterior cord is formed by union of all posterior divisions of the brachial plexus; the upper subscapular and axillary nerves are among its branches, and the radial nerve is a terminal branch. *(Hollinshead, 186–187)*

53. (B) The long thoracic nerve is located on the medial wall of the axilla on the surface of the serratus anterior muscle, which is supplies. This nerve arises from the brachial plexus in the neck before the trunks are formed. None of the other muscles listed are supplied by the long thoracic nerve. *(Hollinshead, p 186)*

54. (D) The trapezius muscle originates from the superior nuchal line on the occipital bone and from the external occipital protuberance. It originates from the ligamentum nuchae of the cervical vertebral spinous processes, from the spinous process of the 7th cervical vertebra, and from all the thoracic vertebral spinous processes and their connecting supraspinous ligaments. This muscle inserts on approximately the distal third of the clavicle and on the acromion and spine of the scapula. *(Hollinshead, p 194)*

55. (C) The thoracodorsal nerve supplies the latissimus dorsi muscle. It leaves the axilla on the costal surface of the muscle and runs downward on this surface with the thoracodorsal artery. None of the other nerves listed supply this muscle. *(Hollinshead, p 195)*

56. (C) The axillary nerve runs deep to the deltoid, circling the surgical neck of the humerus and sending branches into the deltoid. The supraspinatus and infraspinatus are innervated by the suprascapular nerve and the trapezius by the accessory nerve. *(Hollinshead, pp 198–201)*

57. (A) The infraspinatus and teres minor both are lateral rotators of the arm. The supraspinatus primarily is an abductor and is active in supporting the arm against a downward pull. The subscapularis and teres major both are medial rotators, as are the anterior deltoid and latissimus dorsi. The serratus anterior and rhomboidus major have no attachment on the humerus and therefore cannot rotate it. *(Hollinshead, p 201)*

58. (D) The supraspinatus assists the deltoid in abduction of the arm. This muscle arises from the supraspinatous fossa of the scapula and passes laterally over the top of the shoulder to attach to the uppermost of the three facets of the greater tubercle of the humerus. None of the other muscles listed are in a position to accomplish abduction of the arm. *(Hollinshead, p 199)*

59. (E) The transverse cervical artery and the suprascapular artery, typically both branches of the thyrocervical trunk, arise in the neck. The other arteries listed arise from the axillary artery in the axilla. *(Hollinshead, pp 203–204)*

60. (D) All of the muscles listed except the deltoid are intimately related to the shoulder joint. Since most of them are rotators, the musculotendinous cuff also is called the rotator cuff. The deltoid muscle completely covers the shoulder joint and the muscles of the rotator cuff. *(Hollinshead, p 204)*

61. (D) The coracohumeral ligament apparently prevents downward displacement of the humeral head when the arm is by the side. With the arm abducted, the ligament is lax, and the strength of the joint depends entirely on the musculotendinous cuff. The glenoid fossa is shallow and does not offer a stable articulating surface for the relatively large head of the humerus. The other ligaments listed do not appear to be of importance. *(Hollinshead, p 205)*

62. (A) The biceps brachii muscle, along with the coracobrachialis and the brachialis muscles, is located on the anterior arm. The biceps is the only one of this group that originates on the supraglenoid tubercle of the scapula. The biceps has a short head originating on the coracoid process, the site of origin of the coracobrachialis. The brachialis is the only one of the group originating on the anterior surface of the humerus and inserting on the ulnar tuberosity. All of these muscles are innervated by the musculocutaneous nerve. *(Hollinshead, p 209)*

63. (B) The median nerve runs down the arm on the axillary and brachial arteries. It gives off no branches to structures of the arm. The musculocutaneous nerve is a derivative of the lateral cord of the brachial plexus. The ulnar nerve is a derivative of the medial cord of the plexus. The radial nerve does not innervate the coracobrachialis muscle, and the lateral antebrachial cutaneous nerve, a continuation of the musculocutaneous nerve, continues into the forearm. *(Hollinshead, pp 212–213)*

64. (E) When the extended thumb is separated widely from the index finger, two ridges are raised by tendons that enclose a depression between them distal to the end of the radius. This depression is named the anatomical snuffbox because of the use to which it was once put. The abductor pollicis longus and extensor pollicis brevis tendons form the anterior boundary of the anatomical snuffbox; the extensor pollicis longus tendon forms its posterior border. It is located laterally, not medially, to the extensor pollicis longus and has no relation to the extensor indicis tendon. *(Hollinshead, pp 220,241–243)*

65. (C) Of the structures listed, the styloid process is the only one located at the distal end of the ulna. The olecranon, trochlear notch, ulnar tuberosity, and coronoid process are all at or near the proximal end of the ulna. *(Hollinshead, p 223)*

66. (D) The brachialis muscle inserts on the ulna, not the radius. The biceps, supinator, brachioradialis, and pronator quadratus all have insertions on the radius. *(Hollinshead, p 223)*

67. (A) The lunate is the only bone listed that is found in the proximal row of carpals. All of the others listed are found in the distal row of carpals. *(Hollinshead, p 226)*

68. (C) The radial nerve is accompanied in the arm by the first major branch of the brachial artery, the profunda brachii. The radial nerve ends by dividing into superficial and deep branches. The superficial branch gives cutaneous nerves to the posterior forearm and much of the dorsum of the hand. The deep branch of the radial nerve gives motor fibers to the extensor muscles of the arm and forearm. This nerve is a terminal branch of the posterior cord of the brachial plexus. It does not innervate the biceps or the flexor carpi ulnaris muscles. *(Hollinshead, pp 214,232,245)*

69. (A) The flexor digitorum superficialis arises by two heads. The humeroulnar head arises from the medial epicondyle of the humerus and from the medial border of the base of the coronoid process of the ulna; the radial head arises from the upper part of the anterior border of the radius. The flexor carpi radialis arises from the medial epicondyle of the humerus, as does the palmaris longus. The flexor pollicis longus arises from the anterior surface of the radius and adjacent interosseous membrane; it does not originate on the humerus. Neither does the flexor digitorum profundus reach the humerus, originating only below the elbow on the ulna. *(Hollinshead, pp 250–251,260–261)*

70. (C) The radial artery usually gives off a superficial palmar branch that enters the thenar muscles; this artery frequently joins the superficial palmar arch. The radial artery arises as the lateral terminal branch of the brachial artery. All of the other items involve the ulnar artery, which gives rise to the common interosseous and provides the major components of the superficial palmar arch from which arise common digital arteries. *(Hollinshead, pp 255,257)*

71. (D) The muscular branch of the median nerve turns laterally into the thenar muscles, where it usually is distributed to about two and one-half muscles. The radial nerve gives rise to the posterior interosseous nerve. The median nerve passes deep to the flexor retinaculum; it innervates flexor muscles on the forearm except for the flexor carpi ulnaris and the ulnar side of the flexor digitorum profundus. The median nerve supplies only the 1st and 2nd lumbrical muscles, not all of them. *(Hollinshead, pp 258–259,261)*

72. **(A)**   The median nerve innervates all the short muscles of the thumb except the adductor and the deep head of the short flexor, which typically are innervated by the deep branch of the ulnar nerve. The palmaris brevis also is supplied by the ulnar nerve. Typically, all of the interossei are supplied by the ulnar nerve; perhaps in 10% of cases, the first dorsal interosseous is supplied by the median nerve. The abductor pollicis longus is supplied by the radial nerve. *(Hollinshead, pp 244,266–267,271)*

73. **(A)**   The superficial branch of the ulnar artery forms the superficial palmar arch. The radial artery divides into the deep palmar arch and the princeps pollicis artery. The palmar metacarpal arteries arise from the deep palmar arch and join the common digital arteries from the superficial arch to form the proper digital arteries. Proper digital arteries run on each side of the fingers. *(Hollinshead, pp 251,268–270)*

74. **(C)**   The biceps brachii is both a flexor at the elbow and a strong supinator when the arm is flexed or more power is demanded. The brachialis is a flexor of the elbow and primarily is responsible for maintaining a flexed position. The flexor carpi radialis only assists in flexion at the elbow. The brachioradialis contracts if the movement is a quick one or if resistance is offered to flexion while the forearm is pronated. The supinator participates in all supination and is equally effective whether the forearm is flexed or extended. *(Hollinshead, pp 273–274)*

75. **(E)**   Anomalous innervation of hypothenar muscles apparently is never a result of the median nerve sending a direct branch across the palm to the hypothenar muscles. Recent electromyographic clinical evidence is said to show all the other anomalous innervations listed. *(Hollinshead, p 280)*

76–79.   **76. (E), 77. (D), 78. (C), 79. (B)** The axillary and radial nerves are terminal branches of the posterior division of the brachial plexus. The axillary nerve supplies the deltoid and the skin covering the deltoid. The coracobrachialis, the biceps,

and the brachialis all are supplied by the musculocutaneous nerve, the continuation of the lateral cord of the brachial plexus. All the interossei muscles are innervated by the ulnar nerve, the continuation of the medial cord of the brachial plexus. The recurrent branch of the median nerve supplies the abductor pollicis brevis. *(Basmajian, pp 341,357, 377–379,393)*

80–81.   **80. (C), 81. (D)** The origin of the superficial palmar arch is the ulnar artery. The ulnar artery is the larger terminal branch of the brachial artery. As the ulnar artery enters the hand, it gives off a small, deep branch into the hypothenar muscles and then continues as the superficial palmar arch. The origin of the deep palmar arch is the radial artery. *(Hollinshead, pp 254–256,266,268–269)*

82. **(E)**   The distal end of the radius and the articular disk of the distal radioulnar joint articulate with the proximal row of carpal bones (scaphoid, lunate, and triquetrum). The articular nerves are derived from the anterior interosseous nerve, a branch of the median nerve. The head of the ulna articulates with the ulnar notch in the distal end of the radius to form the distal radioulnar joint. The articular disk binds the lower end of the ulna and radius together and is the main uniting structure of the radioulnar joint. The radiocarpal joint is a ball-and-socket type of synovial joint. *(Moore, p 625)*

83. **(E)**   The brachial artery divides into two terminal branches, the radial artery and the large ulnar artery. The ulnar artery gives off the anterior ulnar recurrent branch just below the elbow; it also gives off the common interosseous artery that branches into anterior and posterior interosseous arteries. The pulsation of the ulnar artery can be felt where it passes anterior to the head of the ulna. It leaves the forearm by passing superficial to the flexor retinaculum. *(Moore, p 581)*

84. **(A)**   In the syndesmosis, the apposed bones are simply joined together by intervening fibrous tissue. The synchondroses and symphysis are cartilaginous joints. Both the ginglymus and trochoidal are examples of synovial joints. *(Woodburne, pp 46–47)*

85. **(B)**   The spheroidal or ball-and-socket joint is the articulation of greatest freedom of motion. The ball-and-socket character allows motion in an almost infinite number of axes passing near the center of the "ball." *(Woodburne, p 48)*

The Lower Limbs
Questions

1. The iliac crest is palpable at the level of which of the vertebrae?

    (A) the 12th thoracic
    (B) the 2nd lumbar
    (C) the 4th lumbar
    (D) the 1st sacral
    (E) the 5th sacral

2. All of the following statements concerning the posterior superior iliac spine are correct EXCEPT

    (A) the iliac crest ends posteriorly in the posterior superior iliac spine
    (B) it is often located in the depths of a dimple of skin
    (C) it lies at the level of the 2nd sacral spine
    (D) it lies opposite the middle of the sacroiliac articulation
    (E) it is palpable at the lower end of the inguinal ligament

3. The sciatic nerve leaves the gluteal region for the thigh midway between the

    (A) pubic tubercle and the posterior superior iliac spine
    (B) greater trochanter and the ischial tuberosity
    (C) anterior superior iliac spine and the pubic tubercle
    (D) ischial tuberosity and the pubic tubercle
    (E) pubic symphysis and the ischial tuberosity

4. The patella is located in the tendon of which of the following muscles?

    (A) adductor magnus
    (B) sartorius
    (C) biceps femoris
    (D) quadriceps femoris
    (E) semitendinosus

5. The tendons of which of the following muscles form the lateral margin of the popliteal fossa?

    (A) semitendinosus
    (B) semimembranosus
    (C) biceps femoris
    (D) gracilis
    (E) sartorius

6. All of the following statements concerning the lesser saphenous are correct EXCEPT

    (A) it enters the leg in front of the lateral malleolus
    (B) it enters the leg on the lateral side of the calcaneal tendon
    (C) it ascends over the middle of the calf
    (D) it perforates the crural fascia
    (E) it ends in the popliteal vein

7. Which of the following statements concerning the lateral malleolus is correct?

    (A) the tip of the lateral malleolus is approximately 1.5 cm lower than the tip of the medial malleolus
    (B) it is the distal end of the tibia
    (C) it is posterior to the lesser saphenous vein
    (D) it is located on the same side as the sustentaculum tali of the calcaneus
    (E) it is located on the same side as the tuberosity of the navicular

8. All of the following statements concerning the greater saphenous vein are correct EXCEPT

    (A) it receives the superficial epigastric vein
    (B) it is joined to the femoral vein by perforating communications
    (C) it contains no valves
    (D) it receives the superficial circumflex iliac vein
    (E) it is the longest vein of the body

9. Which of the statements concerning the superficial inguinal lymph nodes is correct?

    (A) they receive lymph from the upper abdominal wall
    (B) they send their efferent channels mainly to the deep inguinal nodes
    (C) they form a chain parallel to and about 1 cm below the inguinal ligament
    (D) they receive lymph from the uterus
    (E) they receive lymph from the prostate gland

10. The saphenous nerve is a terminal branch of which of the following nerves?

    (A) femoral
    (B) obturator
    (C) genitofemoral
    (D) ilioinguinal
    (E) sciatic

11. All of the following statements concerning the medial sural cutaneous nerve are correct EXCEPT

    (A) it arises from the femoral nerve
    (B) it arises in the popliteal fossa
    (C) it descends in the groove between the two heads of the gastrocnemius muscle
    (D) it is joined by the fibular (peroneal) communicating branch to form the sural nerve
    (E) it supplies the heel and foot area

12. Which of the following structures is located in the saphenous opening?

    (A) sural nerve
    (B) gluteal aponeurosis
    (C) iliotibial tract
    (D) fascia cribrosa
    (E) saphenous nerve

13. All of the following statements concerning the femoral triangle are correct EXCEPT

    (A) the floor of the triangle is represented medially by the pectineus and adductor longus muscle
    (B) laterally, the floor is represented by the lateral border of the sartorius

    (C) it is the subfascial space of the upper one-third of the thigh
    (D) the triangle is bounded above by the inguinal ligament
    (E) the femoral artery bisects the triangle in a vertical direction

14. Which of the following statements concerning the femoral sheath is correct?

    (A) it is a diverticulum of the superficial fascia
    (B) it extends approximately 6 to 8 cm beyond the inguinal ligament
    (C) the extraperitoneal connective tissue of the abdomen subdivides the sheath into four compartments
    (D) it blends with the adventitia of the blood vessels as its termination
    (E) it contains the rectus femoris muscle

15. Which of the following structures is located in the medial femoral compartment?

    (A) femoral artery
    (B) femoral vein
    (C) femoral canal
    (D) femoral nerve
    (E) obturator nerve

16. Which of the following nerves traverses the adductor canal?

    (A) femoral
    (B) obturator
    (C) saphenous
    (D) sciatic
    (E) genitofemoral

17. All of the following statements concerning the popliteal space are correct EXCEPT

    (A) this space is triangular
    (B) the superior borders are produced by the hamstring tendons
    (C) the inferior borders are produced by the medial and lateral heads of the gastrocnemius muscle
    (D) the tibial nerve runs through the fossa in a vertical direction
    (E) the posterior femoral cutaneous nerve descends across the fossa in the midline

18. Which of the following statements concerning the lateral femoral (gluteal) muscles is correct?

    (A) they include strong abductors
    (B) they include strong medial rotators

(C) they extend the leg at the knee

(D) they are innervated by the obturator nerve

(E) they include the sartorius

19. The lateral femoral (gluteal) muscles include all of the following muscles EXCEPT the

(A) quadratus femoris

(B) obturator internus

(C) piriformis

(D) tensor fascia latae

(E) pectineus

20. Which of the following statements concerning the anterior femoral muscles is correct?

(A) they are preaxial

(B) they are innervated by the obturator nerve

(C) they include the longest muscle in the body

(D) they include the gracilis

(E) they adduct the thigh

21. All of the following statements concerning the "hamstring" muscles are correct EXCEPT

(A) they are located in the posterior femoral group

(B) they arise primarily from the ischial tuberosity

(C) they are primary preaxial

(D) they are all supplied by the femoral nerve

(E) they flex the leg and extend the thigh

22. The adductor tubercle is located on the

(A) greater trochanter

(B) medial epicondyle

(C) intertrochanteric crest

(D) proximal end of the femur

(E) linea aspera

23. All of the following statements concerning the obturator artery are correct EXCEPT

(A) it is a branch of the external iliac artery

(B) it distributes largely outside the pelvis

(C) it passes through the obturator canal

(D) it divides into posterior and anterior branches

(E) it gives off an acetabular branch

24. All of the following statements concerning the course of the femoral artery are correct EXCEPT

(A) it descends into the lower limb by passing under the inguinal ligament

(B) it descends into the lower limb midway between the anterior superior spine of the ilium and the pubic symphysis

(C) it descends through the femoral triangle

(D) it descends through the adductor canal

(E) it descends through the femoral canal

25. All of the following statements concerning the obturator nerve are correct EXCEPT

(A) it is the principal preaxial nerve of the lumbar plexus

(B) it arises from the anterior branches of lumbar nerves 2, 3, and 4

(C) it descends along the lateral border of the psoas muscle

(D) it enters the thigh through the obturator canal

(E) it divides into an anterior and a posterior branch

26. Which of the following statements concerning the femoral nerve is correct?

(A) it is the largest branch of the lumbar plexus

(B) it is a preaxial nerve

(C) it is formed by anterior branches of the 2nd, 3rd, and 4th lumbar nerves

(D) it passes under the inguinal ligament medial to the psoas muscle

(E) it has no cutaneous branches

27. All of the following statements concerning the sciatic nerve are correct EXCEPT

(A) it arises from spinal cord segments L4 through S3

(B) it leaves the pelvis through the lower part of the greater sciatic foramen

(C) it extends from the inferior border of the piriformis muscle to the lower one-third of the thigh

(D) inferiorly, the nerve lies against the anterior surface of the adductor magnus

(E) it is crossed obliquely by the long head of the biceps femoris muscle

28. All of the following statements concerning the muscles of the superficial posterior compartment of the leg are correct EXCEPT

(A) the muscles are preaxial

(B) the muscles insert onto the tuberosity of the calcaneus

(C) the contraction of these muscles produces flexion of the toes

(D) the tibial nerve innervates these muscles

(E) the plantaris muscle is located in this compartment

29. Which of the following statements concerning the tibialis posterior is correct?

    (A) it is a postaxial muscle
    (B) it is innervated by the peroneal nerve
    (C) it inserts into the tuberosity of the navicular
    (D) it everts the foot
    (E) it is located in the same compartment as the tibialis anterior

30. Which of the following statements concerning the posterior tibial artery are correct?

    (A) it is the direct continuation of the popliteal artery
    (B) it descends in the lateral compartment of the leg
    (C) it passes behind the lateral malleolus
    (D) it gives rise to the dorsalis pedis artery
    (E) it descends between the tibialis anterior and the extensor digitorum longus muscles

31. All of the following statements concerning the quadratus plantae are correct EXCEPT

    (A) it is an accessory muscle to the long digital flexor
    (B) it lies on the superior aspect of the flexor digitorum brevis muscle
    (C) it inserts into the tendon of the flexor digitorum longus muscle
    (D) it arises by heads that are separated from each other by the long plantar ligament
    (E) it gives rise to the plantar aponeurosis

32. All of the following statements concerning the central compartment of the foot are correct EXCEPT

    (A) it is deep to the plantar aponeurosis
    (B) it is bounded by the lateral intermuscular and medial intermuscular septa at its border
    (C) it contains the dorsal interosseous muscles
    (D) it contains the flexor digitorum brevis
    (E) it contains the quadratus plantae

33. All of the following statements concerning the iliofemoral ligament are correct EXCEPT

    (A) it is y-shaped
    (B) it attaches to the intertrochanteric line
    (C) it becomes taut in full extension
    (D) it is attached to the anterior superior iliac spine
    (E) it helps to maintain the erect posture

34. All of the following statements concerning the ligamentum capitis femoris are correct EXCEPT

    (A) it is intracapsular
    (B) it ends in the fovea of the head of the femur
    (C) it is covered by a sleeve of synovial membrane
    (D) it becomes taut in abduction of the femur
    (E) it arises from the acetabular notch and the transverse ligament of the acetabulum

35. Which of the following structures separates the tibial collateral ligament from the overlying insertions of the sartorius, gracilis, and semitendinosus?

    (A) ligamentum patellae
    (B) deep infrapatellar space
    (C) subcutaneous infrapatellar bursa
    (D) bursa anserina
    (E) oblique popliteal ligament

36. All of the following statements concerning the medial meniscus are correct EXCEPT

    (A) it is fibrocartilage
    (B) it is thicker at its external margins
    (C) it attaches in the anterior intercondylar area of the tibia in front of the anterior cruciate ligament
    (D) its posterior attachment is in the corresponding posterior fossa posterior to the origin of the posterior cruciate ligament
    (E) it is crescent-shaped

37. Which of the following statements concerning the lateral meniscus is correct?

    (A) it attaches to the anterior intercondylar area lateral to and in front of the anterior cruciate ligament
    (B) its posterior termination is in the posterior intercondylar area behind the end of the medial meniscus
    (C) it frequently gives rise to the posterior meniscofemoral ligament
    (D) it is elastic cartilage
    (E) it covers a somewhat smaller surface of the tibia than does the medial meniscus

38. All of the following statements concerning the anterior cruciate ligament are correct EXCEPT

    (A) it arises from the nonarticular area in front of the intercondylar eminence of the tibia
    (B) it extends backward to attach on the medial aspect of the lateral femoral condyle
    (C) it prevents posterior displacement of the tibia
    (D) it is somewhat taut in all positions of flexion
    (E) it is tightest in full extension and full flexion

39. Which of the following statements concerning the posterior cruciate ligament is correct?

 (A) it attaches to the medial aspect of the lateral femoral condyle
 (B) it prevents posterior displacement of the tibia
 (C) it is loose in full extension and full flexion
 (D) it is extracapsular
 (E) it gives rise to the posterior meniscofemoral ligament

40. The deltoid ligament involves all of the following bones EXCEPT the

 (A) medial malleolus
 (B) sustentaculum tali
 (C) navicular
 (D) medial cuneiform
 (E) talus

41. All of the following statements concerning the talus are correct EXCEPT

 (A) it articulates with the tibia and fibula above
 (B) it articulates with the navicular in front
 (C) it articulates with the calcaneus below
 (D) it is the largest and strongest bone of the foot
 (E) its upper portion is called the trochlea

42. All of the following statements concerning the metatarsal bones are correct EXCEPT

 (A) the first metatarsal bone is the shortest, broadest, and most massive of the metatarsals
 (B) the 2nd metatarsal bone is the longest
 (C) the tuberosity of the 5th metatarsal gives insertion to the peroneus brevis tendon
 (D) the tuberosity of the 1st metatarsal provides insertion for the peroneus longus
 (E) the bodies are narrow and tend to be rectangular in cross-section

43. All of the following statements concerning the adductor hallucis muscle are correct EXCEPT

 (A) it inserts into the lateral side of the base of the proximal phalanx of the great toe
 (B) it arises by oblique and transverse heads
 (C) it is innervated by the medial plantar nerve
 (D) it adducts the great toe
 (E) it aids in maintaining the arches of the foot

44. All of the following statements concerning the fibular collateral ligament are correct EXCEPT

 (A) it prevents hyperextension
 (B) it prevents abduction angulation of the bones
 (C) it prevents adduction angulation of the bones

 (D) the tendon of the popliteus muscle passes deep to the fibular collateral ligament
 (E) the tendon of the biceps femoris muscle passes deep to the fibular collateral ligament

45. Which of the following structures pass between the capsule of the knee joint and the fibular collateral ligament?

 (A) inferior genicular blood vessels
 (B) anterior tibial artery
 (C) posterior tibial artery
 (D) common peroneal nerve
 (E) fibular artery

46. Which of the following ligaments is known as the "spring ligament"?

 (A) long plantar
 (B) plantar calcaneocuboid
 (C) deltoid
 (D) plantar calcaneonavicular
 (E) plantar cuneonavicular

47. All of the following statements concerning the lateral ligaments of the ankle joint are correct EXCEPT

 (A) these ligaments are weaker than the deltoid ligament
 (B) the anterior talofibular ligament stretches from the lateral malleolus to the talus
 (C) the calcaneofibular ligament stretches from the lateral malleolus to the sustentaculum tali
 (D) the posterior talofibular ligament is almost horizontal
 (E) the lateral ligaments are separate ligaments

48. The flexor retinaculum covers all of the following structures that pass behind the medial malleolus EXCEPT the

 (A) tendon of the tibialis posterior muscle
 (B) tendon of the flexor digitorum longus muscle
 (C) posterior tibial artery
 (D) tibial nerve
 (E) tendon of the flexor hallucis brevis

49. The uppermost limits of the lower limb include all of the following EXCEPT the

 (A) iliac crest
 (B) inguinal ligament
 (C) ischial tuberosity
 (D) symphysis pubis
 (E) acetabulum

50. Which of the following muscles insert into the base and inferolateral border of the first metatarsal bone?

(A) soleus

(B) extensor hallucis longus

(C) peroneus longus

(D) plantaris

(E) tibialis posterior

51. Parts and regions of the lower limb are defined correctly by which of the following?

(A) malleolus, the knee

(B) clunis, the gluteals

(C) tarsus, the calf

(D) sura, the ankle

(E) hallux, digit 5

52. The skeleton of the lower limb can be described correctly by all of the following EXCEPT

(A) the pelvic girdle is attached firmly to the vertebral column

(B) the bones that compose the pelvic girdle fuse together in development

(C) the two coxal bones are firmly articulated with each other at the midline

(D) the fibula does not enter into the knee joint

(E) the hip joint is identical in all respects to the shoulder joint

53. The lumbar plexus can be described correctly by which of the following statements?

(A) the 2nd, 3rd, and 4th lumbar nerves contribute to its branches

(B) it gives rise to the sciatic nerve

(C) most of its branches enter the buttock

(D) it gives rise to the tibial nerve

(E) it sends innervation to the muscles of the calf

54. In relation to vessels of the lower limb, which of the following statements is true?

(A) the popliteal artery is a branch of the external iliac artery

(B) the anterior tibial artery is a direct branch of the deep femoral artery

(C) the superficial veins rarely become varicose

(D) their arterial stem is the femoral artery

(E) communicating veins normally conduct blood from the deep veins to the superficial veins

55. Which of the following statements concerning veins and lymphatics of the lower limb is correct?

(A) large superficial veins originate on the sole of the foot

(B) the great saphenous vein is seen on the lateral side of the knee

(C) the small saphenous vein commonly ends in the popliteal vein

(D) there are many deep lymph nodes

(E) the general direction of superficial lymphatics is toward the foot

56. All of the following statements about nerves and vessels of the thigh are correct EXCEPT

(A) the femoral artery terminates in the anterior thigh

(B) the obturator nerve is distributed almost entirely to the thigh

(C) arteries entering the buttock are distributed almost entirely to the buttock

(D) the sciatic nerve supplies all the posterior muscles of the leg

(E) through its branches, the sciatic nerve supplies all muscles of the foot

57. Which of the following statements is true in relation to pelvic girdle bones?

(A) their ossification is complete by 2 years of age

(B) the pubis forms the lateral part of the acetabulum

(C) the ischium forms the medial inferior part of the acetabulum

(D) the ilium forms the upper part of the acetabulum

(E) the acetabular notch is found on the superior wall of the acetabulum

58. Structures adding strength to the pelvic girdle consist of all the following EXCEPT the

(A) transverse acetabular ligament

(B) sacroiliac ligaments

(C) sacrotuberous ligament

(D) sacrospinous ligament

(E) iliolumbar ligament

59. Blood supply to the upper end of the femur is derived mostly from the

(A) artery of the ligament of the head of the femur

(B) inferior gluteal artery

(C) medial femoral circumflex artery

(D) superior gluteal artery

(E) superficial iliac circumflex artery

60. The gluteus maximus can be described correctly by which of the following statements?

(A) it passes through the greater sciatic foramen
(B) it inserts into the head of the femur
(C) it is innervated by the superior gluteal nerve
(D) it has a chief action of abduction at the hip joint
(E) it arises partly from the sacrotuberous ligament

61. The chief action of the gluteus medius is

(A) extension at the hip joint
(B) flexion at the hip joint
(C) medial rotation of the femur
(D) abduction at the hip joint
(E) adduction at the hip joint

62. Distribution of which of the following arteries is primarily confined to the buttock?

(A) internal pudendal
(B) inferior gluteal
(C) femoral
(D) profunda femoris
(E) lateral femoral circumflex

63. The gluteus medius and gluteus minimus muscles have similar characteristics EXCEPT

(A) both arise from the ilium
(B) both insert on the greater trochanter of the femur
(C) both are supplied by the superior gluteal nerve
(D) both are particularly important in walking
(E) both are strong flexors and medial rotators

64. Which of the following statements is true in regard to the sciatic nerve?

(A) it consists of two nerves
(B) it passes anterior to the obturator internus
(C) it gives off several fibers to the buttock
(D) it runs superficial to the thigh muscles that arise from the ischial tuberosity
(E) it generally runs through the piriformis muscle

65. All of the following statements correctly describe the fascia lata of the thigh EXCEPT

(A) it consists of dense deep fascia
(B) it is reinforced by a strong medial part, the iliotibial tract
(C) it splits to cover both sides of the tensor fasciae latae muscle

(D) at the knee it blends with expansions from muscle tendons
(E) just below the inguinal ligament, it presents the saphenous hiatus

66. Which of the following statements is correct in relation to extension at the knee joint with the hip extended?

(A) the sartorius begins the movement
(B) the rectus femoris is the most efficient actor
(C) the vastus medialis does not assist in the movement
(D) the vastus lateralis does not participate
(E) the articularis genus muscle is a primary actor

67. Correct description of the femoral nerve includes which of the following?

(A) it supplies no cutaneous branches
(B) usually it contains fibers from L5, S1, and S2
(C) in the femoral triangle, it lies medial to the femoral vessels
(D) it supplies the adductor magnus muscle
(E) it supplies the rectus femoris muscle

68. All of the following muscles arise from the ischial tuberosity EXCEPT the

(A) short head of the biceps femoris
(B) semitendinosus
(C) long head of the biceps femoris
(D) semimembranosus
(E) posterior adductor magnus

69. All of the following muscles cross the knee joint EXCEPT the

(A) gracilis
(B) adductor magnus
(C) sartorius
(D) biceps femoris
(E) semitendinosus

70. The thigh muscle that receives innervation from both tibial and common peroneal nerves is the

(A) semimembranosus
(B) biceps femoris
(C) adductor magnus
(D) semitendinosus
(E) gracilis

71. Which of the following muscles can extend the thigh at the hip without at the same time producing flexion at the knee?

    (A) biceps femoris, long head
    (B) semitendinosus
    (C) biceps femoris, short head
    (D) adductor magnus
    (E) semimembranosus

72. Which of the following is the most anterior of the structures in the popliteal fossa?

    (A) popliteal artery
    (B) popliteal vein
    (C) common peroneal nerve
    (D) sciatic nerve
    (E) tibial nerve

73. Which of the following statements is correct regarding the tarsal bones?

    (A) the cuboid lies medially in the foot
    (B) the calcaneus is the smallest tarsal bone
    (C) the navicular lies just in front of the cuneiforms
    (D) the cuneiforms lie lateral to the cuboid
    (E) the talus lies above the calcaneus

74. All of the following statements regarding the arches of the foot are correct EXCEPT

    (A) the medial part of the longitudinal arch is higher than the lateral part
    (B) the lateral longitudinal arch passes forward from the calcaneus through the cuboid to the heads of the two lateral metatarsals
    (C) the transverse arch lies at the level of the proximal row of tarsals
    (D) the two arches interlock to form a functional single arch
    (E) the arch is loaded from the top through the talus

75. Which is the primary movement that occurs at the talocrural joint?

    (A) inversion and eversion
    (B) flexion and extension
    (C) eversion and abduction
    (D) inversion and adduction
    (E) equinovarus

76. Cutaneous innervation of the leg includes all of the following nerves EXCEPT the

    (A) saphenous
    (B) superficial peroneal
    (C) lateral sural cutaneous
    (D) obturator
    (E) posterior femoral cutaneous

77. Which of the following muscles is both a dorsiflexor and an inverter of the foot?

    (A) peroneus brevis
    (B) peroneus longus
    (C) extensor hallucis longus
    (D) peroneus tertius
    (E) extensor digitorum longus

78. Muscles that originate predominantly on the fibula consist of all of the following EXCEPT the

    (A) tibialis anterior
    (B) extensor hallucis longus
    (C) peroneus brevis
    (D) extensor digitorum longus
    (E) peroneus tertius

79. Muscles innervated by the deep peroneal nerve include all of the following EXCEPT the

    (A) tibialis anterior
    (B) extensor digitorum longus
    (C) extensor hallucis longus
    (D) peroneus brevis
    (E) peroneus tertius

80. Which of the following arteries is the continuation of the anterior tibial artery in the foot?

    (A) recurrent
    (B) dorsalis pedis
    (C) medial plantar
    (D) posterior tibial
    (E) peroneal

81. Which of the following muscles is not a plantar flexor at the ankle?

    (A) gastrocnemius
    (B) soleus
    (C) peroneus longus
    (D) peroneus tertius
    (E) posterior tibial

82. Which of the following arteries is a terminal branch of the popliteal artery?

    (A) anterior tibial
    (B) dorsalis pedis
    (C) peroneal
    (D) medial superior genicular
    (E) sural

83. A branch of the femoral artery that enters into collateral circulation around the knee is the

    (A) lateral femoral circumflex
    (B) lateral superior genicular
    (C) descending genicular
    (D) anterior tibial
    (E) anterior tibial recurrent

84. Which of the following statements correctly describes the triceps surae?

    (A) it includes the anterior tibialis muscle
    (B) it includes the plantaris muscle
    (C) it inserts into the tendo calcaneus
    (D) it includes the posterior tibialis muscle
    (E) it is innervated by the common peroneal nerve

85. All of the following statements concerning the profunda femoris artery are correct EXCEPT

    (A) it branches from the femoral artery
    (B) it gives off the lateral femoral circumflex artery
    (C) it gives off the medial femoral circumflex artery
    (D) it usually gives off four perforating branches
    (E) it gives rise to the superficial epigastric

ANSWERS AND EXPLANATIONS

1. **(C)** The iliac crest is palpable throughout its entire length. The highest point of its curvature is at the level of the 4th lumbar vertebra. *(Woodburne, p 563)*

2. **(E)** The iliac crest ends posteriorly in the posterior superior iliac spine, which is often in the depths of a dimple of skin. It lies at the level of the 2nd sacral spine and opposite the middle of the sacroiliac articulation. The pubic tubercle is palpable at the lower end of the inguinal ligament. *(Woodburne, p 563)*

3. **(B)** The sciatic nerve leaves the gluteal region for the thigh midway between the greater trochanter and the ischial tuberosity. The nerve descends from this point toward the middle of the back of the knee. *(Woodburne, p 563)*

4. **(D)** About the knee, the skin is thick. In front of the knee, it is lax and freely movable, contributing to easy movement of the joint. The bony prominence anteriorly is the patella, a sesamoid bone in the quadriceps femoris tendon. *(Woodburne, p 564)*

5. **(C)** The hollow behind the knee is the popliteal fossa. The heavy cordlike tendons which form its boundaries are the tendon of the biceps femoris muscle laterally and the tendons of the semitendinosus and semimembranosus muscles medially. *(Woodburne, p 564)*

6. **(A)** The lesser saphenous vein leaves the foot behind the lateral malleolus, enters the leg on the lateral side of the calcaneal tendon, and ascends over the middle of the calf. It perforates the crural fascia, ending in the popliteal vein. *(Woodburne, p 565)*

7. **(A)** The tip of the lateral malleolus is 1.5 cm lower than the tip of the medial malleolus. Several centimeters below the tip of the medial malleolus, one can palpate the sustentaculum tali of the calcaneus and, an equal distance in front of the sustentaculum, the tuberosity of the navicular bone. *(Woodburne, p 565)*

8. **(C)** The greater saphenous vein, the longest vein of the body, turns deeply through the saphenous opening to empty into the femoral vein. Just before it turns through the saphenous opening, the greater saphenous vein receives the superficial epigastric, the superficial circumflex iliac, and the superficial external pudendal veins. The valves in the greater saphenous vein vary from 10 to 20 in number. Perforating communications interconnect the superficial and deep veins. *(Woodburne, pp 565–566)*

9. **(C)** The superficial inguinal nodes form a chain parallel to and about 1.5 cm below the inguinal ligament. These nodes receive lymph from the lower abdominal wall, the buttocks, the penis and scrotum (or the labia majora), and the perineum. The superficial inguinal nodes send their efferent mainly to the external iliac nodes. Only a few reach the deep inguinal nodes. *(Woodburne, p 567)*

10. **(A)** The saphenous nerve is the terminal branch of the femoral nerve. Arising from the femoral nerve in the femoral triangle, it enters the adductor canal, where it crosses the femoral vessels anteriorly from their lateral to their medial side. It descends in the leg in company with the greater saphenous vein. *(Woodburne, p 570)*

11. **(A)** The medial sural cutaneous nerve arises from the tibial nerve in the popliteal fossa. It descends in the groove between the two heads of the gastrocnemius muscle as far as the middle of the leg. Here, it pierces the deep fascia and is joined by the fibular (peroneal) communicating branch to form the sural nerve. It supplies the heel and foot areas. *(Woodburne, pp 570–571)*

12. **(D)** The fascia cribrosa, derived from subcutaneous connective tissue, fills the saphenous opening. *(Woodburne, p 573)*

13. **(B)** The femoral triangle is the subfascial space of the upper one-third of the thigh. It contains the first portion of the femoral vessels and branches of the femoral nerve. The triangle is bounded above by the inguinal ligament; laterally, by the medial border of the sartorius muscle; and medially, by the medial border of the adductor longus muscle. The crossing of the adductor longus by the sartorius closes the triangle below. The floor of the triangle is also muscular; it is represented medially by the pectineus and adductor longus muscles and, laterally, by the iliopsoas. The femoral artery bisects the triangle in a vertical direction. *(Woodburne, p 573)*

14. **(D)** The femoral sheath is a diverticulum of the transversalis fascia, which is prolonged along the femoral vessels and covers them on all sides for about 2 to 3 cm beyond the inguinal ligament. At its termination, its fibers blend with the adventitia of the blood vessels. The extraperitoneal connective tissue of the abdomen extends along the vessels and contributes to the three subdivisions of the sheath. *(Woodburne, p 574)*

15. **(C)** The femoral sheath is subdivided into three compartments by the extraperitoneal connective tissue—a lateral one for the artery, a middle one for the vein, and a medial one that lodges one or more deep inguinal lymph nodes and fat. The medial compartment is designated as the femoral canal. *(Woodburne, p 574)*

16. **(C)** The saphenous nerve enters the adductor canal lateral to the vessels, crosses them anteriorly, and lies medial to them at the lower end of the canal. The adductor canal is a facial compartment that conducts the femoral vessels through the middle one-third of the thigh. It begins about 15 cm below the inguinal ligament at the crossing of the sartorius muscle over the adductor longus muscle. The canal ends at the upper limit of the adductor hiatus where the femoral vessels pass to the back of the knee. *(Woodburne, p 574)*

17. **(A)** The popliteal fossa lies above and behind the knee. The space is diamond-shaped. The lateral and medial heads of the gastrocnemius muscle of the leg form the inferior sides of the diamond. The superior borders of the figure are produced by the diverging hamstring tendons. The posterior femoral cutaneous nerve and the tibial and common fibular (peroneal) divisions of the sciatic nerve cross the fossa. The tibial nerve runs through the fossa in a vertical direction. *(Woodburne, p 576)*

18. **(A)** The lateral femoral muscles lies in the gluteal region and include strong abductors and lateral rotators of the thigh. The medial femoral muscles are known as the adductor group and have adduction as their principal function. They are medial rotators. The anterior femoral muscles extend the leg at the knee. The medial femoral muscles are innervated by the obturator nerve. The sartorius is part of the anterior femoral group. *(Woodburne, pp 576–579)*

19. **(E)** The pectineus is a preaxial muscle and is included with the medial femoral muscles. The tensor fascia latae, piriformis, obturator internus, quadratus femoris, gemelli, and gluteal muscles are all located in the lateral femoral group. *(Woodburne, pp 576–579)*

20. **(C)** The anterior femoral muscles are all postaxial and are innervated by the femoral nerve. They include the sartorius (largest muscle in the body), the quadriceps femoris, and the articularis genu. The gracilis is located in the medial femoral muscles group. *(Woodburne, pp 579–581)*

21. **(D)** The posterior femoral muscles compose the "hamstring" group. They arise from the ischial tuberosity (preaxial) and are supplied by the tibial division of the sciatic nerve. The biceps femoris muscle, however, has a supplement origin from the femur, and this portion of the muscle (postaxial) is corresponding, supplied by the common fibular (peroneal) portion of the sciatic nerve. The "hamstring" muscles flex the leg and extend the thigh. *(Woodburne, pp 584–585)*

22. **(B)** The adductor tubercle is located on the medial epicondyle as a pointed projection on which the tendon of the adductor magnus muscle inserts. The linea aspera is a thickened ridge along the posterior middle one-third of the femur. The trochanters are joined behind by the intertrochanteric crest. *(Woodburne, p 587)*

23. **(A)** The obturator artery is a branch of the internal iliac artery that distributes largely outside the pelvis. Having passed through the obturator canal, the obturator artery divides at the upper margin of the obturator foramen into anterior and posterior branches. The posterior branch supplies the origin of the adductor magnus and gives off an acetabular branch. *(Woodburne, p 588)*

24. **(E)** The femoral artery enters the lower limb by passing under the inguinal ligament midway between the anterior superior spine of the ilium and the pubic symphysis. It descends through the femoral triangle and, at its apex, enters the adductor canal. The femoral canal contains only lymph

nodes and fat. The femoral artery does not pass through the femoral canal. *(Woodburne, pp 574,588)*

25. **(C)** The obturator nerve is the principal preaxial nerve of the lumbar plexus. It arises from the anterior branches of lumbar nerves 2, 3, and 4 and descends along the medial border of the psoas muscle. It enters the thigh through the obturator canal; the nerve divides into an anterior and a posterior branch. *(Woodburne, p 593)*

26. **(A)** The femoral nerve is the largest branch of the lumbar plexus. It is a postaxial nerve, formed by the posterior branches of the 2nd, 3rd, and 4th lumbar nerves. It passes under the inguinal ligament in the groove formed by the adjacent margins of the psoas and iliacus muscles and then enters the femoral triangle. It gives rise to the anterior femoral cutaneous and the saphenous. *(Woodburne, p 594)*

27. **(D)** The sciatic nerve arises from spinal cord segments L4 through S3. The sciatic nerve leaves the pelvis through the lower part of the greater sciatic foramen and extends from the inferior border of the piriformis muscle to the lower one-third of the thigh. Inferiorly, the nerve lies against the posterior surface of the adductor magnus muscle and is crossed obliquely by the long head of the biceps femoris muscle. *(Woodburne, p 595)*

28. **(C)** The muscles of the superficial posterior compartment are preaxial. They insert onto the tuberosity of the calcaneous and their contraction produces plantar flexion of the foot, not flexion of the toes. This compartment includes the gastrocnemius, soleus, and plantaris. *(Woodburne, pp 597–601)*

29. **(C)** The tibialis posterior is located in the deep posterior compartment, and the tibialis anterior is located in the anterior compartment. The tibialis posterior inserts into the tuberosity of the navicular and into the underside of the medial cuneiform bone. It is innervated by the tibial nerve, and it is a powerful adductor and inverter of the foot. *(Woodburne, pp 602–603)*

30. **(A)** The posterior tibial artery is the direct continuation of the popliteal artery. It descends in the deep posterior compartment of the leg and passes behind the medial malleolus at the ankle. Entering the foot, the artery divides beneath the origin of the adductor hallucis muscle into the medial plantar and lateral plantar arteries. The anterior tibial artery descends between the tibialis anterior and the extensor digitorum longus. It crosses the ankle to enter the dorsum of the foot as the dorsalis pedis artery.

31. **(E)** The plantar fascia forms a thickened plantar aponeurosis. The quadratus plantae lies on the superior aspect of the flexor digitorum brevis muscle. The quadratus plantae is an accessory muscle to the long digital flexor. It arises by two heads that are separated from each other by the long plantar ligament. The quadratus has a flattened band that inserts into the tendon of the flexor digitorum longus muscle. *(Woodburne, pp 614,618)*

32. **(C)** The central compartment, deep to the plantar aponeurosis, is bounded by the lateral intermuscular and medial intermuscular septa at its borders. It is occupied by the flexor digitorum brevis, the muscles associated with the tendons of the flexor digitorum longus muscle—quadratus plantae and the four lumbricals. The dorsal interosseous muscles are located in the interosseous adductor compartment. *(Woodburne, pp 616–619)*

33. **(D)** The iliofemoral ligament lies on the anterior surface of the articular capsule. It has the form of an inverted y. The stem of the inverted y is attached by its apex to the lower part of the anterior inferior iliac spine. The diverging fibers of the ligament attach to the entire length of the intertrochanteric line. The iliofemoral ligament becomes taut in full extension and thus helps to maintain the erect posture. *(Woodburne, p 622)*

34. **(D)** The ligamentum capitis femoris is intracapsular. It arises from the acetabular notch and the transverse ligament of the acetabulum. It is approximately 3.5 cm in length and ends in the fovea of the head of the femur. It is covered by a sleeve of synovial membrane and becomes taut in adduction of the femur. *(Woodburne, p 622)*

35. **(D)** Only the bursa anserina separates the tibial collateral ligament from the overlying insertions of the sartorius, gracilis, and semitendinosus muscles. The ligamentum patellae is the continuation of the tendon of the quadriceps femoris. A deep, infrapatellar bursa intervenes between the ligament and the bone immediately superior to the insertion. A large subcutaneous infrapatellar bursa is developed in the subcutaneous tissue over the ligament. *(Woodburne, pp 624–625)*

36. **(D)** The medial meniscus is a crescent-shaped wafer of fibrocartilage that is thicker at its external margins. It attaches in the anterior intercondylar area of the tibia in front of the anterior cruciate ligament. Its posterior attachment is in the corresponding posterior fossa in front of the origin of the posterior cruciate ligament. *(Woodburne, p 626)*

37. **(C)** The lateral meniscus is fibrocartilage that covers a somewhat greater proportion of the tibial

surface than does the medial meniscus. Its anterior end is attached in the anterior intercondylar area lateral to and behind the end of the anterior cruciate ligament. Its posterior termination is in the posterior intercondylar area in front of the end of the medial meniscus. Close to its posterior attachment, it frequently sends off a collection of fibers, the posterior meniscofemoral ligament. *(Woodburne, p 626)*

38. **(C)** The anterior cruciate ligament arises from the rough, nonarticular area in front of the intercondylar eminence of the tibia and extends upward and backward to the posterior part of the medial aspect of the lateral femoral condyle. The anterior cruciate ligament prevents anterior displacement of the tibia. It is somewhat taut in all positions of flexion but becomes tightest in full extension and full flexion. *(Woodburne, p 626)*

39. **(B)** The posterior cruciate ligament extends from the area behind the tibial intercondylar eminence to the lateral side of the medial condyle of the femur. The posterior cruciate ligament prevents posterior displacement of the tibia. It is taut in all positions of flexion but becomes tightest in full extension and full flexion. The cruciate ligaments lie within the capsule of the knee joint. *(Woodburne, p 626)*

40. **(D)** The deltoid ligament is a strong triangular ligament that is attached by its apex to the anterior and posterior borders and the tip of the medial malleolus. The ligament broadens below to form a continuous attachment to the bones of the foot. The anterior and posterior tibiotalar ligaments extend to the talus. The tibionavicular extends to the navicular bone, and the tibiocalcaneal ligament attaches to the sustentaculum tali of the calcaneus. *(Woodburne, p 630)*

41. **(D)** The talus articulates with many bones—the tibia and the fibula above and at the sides, the calcaneus below, and the navicular in front. It does not provide attachment for muscles but does receive ligaments. Its upper portion is known as the trochlea. The calcaneus is the largest and strongest bone of the foot. *(Woodburne, pp 632–633)*

42. **(E)** The first metatarsal bone is the shortest, broadest, and most massive of the series. The tuberosity of the 1st metatarsal bone provides an insertion for the peroneus longus muscle. The 2nd metatarsal bone is the longest. The tuberosity of the 5th metatarsal gives insertion to the peroneus brevis tendon. The bodies are narrow and tend to be triangular in cross-section. *(Woodburne, p 634)*

43. **(C)** The adductor hallucis muscle arises by oblique and transverse heads. The tendons of both heads insert into the lateral side of the base of the proximal phalanx of the great toe. The lateral plantar nerve supplies the abductor digiti minimi, flexor digiti minimi brevis, quadratus plantae, adductor hallucis, the dorsal and plantar interosseous, and the lateral three lumbrical muscles. The adductor hallucis adducts the great toe and aids in maintaining the arches of the foot. *(Woodburne, pp 618–621)*

44. **(E)** The fibular collateral ligament becomes taut in extension and prevents hyperextension. It also prevents an abduction or adduction angulation of the bones. The tendon of the popliteus muscle passes deep to the fibular collateral ligament, and the tendon of the biceps femoris muscle divides on either side of its lower attachment. *(Woodburne, p 625)*

45. **(A)** The inferior genicular blood vessels pass between the collateral ligaments and the capsule of the knee joint. The tendon of the popliteus muscle passes deep to the fibular collateral ligament. *(Woodburne, p 625)*

46. **(D)** Notable on the sole of the foot are the long plantar ligament, and the plantar calcaneocuboid and plantar calcaneonavicular ligaments. The elasticity of the latter and its support of the head of the talus have led to its being called the "spring ligament." *(Woodburne, p 639)*

47. **(C)** The lateral ligaments are the anterior talofibular, the calcaneofibular, and the posterior talofibular. These are separate ligaments and do not constitute so strong a ligamentous connection as does the deltoid ligament on the medial side. The anterior and posterior talofibular ligaments connect the lateral malleolus to the talus. The posterior talofibular ligament is almost horizontal as it passes medially from the lateral malleolus to the posterior process of the talus. The calcaneofibular ligament extends from the lateral malleolus to the lateral side of the calcaneus, not to the medial surface where the sustentaculum tali is located. *(Woodburne, pp 630–631)*

48. **(E)** The flexor retinaculum covers a number of structures that pass behind the medial malleolus—the tendon of the tibialis posterior muscle, the tendon of the flexor digitorum longus muscle, the tendon of the flexor hallucis longus muscle, the posterior tibial artery and veins, and the tibial nerve. *(Woodburne, p 611)*

49. **(E)** The lower limb is separated from the pelvic portion of the trunk by the external borders of the pelvic bones, together with their associated ligaments. Thus, the uppermost limits of the limb are the iliac crest, the inguinal ligament, the symphysis pubis, the ischiopubic ramus, the ischial tuberosity, the sacrotuberal ligament, and the dorsum of the sacrum and the coccyx. *(Woodburne, p 563)*

50. **(C)** The peroneus longus inserts into the inferolateral surface of the medial cuneiform bone and on the base and inferolateral border of the first metatarsal bone. The soleus and plantaris insert into the calcaneus. The tibialis posterior inserts into the tuberosity of the navicular and into the underside of the medial cuneiform bone. *(Woodburne, pp 600–601)*

51. **(B)** The gluteal region is the natis, clunis, or buttock. The malleoli are bony projections of the ankle. Sura is the calf of the leg; tarsus is the region of the ankle; and hallux is the big toe. *(Hollinshead, p 334)*

52. **(E)** All the items are correct except E. The hip joint is not at all identical to the shoulder joint, as it is far stronger structurally than the shoulder. The upper end of the femur fits into a deep, cup-like cavity, the acetabulum, while the glenoid cavity is shallow and does not hold the head of the humerus tightly. The femur, corresponding to the humerus, is the largest bone of the body. The pelvic girdle is directly and firmly attached to the vertebral column, and the two coxal bones firmly articulate with each other at the midline. *(Hollinshead, p 336)*

53. **(A)** The 2nd, 3rd, and 4th lumbar nerves typically contribute to the two major branches of the lumbar plexus. The sacral plexus, not the lumbar plexus, gives rise to the sciatic nerve. Most of the branches of the sacral, not the lumbar plexus, enter the buttock. The sacral plexus gives rise to the tibial nerve, a component of the sciatic nerve, that is distributed to muscles of the calf and the plantar aspect of the foot. *(Hollinshead, pp 339–340)*

54. **(D)** The arterial stem of the lower limb is the femoral artery, the continuation of the external iliac artery at the inguinal ligament. The popliteal artery is the continuation of the femoral artery as it passes into the posterior aspect of the thigh behind the knee. The anterior and posterior tibial arteries are branches of the popliteal artery. Superficial veins are subject to becoming varicose. Communicating veins normally conduct blood from superficial into deep veins. *(Hollinshead, pp 343–345)*

55. **(C)** The small saphenous vein begins along the lateral margin of the foot, passes upward along the posterior aspect of the calf, and commonly ends in the popliteal vein. The superficial veins (greater and lesser saphenous veins) originate on the dorsum, not the sole, of the foot. The great saphenous vein runs up the medial side of the limb, not the lateral side; it can be seen on the medial side of the knee. The deep lymphatic vessels follow blood vessels, and there are few deep lymph nodes. The superficial lymphatics are numerous and run up all surfaces of the leg. *(Hollinshead, p 345)*

56. **(A)** The femoral artery continues into the leg and foot, but the anterior nerves, chiefly femoral and obturator, are distributed almost entirely to the thigh. Arteries entering the buttock are distributed almost entirely to this part, but the sciatic nerve continues through the buttock and the thigh to supply all the muscles of the leg and foot and most of the skin of these parts. *(Hollinshead, pp 349–350)*

57. **(D)** Ossification of the coxal bone occurs from three primary centers, one each for the ilium, ischium, and pubis. These centers fuse over a considerable range of time, but usually ossification of the coxal bone is complete by age 20 to 21 years. The ilium forms the upper part of the acetabulum. The pubis forms the anterior part of the acetabulum and the anteromedial part of the hip bone. The ischium forms the posterior inferior part of the acetabulum and the lower posterior part of the hip bone. The acetabular notch is in the inferior, not the superior, wall of the acetabulum. *(Hollinshead, pp 350,353)*

58. **(A)** The continuation of the labrum of the acetabulum across the acetabular notch is called the transverse acetabular ligament. Between it and the edge of the notch is loose connective tissue, through which one or more acetabular arteries enter the joint. The transverse acetabular ligament does not add to stability of the joint. The sacroiliac joint is reinforced by heavy ligaments. The sacrotuberous ligament is a particularly strong bracing ligament of the sacroiliac joint; it forms the medial border of both the greater and lesser sciatic foramina. The sacrospinous ligament runs between the sacrum and coccyx and the ischial spine; it separates the greater sciatic foramen from the lesser sciatic foramen. The sacrotuberous and sacro-spinous ligaments are so placed as to resist rotation of the sacrum between the coxal bones. The iliolumbar ligament attaches to the anterior or pelvic surface of the ilium and sacrum. *(Hollinshead, pp 353–356,395–396)*

59. **(C)** The arteries to the upper end of the femur are derived mostly from the medial and lateral femoral circumflex arteries, the two largest branches of the profunda femoris artery. The artery of the ligament of the head of the femur, derived from the obturator or the medial femoral circumflex artery, enters the head through the liga-

ment of the head and supplies a variable amount of bone adjacent to the fovea. Otherwise, the head and neck are supplied by branches of the two circumflex arteries. *(Hollinshead, pp 359–360,388)*

60. **(E)**   The gluteus maximus muscle arises from the outer surface of the ilium behind the posterior gluteal line, from the dorsal surface of the sacrum and coccyx, and from the adjacent sacrotuberous ligament. It is inserted into both the iliotibial tract and the gluteal tuberosity of the femur. It receives its nerve supply from the inferior gluteal nerve, and its primary action is extension at the hip joint. It does not pass through the greater sciatic foramen. *(Hollinshead, pp 362–365)*

61. **(D)**   The chief action of the gluteus medius is abduction of the free limb. More importantly, together with the gluteus minimus, it keeps the contralateral side of the pelvis from sagging markedly when the weight of the body is put upon one limb; therefore, these muscles are exceedingly important in walking. Only the gluteus minimus is active in flexion and medial rotation of the femur. Apparently, the gluteus medius assists with extension and lateral rotation of movements. It is not a chief actor in the movements of adduction, medial rotation, or flexion at the hip joint. *(Hollinshead, p 365)*

62. **(B)**   The distribution of the superior and inferior gluteal vessels primarily is confined to the buttock. The internal pudendal artery primarily passes through the buttock to another distribution. The femoral artery and its branch, the profunda femoris, are not vessels of the gluteal region. *(Hollinshead, pp 366,387)*

63. **(E)**   Neither of the muscles—gluteus medius or gluteus minimus—is a strong flexor at the hip joint, although the gluteus minimus may act in the movement. The gluteus minimus also has been shown by electromyography to be active in medial rotation of the thigh, while the gluteus medius apparently is active only in lateral rotation and extension of the thigh. These muscles are similar in all the other choices listed. *(Hollinshead, pp 363–365)*

64. **(A)**   The sciatic nerve consists of two nerves—the tibial and common peroneal—that are bound together closely by connective tissue. The sciatic nerve normally emerges below the piriformis muscle, although it may come through the muscle, or the nerve may be divided by the muscle. It always runs across the posterior surfaces of the obturator internus, gemelli, and quadratus femoris muscles. It gives off no fibers to muscles of the buttock. As it runs down the thigh, it disappears deep to the hamstring muscles that arise from the ischial tuberosity. *(Hollinshead, p 368)*

65. **(B)**   The fascia lata of the thigh consists of dense, deep fascia reinforced by a particularly strong lateral band, the iliotibial tract. The fascia lata is rather weak over the medial adductor muscles but is stronger both anteriorly and posteriorly. Laterally, it splits to go on both sides of the tensor fasciae latae muscle. At the knee, in general, the fascia lata loses its identity, for it blends with expansions from the tendons at the knee to help form the patellar retinacula and then becomes continuous with the fascia of the leg. Just below the inguinal ligament, the fascia lata presents a defect, the saphenous hiatus, through which passes the great saphenous vein to enter the femoral vein. *(Hollinshead, pp 372–373)*

66. **(B)**   The quadriceps is the only muscle that can extend the knee; the sartorius can only flex it. Of the quadriceps group, the rectus femoris is most efficient as a knee extensor when the hip is extended because it attaches above the hip joint. It does not, however, assist in the last 10 to 15 degrees or more of knee extension, leaving this to the vasti. The vastus medialis, vastus lateralis, and vastus intermedius all participate in extension at the knee joint. The articularis genus inserts into the suprapatellar bursa of the knee joint and pulls this up as the knee is extended to prevent it getting caught in the joint. *(Hollinshead, p 381)*

67. **(E)**   The femoral nerve usually sends two branches to the rectus femoris muscle. The nerve contains both muscular and cutaneous branches that are given off in no particular order. Its cutaneous branches to the thigh are the anterior femoral cutaneous nerves. The other cutaneous branch of the femoral nerve, the saphenous nerve, runs through most of the length of the adductor canal and is distributed to the leg and the foot. The femoral nerve usually contains fibers from the 2nd, 3rd, and 4th lumbar nerves; it lies lateral to the femoral vessels in the femoral triangle. The obturator nerve supplies the anterior portion of the adductor magnus, and the tibial nerve its posterior portion. *(Hollinshead, pp 384–385)*

68. **(A)**   The short head of the biceps femoris is the muscle listed that does not arise from the ischial tuberosity. Its long head arises from the ischial tuberosity; the short head arises from the lateral lip of the linea aspera of the femur. *(Hollinshead, p 389)*

69. **(B)**   The posterior part of the adductor magnus, arising from the ischial tuberosity, extends vertically downward and reaches the lowest attachment of the muscle, the adductor tubercle on the femur. It, therefore, does not cross the posterior knee but is an extensor of the hip. All of the other

muscles listed have attachments on the tibia below the knee. *(Hollinshead, pp 374,381–382,389)*

70. **(B)**   The biceps femoris muscle receives innervation from both tibial and common peroneal nerves of the sciatic, the long head from the tibial nerve, and the short head from the common peroneal nerve. The semitendinosus and semimembranosus muscles receive innervation from only the tibial nerve. The posterior part of the adductor magnus receives innervation from the tibial nerve; its anterior part is supplied by the obturator nerve. The gracilis receives fibers from neither the tibial or common peroneal nerve; it is innervated by the anterior branch of the obturator nerve. *(Hollinshead, pp 381,383,390)*

71. **(D)**   The posterior part of the adductor magnus can extend the thigh, along with the other muscles arising from the ischial tuberosity. It can extend the thigh without at the same time producing flexion at the knee because it inserts above the knee and, therefore, cannot act over the knee. The long head of the biceps, the semitendinosus, and the semimembranosus all extend the hip and flex the knee. The short head of the biceps can only flex the knee because it arises on the femur below the hip joint. *(Hollinshead, p 392)*

72. **(A)**   The popliteal fossa is the area posterior to the knee. Its lower borders are formed by the two heads of the gastrocnemius muscle that arise from the medial and lateral condyles of the femur and converge to a union in the upper part of the calf. In the upper part of the fossa, the sciatic nerve lies posterolateral to the popliteal vessels. The popliteal vein is next anteriorly, and the popliteal artery is the most anterior, lying directly on the popliteal surface of the femur. The common peroneal nerve diverges laterally to pass around the lateral side of the leg. The tibial nerve descends almost straight down through the fossa. *(Hollinshead, p 392)*

73. **(E)**   The talus lies above the calcaneus and receives body weight from the tibia. The cuboid lies laterally in the foot, in front of the calcaneus. The calcaneus is the largest, not the smallest, tarsal bone. The navicular lies just posterior to the cuneiforms and in front of the talus. The cuneiforms lie medial to the cuboid and in front of the navicular. *(Hollinshead, pp 405–406)*

74. **(C)**   The transverse arch lies at the level of the distal row of tarsals rather than at the proximal row. All of the other statements regarding the arches of the foot are correct. Although it is convenient to describe two arches, longitudinal and transverse, they interlock so that they form a functioning single arch of complex form. Weight is distributed in this arch according to the engineering principle that the distribution of stress throughout an arch is strictly proportional to the relative heights of various parts of the arch. This is true only when the arch is loaded from the top, which is, in the normal foot, the talus. *(Hollinshead, pp 411–412)*

75. **(B)**   Because the trochlea tali is grasped so firmly between the medial and lateral malleoli, little movement is possible at the talocrural joint except flexion and extension. A certain amount of inversion and eversion is possible at the subtalar joint because the calcaneus, underlying the talus, can rock from side to side. Movement occurs also between other tarsal bones, but the greatest amount of movement occurs at the transverse tarsal joint—dorsiflexion, plantar flexion, and two combined movements, one of eversion and abduction and one of inversion and adduction. *(Hollinshead, p 412)*

76. **(D)**   The obturator nerve does not extend down into the leg area and, therefore, does not provide cutaneous innervation to that region. It does give rise to an articular branch to the knee joint that descends along the femoral artery; it also gives rise to the cutaneous branch of the obturator distributed to skin on the medial side of the thigh. The saphenous nerve, from the femoral, the superficial peroneal nerve, the lateral and medial sural cutaneous nerves, and the posterior femoral cutaneous nerve all supply areas of skin of the leg. *(Hollinshead, pp 385–386,413–414)*

77. **(C)**   The extensor hallucis longus primarily is an extensor of the big toe, but it is also in a position to dorsiflex, adduct, and invert the foot. The extensor digitorum longus and the peroneus tertius also dorsiflex the foot but are located more laterally, so that instead of inverting, they evert and abduct the foot. The peroneus longus and brevis both evert the foot. They are also plantar flexors instead of dorsiflexors. *(Hollinshead, pp 416,420,423)*

78. **(A)**   The tibialis anterior does not arise from the fibula but from the lateral surface of the tibia, from the interosseous membrane, from an upper part of its covering fascia, and from an intermuscular septum between it and the extensor digitorum longus. The extensor digitorum longus has some origin from the tibia, but it arises mostly from the fibula and the anterior intermuscular septum. The other muscles listed arise from the fibula. *(Hollinshead, pp 420–421)*

79. **(D)**   All of the muscles listed, except the peroneus brevis, are innervated by the deep peroneal nerve. They are all dorsiflexors of the foot. The peroneus brevis is innervated by the superficial peroneal

nerve and is an abductor and weak plantar flexor of the foot. *(Hollinshead, pp 420,423)*

80.   **(B)**   The dorsalis pedis artery typically is the continuation of the anterior tibial artery after it passes under the inferior extensor retinaculum onto the dorsum of the foot. The dorsalis pedis usually appears just medial to the deep peroneal nerve on the dorsum of the foot. It runs distally toward the interspace between the first and second toes. *(Hollinshead, p 424)*

81.   **(D)**   The peroneus tertius arises from the fibula and the anterior intermuscular septum. This origin is continuous with that of the extensor digitorum longus, and the two tendons pass together across the ankle. The tendon of the peroneus tertius diverges laterally to insert into the dorsal surface of the base of the 5th metatarsal. This muscle, therefore, is placed on the dorsal surface of the foot and becomes a dorsiflexor, not a plantar flexor. The other muscles listed are plantar flexors. *(Hollinshead, pp 421,423,429)*

82.   **(A)**   The popliteal artery, the continuation of the femoral artery when it enters the popliteal fossa, descends through the middle of the popliteal fossa anterior to the popliteal vein; it accompanies the tibial nerve deep to the gastrocnemius and soleus muscles. It ends by dividing into the anterior and posterior tibial arteries; this division usually occurs on the posterior surface of the popliteus muscle. The anterior tibial artery then turns forward below the muscle and above the interosseous membrane to continue down the anterior aspect of the leg. *(Hollinshead, pp 432–433)*

83.   **(C)**   The femoral artery runs downward in the adductor canal. Close to the lower end of the canal, the artery gives off its last named branch, the descending genicular artery; this artery gives off branches on the medial side of the knee that anastomose with branches of arteries on the lateral side of the knee to form a pattern of collateral circulation around this joint. The popliteal artery gives off the medial and lateral superior genicular arteries that run medially and laterally around the femur to help form collateral circulation of the knee joint. Medial and lateral inferior genicular arteries that encircle the leg also help form the anastomoses around the knee. *(Hollinshead, pp 389, 432)*

84.   **(C)**   The gastrocnemius and soleus muscles are referred to as the triceps surae. These two muscles, along with the plantaris muscle, insert into the tendo calcaneus (tendon of Achilles). The posterior and anterior tibial muscles are not a part of the triceps surae. The triceps is innervated by the tibial nerve. *(Basmajian, pp 277–278)*

85.   **(E)**   The superficial epigastric artery arises from the femoral artery, not the profunda femoral. The profunda femoris artery usually branches from the lateral side of the femoral artery about 4 cm below the inguinal ligament. It gives off the lateral and medial femoral circumflex arteries. Usually, it gives off four perforating arteries that encircle the shaft of the femur tightly, perforating any muscle they encounter. *(Basmajian, pp 267–268)*

Clinical Upper Limbs
Questions

DIRECTIONS (Questions 1 through 15): Each of the numbered items or incomplete statements in this section is followed by answers or by completions of the statement. Select the ONE lettered answer or completion that is BEST in each case.

1. The paralysis of which of the following muscles results in a "winged scapula" and inability to elevate the arm above the horizontal?

   (A) infraspinatus
   (B) subscapularis
   (C) deltoid
   (D) serratus anterior
   (E) trapezius

2. Damage to which of the following nerves results in the loss of opposition in the thumb?

   (A) ulnar
   (B) motor branch of the median
   (C) musculocutaneous
   (D) radial
   (E) axillary

3. Dupytren's contracture is a pathological thickening and contracture of fibers of the

   (A) thenar fascia
   (B) palmar aponeurosis
   (C) hypothenar fascia
   (D) superficial transverse metacarpal ligament
   (E) external abdominal aponeurosis

4. Which of the following bones is the most frequently fractured bone of the body?

   (A) humerus
   (B) tibia
   (C) first metacarpal
   (D) axis
   (E) clavicle

5. Fractures of the humerus through its mid or upper shaft carry the danger of serious damage to the

   (A) brachial artery
   (B) radial nerve
   (C) musculocutaneous nerve
   (D) median nerve
   (E) ulnar nerve

6. The fracture of which of the following bones is dangerous because ischemic necrosis may result?

   (A) distal end of the radius
   (B) clavicle
   (C) 5th metacarpal
   (D) scaphoid
   (E) olecranon process

7. Injury to the upper part of the brachial plexus usually results

   (A) from violent separation of head and shoulder
   (B) in spastic paralysis of the upper limb
   (C) in Klumpke's paralysis
   (D) in paralysis of the hand
   (E) in involvement of nerves C8 and T1

8. An injury to the spinal accessory nerve primarily would affect

   (A) adduction of the arm at the glenohumeral joint
   (B) lateral rotation of the arm
   (C) depression of the scapula
   (D) protraction of the scapula
   (E) upward rotation of the scapula

9. In the usual pattern of digital synovial tendon sheaths, infection can travel into the common flexor tendon sheath at the wrist from the

   (A) thumb
   (B) index finger
   (C) middle finger
   (D) ring finger
   (E) little finger

10. Which of the following statements is true of Colles' fracture?

   (A) it occurs more frequently in men than in women
   (B) it involves the distal end of the radius
   (C) it causes displacement of the lunate
   (D) it usually involves the styloid process
   (E) it is the most common type of fracture in young people

11. When the median nerve is severed in the elbow region, there is loss of all of the following EXCEPT

   (A) flexion of the proximal interphalangeal joints of the 2nd and 3rd digits
   (B) flexion of the distal interphalangeal joints of the index and middle fingers
   (C) flexion of the metacarpophalangeal joints of the index and middle fingers
   (D) flexion of the distal interphalangeal joints of the ring and little fingers
   (E) flexion of the proximal interphalangeal joints of the 4th and 5th joints

12. Symptoms of carpal tunnel syndrome may include

   (A) loss of abduction of the thumb
   (B) absence of tactile sensation on the palmar surface of the index finger
   (C) loss of flexion at the distal interphalangeal joint of the 4th and 5th digits
   (D) paresthesia on the palmar surface of the middle finger
   (E) diminished sensation in the digits

13. All of the following characteristics of a cystic, usually nontender swelling of a tendon on the dorsum of the wrist or hand are correct EXCEPT

   (A) flexion of the wrist makes the swelling enlarge
   (B) the swelling is a collection of nerve cells
   (C) the swelling often communicates with the extensor synovial sheaths
   (D) clinically this swelling is called a "ganglion"
   (E) extension of the wrist makes the swelling smaller

14. All of the following locations may be used in measuring the pulse rate EXCEPT

   (A) where the radial artery crosses the distal end of the radius
   (B) in the anatomical snuffbox
   (C) between the tendons of the flexor carpi radialis and abductor pollicis longus muscles
   (D) between the abductor pollicis longus and the extensor pollicis longus posteriorly
   (E) across the medial aspect of the pisiform bone

15. Which of the following muscles is most commonly damaged in rotator cuff injuries?

   (A) supraspinatus
   (B) infraspinatus
   (C) subcapularis
   (D) teres minor
   (E) teres major

ANSWERS AND EXPLANATIONS

1. **(D)** The paralysis of the serratus anterior results in a "winged scapula" and inability to elevate the arm above the horizontal. The serratus anterior is innervated by the long thoracic nerve. (*Woodburne, p 117*)

2. **(B)** The median nerve passes through the wrist under the flexor retinaculum and enters the central compartment of the palm. At the distal border of the flexor retinaculum, a stout branch is given off from its radial side. This motor branch of the median nerve supplies the short abductor, the short flexor, and the opponens muscles of the thumb. Damage to this superficially placed nerve results in the loss of opposition in the thumb. (*Woodburne, pp 153–154*)

3. **(B)** Dupytren's contracture is a pathological thickening and contracture of fibers of the palmar aponeurosis. It produces marked tension on the digits with flexion, the digital tendons becoming like bowstrings; the hand may become practically useless. (*Woodburne, p 157*)

4. **(E)** The clavicle is the most frequently fractured bone of the body and fracture occurs most commonly in its middle third, the region of transition of its curvatures. In such a fracture, the weight of the limb and the pull of the pectoralis major muscle cause the distal portion of the clavicle to drop below the proximal fragment. (*Woodburne, p 177*)

5. **(B)** Fractures of the humerus through its mid or upper shaft carry the danger of serious damage to the radial nerve as it lies in its groove along the

posterior and lateral surfaces of the bone, resulting in "wrist drop" from paralysis of the forearm extensors. A supracondylar fracture may do damage to the vessels and nerves at the elbow. (Woodburne, p 177)

6. **(D)** Fracture of the scaphoid bone of the wrist is not uncommon. This occurs at the isthmus of the bone and nonunion or ischemic necrosis may result if viable blood vessels reach only one of the two fragments. (Woodburne, p 177)

7. **(A)** The brachial plexus is often injured by violent separation of the head and shoulder, as may occur in a fall from a motorcycle. These injuries commonly affect the upper part of the plexus. This is also a common type of birth injury resulting from a difficult delivery. Such lesions involving the upper part of the plexus (especially C5 and C6) are called Erb's or Erb–Duchenne paralysis and especially affect the shoulder and arm. Injuries to the lower part of the plexus (C8 and T1) are frequently called Klumpke's paralysis and especially affect the distal part of the limb. This injury does not result in spastic paralysis, as it is a peripheral, not a central nervous system, injury. (Hollinshead, p 187)

8. **(E)** The spinal accessory nerve innervates the trapezius. This muscle as a whole retracts the scapula, but its upper and lower fibers, acting together, upwardly rotate the scapula (turn the glenoid cavity upward). The other actions listed would not be major results of an injury to the spinal accessory nerve. (Hollinshead, p 195)

9. **(E)** The fibrous digital sheaths end proximally over the metacarpal heads, as do the synovial sheaths, except for the little finger. Therefore, if this usual pattern is present, an infection within the sheath of the little finger can easily travel into the common flexor tendon sheath at the wrist. Infections within the other tendon sheaths must be retained within them or must break through their walls. (Hollinshead, pp 252,264)

The tendon of the flexor pollicis longus usually is not involved in the common flexor synovial tendon sheath, although it also may join the sheath. (Basmajian, p 382)

10. **(B)** Colles' fracture, involving the distal end of the radius, occurs more frequently in women than in men. The distal fragment is usually tilted backward and slightly to the lateral side. This dorsal displacement produces a characteristic hump, described as the "dinner fork" deformity. Usually, Colles' fracture does not involve displacement of the lunate bone. It is more common in persons over 50 years of age. (Moore, p 625)

11. **(D)** When the median nerve is severed in the elbow region, there is loss of flexion of the proximal interphalangeal joints of all the digits; this is because of paralysis of the flexor digitorum superficialis muscle, which flexes at these joints. There is also loss of the median nerve innervation to the flexor digitorum profundus. The ability to flex at the metacarpophalangeal joints of the index and middle fingers is affected because the digital branches of the median nerve supply the 1st and 2nd lumbrical muscles. Flexion of the distal interphalangeal joints of the ring and little fingers is not affected because the part of the flexor digitorum profundus producing these movements is supplied by the ulnar nerve. The ability to flex the metacarpophalangeal joints of the 2nd and 3rd digits will be affected. (Moore, pp 575–576)

12. **(C)** The carpal bones articulate with one another and are bound together with ligaments to form a compact mass with a posterior convexity and an anterior concavity. The carpal sulcus thus formed on the anterior side is converted into an osseofibrous carpal tunnel (canal) by the flexor retinaculum. This tunnel is filled completely by tendons and the median nerve. Any lesion that significantly reduces the size of the carpal tunnel may cause compression of the median nerve, resulting in absence of tactile sensation on the palmar surface of the index finger and paresthesia on the palmar surface of the middle finger; these effects are seen on the palmar skin of the thumb and lateral half of the ring finger. Motor effects are seen in those thumb muscles innervated by the median nerve. Adduction of the thumb is not affected because the pollicis adductor muscle is usually supplied by the ulnar nerve, as is the ulnar portion of the flexor digitorum profundus that flexes at the distal interphalangeal joints of these digits. There is often diminished sensation in the digits. (Moore, p 603)

13. **(B)** Sometimes a cystic, usually nontender swelling of a tendon appears on the dorsum of the wrist or hand. Usually, the swelling is the size of a grape but can be larger. Flexion of the wrist makes the swelliong enlarge, and extension of it tends to make it smaller. Clinically, this type of swelling is called a "ganglion." Anatomically, a ganglion refers to a collection of nerve cells, which is not the case here. These swellings often communicate with the extensor synovial sheaths. (Moore, p 582)

14. **(E)** The most common place for measuring the pulse rate is where the radial artery lies on the anterior surface of the distal end of the radius, lateral to the tendon of the flexor carpi radialis muscle, and medial to the abductor pollicis longus muscle. A radial pulse may also be felt in the

"anatomical snuffbox," which is located between the tendons of the abductor pollicis longus and the extensor pollicis brevis anteriorly and the tendon of the extensor pollicis longus posteriorly. *(Moore, pp 581–582)*

15. **(A)** The supraspinatus tendon is the most commonly torn part of the rotator cuff. This injury is common in baseball pitchers. *(Moore, pp 537–539)*

Clinical Lower Limbs
Questions

DIRECTIONS (Questions 1 through 20): Each of the numbered items or incomplete statements in this section is followed by answers or by completions of the statement. Select the ONE lettered answer or completion that is BEST in each case.

1. Congenital dislocation of the hip is thought to be due to a faulty development of the

    (A) shaft of the femur
    (B) acetabulum
    (C) greater and lesser trochanters
    (D) neck of the femur
    (E) pelvic brim

2. Traumatic dislocation of the hip may include all of the following EXCEPT

    (A) the capsule may be ruptured
    (B) the head of the femur may be in the posterior iliac fossa
    (C) the limb may be shortened
    (D) the limb may be abducted and laterally rotated
    (E) the knee on the affected side tending to overlie the normal knee

3. Which of the following injuries is commonly associated with ischemic degeneration?

    (A) a fracture of the femoral neck
    (B) a fracture of the upper third of the shaft of the femur
    (C) a supracondylar fracture of the lower end of the femur
    (D) congenital dislocation of the hip
    (E) dislocation of the knee

4. All of the following are observed with damage to the common fibular (peroneal) nerve EXCEPT

    (A) footdrop
    (B) the foot turns inward

(C) the patient has a loss of the extensors of the foot
(D) the patient has a loss of the extensors of the toes
(E) the patient cannot plantar flex the ankle

5. All of the following statements concerning a femoral hernia are correct EXCEPT

    (A) the femoral canal is the usual site of the hernia
    (B) it commonly bulges forward under the skin
    (C) it emerges lateral and inferior to the public tubercle
    (D) the inner covering of the femoral hernia is the parietal peritoneum
    (E) the femoral hernia commonly extends into the adductor canal

6. All of the following statements concerning a saphenous varix are correct EXCEPT

    (A) it is a dilation of the great saphenous vein anterior to the medial malleolus
    (B) it is a dilation of the great saphenous vein at its terminal part
    (C) it may be confused with a femoral hernia
    (D) it may result in a swelling in the femoral triangle
    (E) it is located just inferior to the inguinal ligament

7. If it is necessary to ligate the femoral artery, blood is supplied to the lower limb through which of the following vessels?

    (A) great saphenous vein
    (B) cruciate anastomosis
    (C) genicular anastomosis
    (D) malleolar network
    (E) small saphenous vein

8. Gluteal intramuscular injections can be made safely only into which of the areas of the buttock?

   (A) tip of the coccyx
   (B) superomedial area
   (C) superolateral area
   (D) inferomedial area
   (E) level of the gluteal fold

9. In the lower limb, which of the following nerves is most commonly injured?

   (A) sciatic
   (B) femoral
   (C) obturator
   (D) common peroneal
   (E) tibial

10. Which of the following bones is the most common to be fractured and to suffer compound injury?

    (A) femur
    (B) tibia
    (C) fibula
    (D) patella
    (E) ischium

11. Pott's fracture involves the

    (A) lateral malleolus
    (B) greater trochanter
    (C) adductor tubercle
    (D) neck of the femur
    (E) acetabulum

12. The ankle reflex involves which of the following cord segments?

    (A) L2–4
    (B) S1–2
    (C) S3–5
    (D) L4–3
    (E) L1–2

13. All of the following statements concerning the tibial nerve are correct EXCEPT

    (A) it is deep and well protected
    (B) it is commonly injured
    (C) it innervates the plantar flexors of the foot
    (D) posterior dislocation of the knee may damage the nerve
    (E) injury to this nerve may be associated with the development of pressure sores

14. All of the following statements concerning intermittent claudication are correct EXCEPT

    (A) it is characterized by leg cramps
    (B) it is related to ischemia of the leg muscles
    (C) it may develop during walking
    (D) it is caused by sciatic nerve compression
    (E) it usually disappears after rest

15. All of the following statements concerning the patellar reflex (knee reflex) are correct EXCEPT

    (A) it results in flexion of the leg
    (B) this reflex is abnormal whenever the femoral nerve is injured
    (C) damage to the reflex centers in the spinal cord segments (L_2, L_3, and L_4) will affect the patellar reflex
    (D) the vastus medialis muscle is involved in this reflex
    (E) the quadriceps femoris is involved in this reflex

16. Dislocation of the hip most usually occurs as a result of

    (A) a severe blow upon the knee while the hip is flexed
    (B) the body weight landing heavily on one foot as the body falls
    (C) a severe blow on the buttock while the hip is flexed
    (D) severe forced hyperextension of the hip while the knee is extended
    (E) an abnormal stretch upon the adductor muscles as the limb is forced into abduction

17. Which of the following fixed deformities is not characteristic of the typical congenital clubfoot?

    (A) dorsiflexion
    (B) plantarflexion
    (C) inversion
    (D) adduction
    (E) equinovarus

18. The common peroneal nerve is most easily injured

    (A) where it leaves the sciatic nerve in the popliteal fossa
    (B) as it branches into the short head of the biceps femoris
    (C) just behind the head of the fibula
    (D) where it emerges below the piriformis muscle
    (E) at the place it divides into the superficial and deep peroneal nerves

19. A femoral hernia usually passes through the

    (A) intermediate compartment
    (B) lateral compartment
    (C) medial compartment
    (D) adductor canal
    (E) inguinal canal

20. All of the following statements concerning a femoral hernia are correct EXCEPT

    (A) it is a weakness in the abdominal wall at the femoral ring
    (B) it is a protrusion of the intestine through the femoral ring into the femoral triangle
    (C) a possible strangulation may result in impairment of blood supply to the herniated bowel
    (D) it is a palpable mass inferolateral to the pubic tubercle
    (E) it passes through the lateral compartment of the femoral sheath

ANSWERS AND EXPLANATIONS

1. **(B)** Congenital dislocation of the hip is thought to be due to faulty development of the acetabulum, especially of its upper rim. The femoral head may also be poorly developed. The condition is much more common in girls. *(Woodburne, p 639)*

2. **(D)** Traumatic dislocation of the hip is not common except as the sequel of an automobile accident. The capsule will be ruptured, the head of the femur will be in the posterior iliac fossa, and the limb will be shortened, adducted, and medially rotated, the knee on the affected side tending to overlie the normal knee. The position is almost diagnostic and is to be contrasted with the positions in fracture of the femoral neck, when the limb will be shortened also but will be laterally rotated (toes pointing outward). *(Woodburne, p 639)*

3. **(A)** The blood vessels of the head and neck of the femur are branches of the medial circumflex femoral and lateral circumflex femoral arteries and of the posterior branch of the obturator artery. Of particular concern is fracture of the femoral neck, occurring frequently in older women. Such fractures tend to be intracapsular, and thus realigning of the head and neck fragments can be a problem. Furthermore, the blood vessels may be ruptured, resulting in degeneration of the head fragment. The fracture of the upper third of the shaft of the femur exemplifies the effect of muscle pull. *(Woodburne, pp 639–640)*

4. **(E)** Damage to the peroneal nerve results in a paralysis that includes footdrop with loss of the extensors of the foot and toes. The foot turns inward. These effects are due to the paralysis of the muscles of the anterior and lateral compartment of the leg. The muscles of the posterior compartment, innervated by the tibial nerve, control plantar flexion. *(Woodburne, p 643)*

5. **(E)** The small femoral canal is the usual site of a femoral hernia. It is common for a femoral hernia to bulge forward under the skin over the saphenous opening. The coverings of the femoral hernia from within outward include the parietal peritoneum, the extraperitoneal connective tissue, the anterior layer of the femoral sheath, the fascia cribrosa, and the skin. A femoral hernia emerges lateral and inferior to the pubic tubercle. *(Woodburne, p 574)*

6. **(A)** A localized dilation of the terminal part of the great saphenous vein, known as a saphenous varix, causes a swelling in the femoral triangle, located just inferior to the inguinal ligament. A saphenous varix may be confused with other groin swellings, such as femoral hernia. *(Moore, pp 383–385)*

7. **(B)** If it is necessary to ligate the femoral artery, blood is supplied to the lower limb through the cruciate anastomosis, the union of the medial and lateral circumflex femoral arteries with the inferior gluteal artery superiorly and the first perforating artery inferiorly. The genicular anastomosis occurs around the knee, and the malleolar network is located at the ankle. The saphenous veins drain the superficial aspects of the lower limb. *(Moore, p 399)*

8. **(C)** As there are a number of important nerves and blood vessels in the gluteal region, injections can be made safely only into the superolateral area of the buttock, that is, superior to the tubercle of the iliac crest; the needle should go deeply enough to pass through the thick, superficial fascia and enter the gluteus medius muscle where it is not covered by the gluteus maximus muscle. Injections into other areas could endanger and possibly injure the sciatic or other nerves and vessels. *(Moore, pp 417–420)*

9. **(D)** The common fibular (peroneal) nerve is the most commonly injured nerve in the lower limb, mainly because it winds superficially around the neck of the fibula. Even when there is injury to the sciatic nerve, its common fibular division is usually more severely affected than its tibial division. Severance of the common fibular nerve results in paralysis of all the dorsiflexor and eversion muscles of the foot—condition known as "footdrop." *(Moore, p 429)*

10. **(B)** Because the body of the tibia is unprotected anteromedially throughout its course and is relatively slender at the junction of its inferior and middle thirds, it is not surprising that the tibia is the most common long bone to be fractured and to suffer compound injury. *(Moore, p 432)*

11. **(A)** Fractures of the fibula commonly occur 2 to 6 cm proximal to the distal end of the lateral malleolus and are often associated with fracture–dislocations of the ankle joint (Pott's fracture). When a person slips and the foot is forced into an excessively inverted position, the ankle ligaments tear and the talus is forcibly tilted against the lateral malleolus, shearing it off. *(Moore, p 437)*

12. **(B)** The ankle reflex (ankle jerk) is the twitch of the gastrocnemius, soleus, and plantaris, which is induced by striking the tendo calcaneus with a reflex hammer. The reflex center for the ankle reflex is the S1 and S2 segments of the spinal cord. *(Moore, p 451)*

13. **(B)** Because the tibial nerve is deep and well protected, it is not commonly injured. However, lacerations in the popliteal fossa and posterior dislocations of the knee joint may damage this nerve, producing paralysis of all muscles in the posterior compartment of the leg and the intrinsic muscles in the sole of the foot. When the plantar flexors of the foot are paralyzed, the patient is unable to curl the toes or stand on them. In addition, there is loss of sensation in the sole of the foot, making it vulnerable to the development of pressure sores. *(Moore, p 458)*

14. **(D)** Intermittent claudication is caused by ischemia of the leg muscles owing to arteriosclerotic stenosis or occlusion of the leg arteries. Intermittent claudication is characterized by leg cramps that develop during walking and disappear soon after rest. This pain is not associated with nerve compression. *(Moore, p 460)*

15. **(A)** With the leg flexed, the patellar ligament is struck to elicit a knee jerk. This patellar reflex results in extension of the leg. This reflex is blocked by damage to the femoral nerve, which supplies the quadriceps muscles (vastus lateralis, medialis, intermedius, and rectus femoris). Similarly, damage to the reflex center in the spinal cord (L_2, L_3, and L_4) will affect the patellar reflex. *(Moore, p 479)*

16. **(A)** Traumatic dislocation of the hip is not a frequent occurrence because of the deep acetabulum. When it takes place, usually it is the result of a severe blow upon the knee while the hip is flexed. The head of the femur is thus dislocated posteriorly, with a tearing of the posterior part of the capsule. Anterior dislocation is much rarer than posterior dislocation; in this case, the head of the femur passes around the medial edge of the iliofemoral ligament and lodges against the body of the pubis or the obturator foramen. *(Hollinshead, p 399)*

17. **(A)** The term clubfoot is used now to describe a condition of plantar flexion, inversion, and adduction (talipes equinovarus). This is the most common type of deformity seen in congenital clubfoot. The cause is not understood. A dorsiflexion deformity is not seen in this type of deformity. *(Hollinshead, p 412)*

18. **(C)** Of the locations listed, the common peroneal nerve is most likely to be injured as it becomes subcutaneous just behind the head of the fibula. Just before or after it has penetrated the posterior intermuscular septum, it divides into two branches, the deep and superficial peroneal nerves. Extended pressure on the lateral side of the knee, as in keeping the legs crossed for a long time, can result in injury to the common peroneal nerve. *(Hollinshead, p 420)*

19. **(C)** The femoral sheath contains three compartments separated by septa. The lateral compartment contains the femoral artery. The intermediate compartment contains the femoral vein, and the medial compartment is the femoral canal, which contains only a slight amount of loose connective tissue and a few lymphatics and lymph nodes. The upper end of the femoral canal is the femoral ring. A femoral hernia descends through the femoral ring into the femoral canal. *(Hollinshead, p 386)*

20. **(E)** All of the choices listed are characteristic of femoral hernia. The femoral ring is a weak point in the abdominal wall that normally admits the size of the tip of the little finger. A femoral hernia is protrusion of abdominal viscera, often the small intestine, through the femoral ring into the femoral canal. The median compartment of the femoral sheath and not the lateral compartment. Strangulation of a femoral hernia that interferes with the blood supply to the herniated bowel may occur owing to the sharpness and rigidity of the boundaries of the femoral ring. A femoral hernia presents as a mass inferolateral to the pubic tubercle and medial to the femoral vein. *(Moore, pp 459–462,593–594,599,601)*

Developmental Upper and Lower Limbs Questions

DIRECTIONS (Questions 1 through 10): Each of the numbered items or incomplete statements in this section is followed by answers or by completions of the statement. Select the ONE lettered answer or completion that is BEST in each case.

1. When do the limb buds become visible as outpocketings from the ventrolateral body wall?

    (A) 5th week of development
    (B) 8th week of development
    (C) end of the 3rd month of development
    (D) beginning of the 6th month of development
    (E) 3rd week of development

2. Development of the upper and lower limbs is similar except that the morphogenesis of the lower limb is

    (A) approximately 1 or 2 days ahead of that of the upper limb
    (B) approximately 4 weeks behind that of the upper limb
    (C) opposite in a distoproximal direction
    (D) opposite in the directions of rotation
    (E) the absence of the apical ectodermal ridge (AER)

3. The mesenchyme in the limb buds begins to condense and hyaline cartilage can be identified during which of the following times of gestation?

    (A) 6th week
    (B) 3rd week
    (C) 4th month
    (D) 6th month
    (E) 11th week

4. Primary ossification centers are present in all long bones of the limbs by the

    (A) 4th week
    (B) 12th week

    (C) 3rd month
    (D) 6th month
    (E) 2nd week

5. When does complete ossification of the diaphysis of the bone occur?

    (A) during the 5th month of gestation
    (B) during the 4th week of gestation
    (C) during the 2nd year
    (D) during the 3rd year
    (E) at birth

6. All of the following statements concerning the epiphyseal plate are correct EXCEPT

    (A) it plays an important role in the growth in length of the bone
    (B) on both sides of the plate, endochondral ossification proceeds
    (C) the plate is permanent
    (D) the plate is found on each extremity in long bones
    (E) the plate is found only at one extremity in short bones

7. All of the following statements or terms are directly or indirectly related to abnormalities of the extremities EXCEPT

    (A) amelia
    (B) thalidomide
    (C) these abnormalities are common
    (D) a high incidence of children with these limb malformations were born between 1957 and 1962
    (E) micromelia

8. All of the following statements concerning clubfoot are correct EXCEPT

   (A) it is usually seen in combination with sydactyly
   (B) the sole of the foot is turned inward
   (C) the foot is adducted and plantar flexed
   (D) it is seen mainly in females
   (E) it may be hereditary in some cases

9. All of the following statements concerning congenital hip dislocation are correct EXCEPT

   (A) it consists of an underdevelopment of the acetabulum
   (B) it consists of an underdevelopment of the head of the femur
   (C) the condition is rather common
   (D) it occurs mostly in females
   (E) all babies with this abnormality are breech deliveries

10. Useful information of "bone age" in children is obtained from ossification studies in which of the following areas?

   (A) cervical vertebra
   (B) skull
   (C) hands and wrists
   (D) ribs
   (E) long bones

ANSWERS AND EXPLANATIONS

1. **(A)** The limb buds become visible as outpocketings from the ventrolateral body wall at the beginning of the 5th week of development. Initially, they consist of a mesenchymal core, derived from the somatic layer of lateral plate mesoderm, which will form the bones and connective tissues of the limb, covered by a layer of cuboidal ectoderm. *(Sadler, p 145)*

2. **(D)** At the limb tip, ectoderm becomes thickened to form the apical ectodermal ridge (AER), which exerts an inductive influence on the underlying mesenchyme. Development of the upper and lower limbs is similar except that morphogenesis of the lower limb is approximately 1 to 2 days behind that of the upper limb. Also during the 7th week of gestation, the limbs rotate in opposite directions. *(Sadler, pp 145–147)*

3. **(A)** While the external shape is being established, the mesenchyme in the buds begins to condense, and by the 5th week of development the first hyaline cartilage models, foreshadowing the bones of the extremities, can be recognized. *(Sadler, pp 147)*

4. **(B)** The ossification of the bones of the extremities, endochondral ossification, begins by the end of the embryonic period. Primary ossification centers are present in all long bones of the limbs by the 12th week of development. *(Sadler, pp 147–148)*

5. **(E)** At birth, the diaphysis of the bone is usually completely ossified, but the two extremities, known as the epiphyses, are still cartilaginous, shortly thereafter, however, ossification centers arise in the epiphyses. *(Sadler, p 148)*

6. **(C)** A cartilage plate (epiphyseal plate) remains temporarily between the diaphyseal and epiphyseal ossification centers. The plate plays an important role in the growth in the length of the bone. On both sides of the plate, endochondral ossification proceeds. When the bone has acquired its full length, the epiphyseal plates disappear and the epiphyses unite with the shaft of the bone. In the long bones, an epiphyseal plate is found on each extremity and in the smaller bones (phalanges) only one extremity. *(Sadler, pp 148–149)*

7. **(C)** The abnormalities of the extremities vary greatly. In the most extreme form, one or two extremities are absent (amelia) or represented only by hands and feet attached to the trunk (meromelia). Sometimes all segments of the extremities are present but are abnormally short (micromelia). These abnormalities are rare and mainly of hereditary nature. A high incidence of children with these limb malformations born between 1957 and 1962 led to the study of the prenatal histories and discovery that many of the mothers had taken thalidomide as a sleeping pill and antinauseant. *(Sadler, p 149)*

8. **(D)** Clubfoot is usually seen in combination with syndactyly. The sole of the foot is turned inward and the foot adducted and plantar flexed. It is seen mainly in males and in some cases is hereditary. *(Sadler, p 150)*

9. **(E)** Congenital hip dislocation consists of an underdevelopment of the acetabulum and the head of the femur. The condition is rather common and occurs mostly in females. Many babies, but not all, with this abnormality are breech deliveries. *(Sadler, p 151)*

10. **(C)** Knowledge about the appearance of various ossification centers is used by radiologists to determine whether a child has reached its proper maturation age. Useful information of "bone age" is obtained from ossification studies in the hands and wrists of children. *(Sadler, p 149)*

Nervous Upper and Lower Limbs
Questions

DIRECTIONS (Questions 1 through 10): Each of the numbered items or incomplete statements in this section is followed by answers or by completions of the statement. Select the ONE lettered answer or completion that is BEST in each case.

1. Pain that arises in muscles, tendons, ligaments, and bones is probably detected by the

   (A) neuromuscular spindles
   (B) Golgi tendon organs
   (C) free nerve endings
   (D) Merkel endings
   (E) pacinian corpuscles

2. All of the following sensory endings are located in joints EXCEPT

   (A) Ruffini-like cutaneous endings
   (B) small pacinian corpuscles
   (C) Golgi tendon organs
   (D) free nerve endings
   (E) Meissner's tactile corpuscles

3. All of the following statements concerning neuro-muscular spindles are correct EXCEPT

   (A) they lie in the long axis of the muscle
   (B) they are typically located near the tendinous insertions of muscle
   (C) they are especially numerous in the muscles of the back
   (D) each spindle consists of a fusiform capsule of connection tissue
   (E) they are supplied by two afferent nerve fibers

4. All of the following statements concerning a motor end plate are correct EXCEPT

   (A) it is a synaptic structure that consists of a motor neuron and the muscle fibers that it innervates
   (B) the number of muscle fibers in a motor unit varies from a few to several hundred
   (C) it is usually located midway along the length of the muscle fiber
   (D) the axonal endings within the end plate contain large, elongated synaptic vesicles
   (E) the motor units of intrinsic hand muscles include only a few muscle fibers

5. All of the following statements concerning peripheral neuropathy are correct EXCEPT

   (A) it commonly involves degenerative changes in peripheral nerves
   (B) it may produce sensory loss
   (C) it may produce motor weakness
   (D) the proximal portions of nerves are affected first
   (E) diabetes may cause peripheral neuropathy

6. The entrapment syndrome for the median nerve is more likely to occur at the

   (A) brachial plexus
   (B) elbow
   (C) carpal tunnel
   (D) neck
   (E) axillary region

7. All of the following characteristics associated with axon reaction are correct EXCEPT

   (A) chromatolysis occurs
   (B) the nucleus assumes an eccentric position away from the axon hillock
   (C) the cell body swells
   (D) the nucleolus disappears
   (E) recovery takes several months

8. All of the following statements concerning tendon jerks (stretch reflex) are correct EXCEPT

   (A) it is a two-neuron or monosynaptic reflex arc

   (B) a sharp tap on the tendon causes synchronous discharges from the spindles

   (C) exaggerated jerks indicate a lack of inhibition of motor neurons by activity in the descending tracts from the brain

   (D) a diminished or absent tendon jerk indicates disease affecting either the afferent or efferent neurons of the stretch reflex

   (E) the alpha motor neurons stimulate the intrafusal fibers of the muscle spindle

9. Syringomyelia is associated with

   (A) a "yokelike" anesthesia for pain and temperature in the lower limbs

   (B) neuronal degeneration being the primary pathological change

   (C) central cavitations, usually in the cervical region

   (D) wasting of the muscles of the lower limb

   (E) usually, involvement of alpha motor nerve neurons

10. All of the following statements concerning poliomyelitis are correct EXCEPT

    (A) muscle tone is reduced or absent

    (B) tendon-jerk reflexes are weak or absent

    (C) muscle atrophy occurs

    (D) a virus selectively attacks neurons located in the dorsal root ganglion

    (E) flaccid paresis or paralysis occurs

ANSWERS AND EXPLANATIONS

1. **(C)** Pain that arises in muscles, tendons, ligaments, and bones is probably detected by free nerve endings in connective tissue. These nociceptive endings respond to physical injury and to local chemical changes, such as those that may be caused by ischemia. *(Barr, p 42)*

2. **(E)** Four types of sensory endings are recognized within and around the capsules of synovial joints. Encapsulated formations similar to the Ruffini cutaneous endings are present in the capsules of joints. The small pacinian corpuscles respond to acceleration and deceleration. The Golgi tendon organs mediate reflex inhibition of adjacent musculature. The free nerve endings respond to injurious mechanical stresses that cause pain. Meissner's tactile corpuscles are located in the dermal papillary ridges. *(Barr, pp 41–42)*

3. **(C)** Neuromuscular spindles lie in the long axis of the muscle. Spindles are typically located near the tendinous insertions of muscles and are especially numerous in muscles that perform highly skilled movements, such as those of the hand, not the back. Each spindle consists of a fusiform capsule of connective tissue. The spindle is supplied by two afferent nerve fibers. *(Barr, pp 42–43)*

4. **(D)** The motor end plates, or myoneural junctions, are synaptic structures with two components—a motor nerve fiber and the subjacent part of the muscle fiber. The number of muscle fibers in a motor unit varies from fewer than 10 to several hundred. Small muscles, such as the extraocular and intrinsic hand muscles must contract with greater precision, so their motor units include only a few muscle fibers. The end plate is usually located midway along the length of the muscle fiber. The axonal endings within the end plate contain small, spherical synaptic vesicles and mitochrondria. *(Barr, pp 45–46)*

5. **(D)** The peripheral nervous system is subject to various disorders. Peripheral neuropathy (neuritis), the most common of these, consists of degenerative changes in peripheral nerves that produce sensory loss and motor weakness. Distal portions of nerves are affected first, with symptoms in the hands and feet. There are many causes of peripheral neuropathy, including nutritional deficiencies, toxic substances of various kinds, and metabolic disorders, notably diabetes. *(Barr, p 50)*

6. **(C)** A nerve may be pressed where it passes over a bony prominence or through a restricted aperture; for example, the ulnar nerve is subject to pressure at the elbow, and the median nerve, in the carpal tunnel at the wrist. The resulting entrapment syndrome includes motor and sensory disturbance in the area of distribution of the nerve. *(Barr, p 50)*

7. **(D)** The best-known change proximal to the site of axonal transection is the axon reaction. The cell body, in sections stained by a cationic dye (the Nissl method), first shows signs of reaction 24 to 48 hours after interruption of the axon. The coarse clumps of Nissl substance are changed to a finely granulated dispersion. This change is known as chromatolysis. The nucleus assumes an eccentric position away from the axon hillock, and the entire cell body swells. The nucleolus enlarges, and recovery takes several months. *(Barr, p 53)*

8. **(E)** The tendon jerk (stretch reflex) has a two-neuron or monosynaptic reflex arc. Slight stretching of a muscle stimulates the sensory endings in neuromuscular spindles. A sharp tap in the tendon causes synchronous discharges from the spindle in

the muscle, with prompt reflex contraction. A diminished or absent tendon jerk indicates disease affecting either the afferent or the efferent neurons of the stretch reflex. Exaggerated jerks indicate a lack of inhibition of motor neurons by activity in descending tracts from the brain. *(Barr, pp 82–83)*

9. **(C)** Syringomyelia is different from the degenerative diseases because neuronal degeneration is not the primary pathological change. There is central cavitation of the spinal cord, usually beginning in the cervical region with a glial reaction (gliosis) adjacent to the cavity. Decussating fibers for pain and temperature in the ventral white commissure are interrupted early in the disease.

The classical clinical picture is that of "yokelike" anesthesia for pain and temperature over the shoulders and upper limbs and consequently wasting of the muscles of the upper limbs. *(Barr, p 86)*

10. **(D)** The syndrome of a lower motor neuron lesion occurs when a muscle is paralyzed or weakened as a result of disease or injury that affects the cell bodies or axons of the innervating neurons. Typical causes include poliomyelitis, in which a virus selectively attacks ventral horn cells or equivalent neurons in the brain stem. The muscle tone is reduced or absent (flaccid paresis or paralysis). The tendon-jerk reflexes are weak or absent. The muscles show atrophy. *(Barr, pp 350–351)*

Illustrations
Upper Limbs—Questions

UPPER LIMB
(Questions 1 through 13)

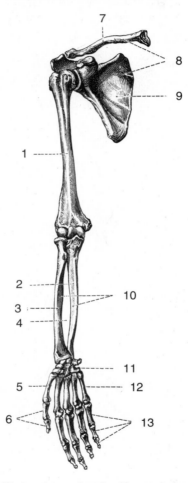

Figure 7–1. Upper limb. (Modified and reproduced, with permission, from Montgomery RL: *Basic Anatomy,* Urban & Schwarzenberg, p. 57, 1980.)

Directions: With reference to the diagram, match the numbered structures with their corresponding lettered items.

(A) interrosseous space

(B) phalanges

(C) shoulder girdle

(D) humerus

(E) carpals

(F) 1st metacarpal

(G) ulna

(H) radius

(I) 5th metacarpal

(J) forearm

(K) clavicle

(L) scapula

COSTAL SURFACE OF SCAPULA
(Questions 14 through 25)

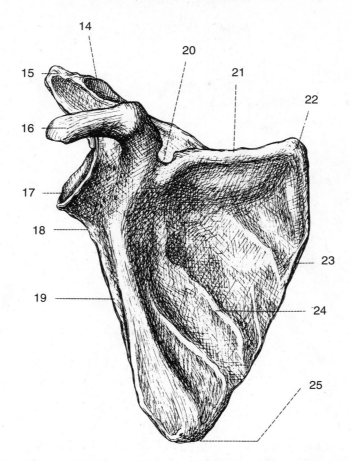

Figure 7–2. Costal surface. (Modified and reproduced, with permission, from Montgomery RL: *Basic Anatomy,* Urban & Schwarzenberg, p. 58, 1980.)

Directions: With reference to the diagram, match the numbered structures with their corresponding lettered items.

(A) lateral border

(B) coracoid process

(C) vertebral border

(D) inferior angle

(E) glenoid fossa

(F) scapular notch

(G) articular facet

(H) superior angle

(I) subscapular fossa

(J) acromion

(K) superior border

(L) infraglenoid tubercle

DORSAL SURFACE OF SCAPULA
(Questions 26 through 42)

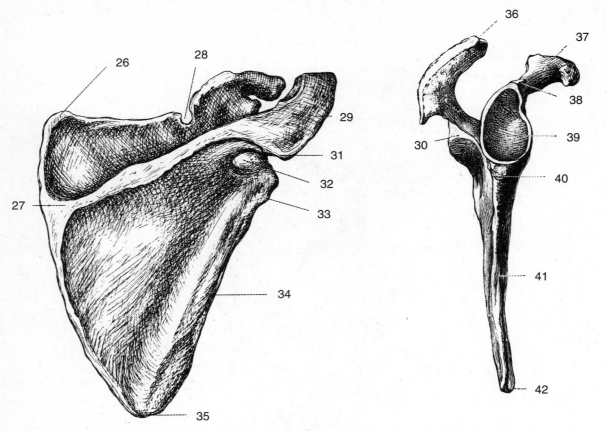

Figure 7–3. Dorsal surface. (Modified and reproduced, with permission, from Montgomery RL: *Basic Anatomy,* Urban & Schwarzenberg, p. 58, 1980.)

Directions: With reference to the diagram, match the numbered structures with their corresponding lettered items.

(A) scapular notch

(B) infraglenoid tubercle

(C) superior angle

(D) lateral border

(E) coracoid process

(F) supraglenoid tubercle

(G) acromion

(H) neck of scapula

(I) inferior angle

(J) scapular spine

(K) glenoid fossa

(L) angle of acromion

SUPERFICIAL MUSCLES OF THE UPPER ARM AND CHEST
(Questions 43 through 53)

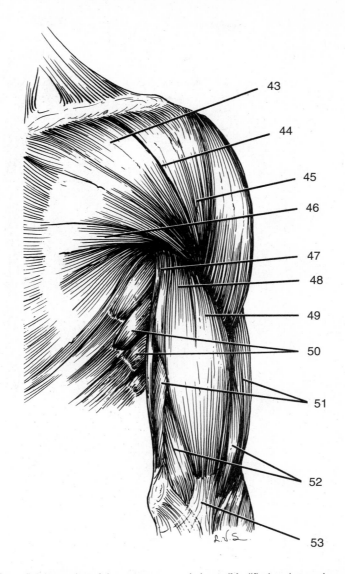

Figure 7–4. Superficial muscles of the upper arm and chest. (Modified and reproduced, with permission, from Lindner HH: *Clinical Anatomy,* Appleton & Lange, p. 537, 1989.)

Directions: With reference to the diagram, match the numbered structures with their corresponding lettered items.

(A) deltoid

(B) coracobrachialis

(C) long head of biceps brachii

(D) brachialis

(E) clavicular portion of pectoralis major

(F) triceps

(G) bicipital aponeurosis

(H) pectoralis major

(I) short head of biceps brachii

(J) serratus anterior

(K) deltopectoral groove

DORSAL MUSCULATURE OF THE SCAPULA
(Questions 54 through 63)

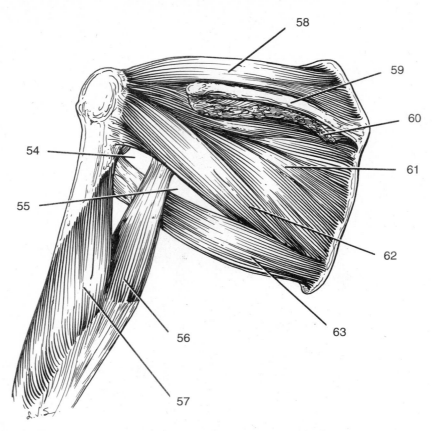

Figure 7–5. The dorsal musculature of the scapula showing formation of triangular and quadrangular spaces. The deltoid muscle has been cut, and the acromion and the lateral portion of the spine of the scapula have been removed. (Modified and reproduced, with permission, from Lindner HH: *Clinical Anatomy,* Appleton & Lange, p. 538, 1989.)

Directions: With reference to the diagram, match the numbered structures with their corresponding lettered items.

(A) long head of triceps

(B) teres major

(C) supraspinatus muscle

(D) quadrangular space

(E) scapular spine

(F) teres minor

(G) infraspinatus muscle

(H) deltoid muscle

(I) triangular space

(J) lateral head of triceps

HUMERUS
(Questions 64 through 86)

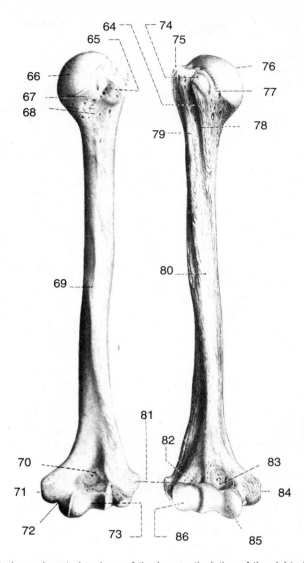

Figure 7–6. Anterior and posterior views of the bony articulation of the right elbow joint. (Modified and reproduced, with permission, from Montgomery RL: *Basic Anatomy,* Urban & Schwarzenberg, p. 59, 1980.)

Directions: With reference to the diagram, match the numbered structures with their corresponding lettered items.

(A) radial notch
(B) crest of lesser tubercle
(C) head of humerus
(D) shaft of humerus
(E) intertubercle groove
(F) lateral epicondyle
(G) crest of greater tubercle
(H) greater tubercle
(I) surgical neck

(J) medial epicondyle
(K) lesser tubercle
(L) radial fossa
(M) olecranon fossa
(N) coronoid fossa
(O) anatomical neck
(P) trochlear
(Q) ulnar nerve groove
(R) capitulum

BONES OF THE FOREARM
(Questions 87 through 111)

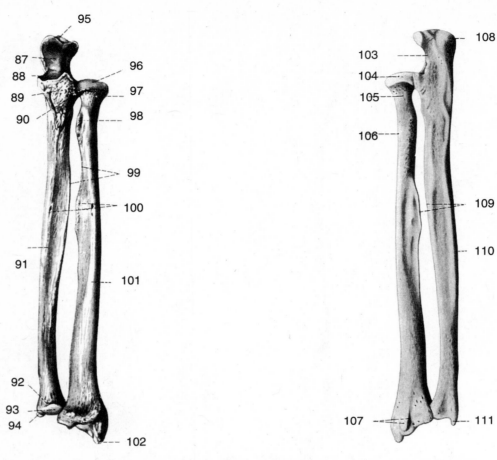

Figure 7–7. Bones of the forearm. (Modified and reproduced, with permission, from Montgomery RL: *Basic Anatomy,* Urban & Schwarzenberg, p. 60, 1980.)

Directions: With reference to the diagram, match the numbered structures with their corresponding lettered items.

(A) styloid process
(B) articular surface
(C) radial tuberosity
(D) nutrient foramen
(E) head of ulna
(F) radius
(G) ulna
(H) extensor tendon sulcus

(I) ulnar tuberosity
(J) head of radius
(K) radial notch
(L) olecranon
(M) coronoid process
(N) interosseous margins
(O) trochlear notch
(P) neck of radius

CARPALS, METACARPALS, AND PHALANGES
(Questions 112 through 133)

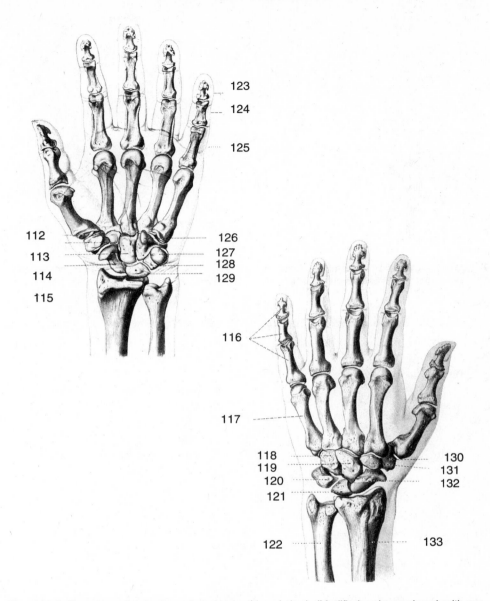

Figure 7–8 Carpals, metacarpals, and phalanges (dorsal view). (Modified and reproduced, with permission, from Montgomery RL: *Basic Anatomy,* Urban & Schwarzenberg, p. 61, 1980.)

Directions: With reference to the diagram, match the numbered structures with their corresponding lettered items.

(A) metacarpals

(B) hamate

(C) ulna

(D) trapezium

(E) radius

(F) triquetrum

(G) proximal phalanx

(H) trapezoid

(I) intermediate phalanx

(J) pisiform

(K) capitate

(L) lunate

(M) scaphoid

(N) distal phalanx

(O) phalanges

ARTICULATION OF THE ELBOW
(Questions 134 through 145)

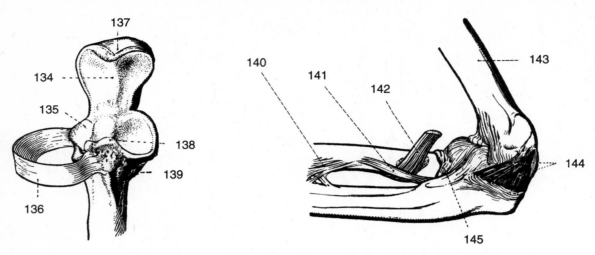

Figure 7–9. Articulation of the elbow. (Modified and reproduced, with permission, from Montgomery RL: *Basic Anatomy,* Urban & Schwarzenberg, p. 76, 1980.)

Directions: With reference to the diagram, match the numbered structures with their corresponding lettered items.

(A) coronoid process

(B) annular radial ligament

(C) oblique ligament

(D) humerus

(E) biceps brachii

(F) trochlear notch

(G) ulnar tuberosity

(H) interosseous membrane

(I) radial notch

(J) olecranon

(K) articular capsule

(L) ulnar collateral ligament

ACROMIOCLAVICULAR AND SHOULDER JOINT ARTICULATIONS
(Questions 146 through 160)

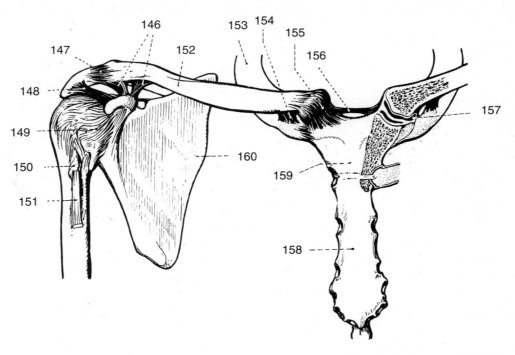

Figure 7–10. Acromioclavicular and shoulder joint articulations. (Modified and reproduced, with permission, from Montgomery RL: *Basic Anatomy,* Urban & Schwarzenberg, p. 75, 1980.)

Directions: With reference to the diagram, match the numbered structures with their corresponding lettered items.

(A) long head biceps brachii

(B) anterior sternoclavicular ligament

(C) articular disk of sternoclavicular articulation

(D) clavicle

(E) coracoclavicular ligament

(F) scapula

(G) manubrium

(H) acromioclavicular articulation

(I) 1st rib

(J) costoclavicular ligament

(K) coracoacromial ligament

(L) sternum

(M) articular capsule

(N) interclavicular ligament

(O) synovial sheath

LIGAMENTS OF THE WRIST (DORSAL VIEW)
(Questions 161 through 169)

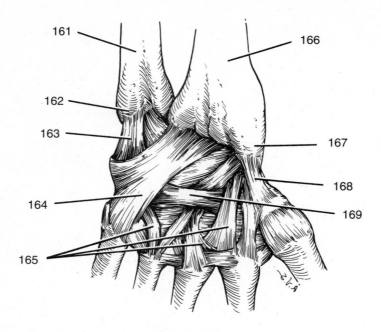

Figure 7–11. Ligaments, dorsal view. (Modified and reproduced, with permission, from Lindner HH: *Clinical Anatomy,* Appleton & Lange, p. 565, 1989.)

Directions: With reference to the diagram, match the numbered structures with their corresponding lettered items.

(A) styloid process (ulna)

(B) dorsal radiocarpal ligament

(C) radial collateral ligament

(D) dorsal intercarpal ligament

(E) radius

(F) styloid process (radius)

(G) ulnar collateral ligament

(H) dorsal carpometacarpal ligaments

(I) ulna

Upper Limbs—Answers

UPPER LIMB

1.	(D)	8.	(C)
2.	(G)	9.	(L)
3.	(H)	10.	(J)
4.	(A)	11.	(E)
5.	(F)	12.	(I)
6.	(B)	13.	(B)
7.	(K)		

COSTAL SURFACE OF SCAPULA

14.	(G)	20.	(F)
15.	(J)	21.	(K)
16.	(B)	22.	(H)
17.	(E)	23.	(C)
18.	(L)	24.	(I)
19.	(A)	25.	(D)

DORSAL SURFACE OF SCAPULA

26.	(C)	35.	(I)
27.	(J)	36.	(G)
28.	(A)	37.	(E)
29.	(G)	38.	(F)
30.	(J)	39.	(K)
31.	(L)	40.	(B)
32.	(H)	41.	(D)
33.	(B)	42.	(I)
34.	(D)		

SUPERFICIAL MUSCLES OF THE UPPER ARM AND CHEST

43.	(E)	49.	(C)
44.	(K)	50.	(J)
45.	(A)	51.	(F)
46.	(H)	52.	(D)
47.	(B)	53.	(G)
48.	(I)		

DORSAL MUSCULATURE OF THE SCAPULA

54.	(D)	59.	(E)
55.	(I)	60.	(H)
56.	(A)	61.	(G)
57.	(J)	62.	(F)
58.	(C)	63.	(B)

HUMERUS

64.	(E)	76.	(C)
65.	(H)	77.	(O)
66.	(C)	78.	(I)
67.	(O)	79.	(G)
68.	(I)	80.	(D)
69.	(A)	81.	(F)
70.	(M)	82.	(L)
71.	(J)	83.	(N)
72.	(Q)	84.	(J)
73.	(P)	85.	(P)
74.	(K)	86.	(R)
75.	(H)		

BONES OF THE FOREARM

87.	(O)	100.	(D)
88.	(M)	101.	(F)
89.	(K)	102.	(A)
90.	(I)	103.	(O)
91.	(G)	104.	(J)
92.	(E)	105.	(P)
93.	(B)	106.	(F)
94.	(A)	107.	(H)
95.	(L)	108.	(L)
96.	(J)	109.	(N)
97.	(P)	110.	(G)
98.	(C)	111.	(A)
99.	(N)		

CARPALS, METACARPALS, AND PHALANGES

112.	(D)	123.	(N)
113.	(H)	124.	(I)
114.	(K)	125.	(G)
115.	(M)	126.	(B)
116.	(O)	127.	(J)
117.	(A)	128.	(F)
118.	(B)	129.	(L)
119.	(K)	130.	(D)
120.	(F)	131.	(H)
121.	(L)	132.	(M)
122.	(C)	133.	(E)

ARTICULATION OF THE ELBOW

134.	(F)	140.	(H)
135.	(I)	141.	(C)
136.	(B)	142.	(E)
137.	(J)	143.	(D)
138.	(A)	144.	(L)
139.	(G)	145.	(K)

ACROMIOCLAVICULAR AND SHOULDER JOINT ARTICULATIONS

146.	(E)	154.	(J)
147.	(H)	155.	(B)
148.	(K)	156.	(N)
149.	(M)	157.	(C)
150.	(O)	158.	(L)
151.	(A)	159.	(G)
152.	(D)	160.	(F)
153.	(I)		

LIGAMENTS OF THE WRIST (DORSAL VIEW)

161.	(I)	166.	(E)
162.	(A)	167.	(F)
163.	(G)	168.	(C)
164.	(B)	169.	(D)
165.	(H)		

Lower Limbs—Questions

SACROILIAC, SYMPHYSIS PUBIS, AND HIP ARTICULATION (ANTERIOR VIEW)
(Questions 170 through 191)

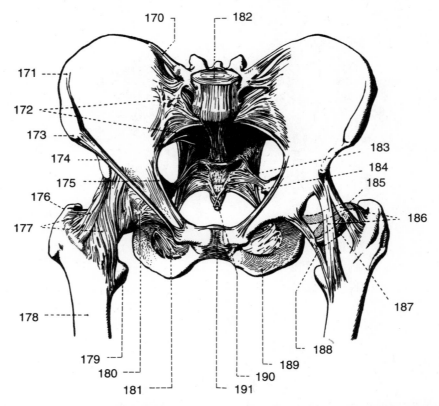

Figure 7–12. Sacroiliac, symphysis pubis, and hip articulation (anterior view). (Modified and reproduced, with permission, from Montgomery RL: *Basic Anatomy,* Urban & Schwarzenberg, p. 78, 1980.)

Directions: With reference to the diagram, match the numbered structures with their corresponding lettered items.

(A) anterior sacroiliac ligaments

(B) inguinal ligament

(C) iliolumbar ligament

(E) greater trochanter

(F) iliac crest

(G) femur

(H) anterior superior iliac spine

(I) 5th lumbar vertebra

(J) sacrotuberous ligament

(K) pelvic brim

(L) sacrospinous ligament

(M) iliofemoral ligament

(N) ischial tuberosity

(O) coccyx

(P) lesser trochanter

(Q) pubic symphysis

(R) pubofemoral ligament

(S) neck of femur

(T) obturator membrane

SACROILIAC, SYMPHYSIS PUBIS, AND HIP ARTICULATIONS
(POSTERIOR VIEW)
(Questions 192 through 208)

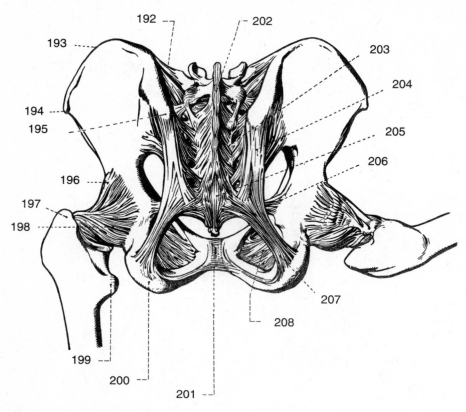

Figure 7–13. Sacroiliac, symphysis pubis, and hip articulation (posterior view). (Modified and reproduced, with permission, from Montgomery RL: *Basic Anatomy,* Urban & Schwarzenberg, p. 79, 1980.)

Directions: With reference to the diagram, match the numbered structures with their corresponding lettered items.

(A) lesser trochanter
(B) iliolumbar ligament
(C) ischial tuberosity
(D) arcuate ligament of pubis
(E) iliac crest
(F) posterior sacrococcygeal ligament
(G) sacrotuberous ligament
(H) anterior superior iliac spine
(I) obturator membrane

(J) sacrospinal ligament
(K) posterior superior iliac spine
(L) posterior sacroiliac ligament
(M) intermediate sacral crest
(N) iliofemoral ligament
(O) supraspinal ligament
(P) greater trochanter
(Q) ischiofemoral ligament

FEMUR
(Questions 209 through 229)

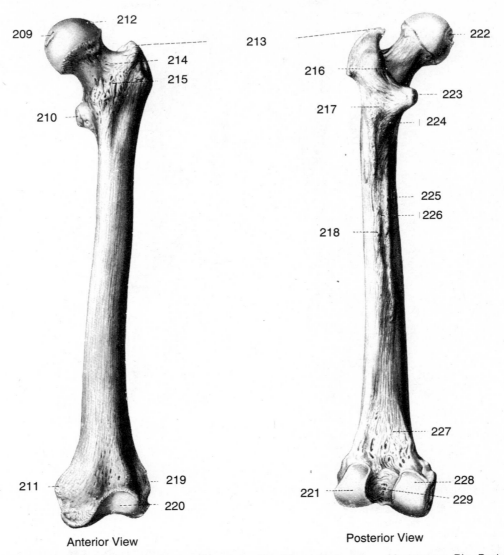

Anterior View   Posterior View

Figure 7–14. Femur. (Modified and reproduced, with permission, from Montgomery RL: *Basic Anatomy,* Urban & Schwarzenberg, p. 65, 1980.)

Directions: With reference to the diagram, match the numbered structures with their corresponding lettered items.

(A) medial epicondyle

(B) greater trochanter

(C) fovea head of femur

(D) gluteal tuberosity

(E) lateral line of linea aspera

(F) intertrochanteric line

(G) lesser trochanter

(H) neck of femur

(I) intertrochanteric crest

(J) patellar facet

(K) linea pectinea

(L) lateral epicondyle

(M) head of femur

(N) lateral condyle

(O) medial line of linea aspera

(P) linea aspera

(Q) intercondylar fossa

(R) medial condyle

(S) popliteal facet

MUSCLES OF THE RIGHT THIGH AND LEG
(Questions 230 through 256)

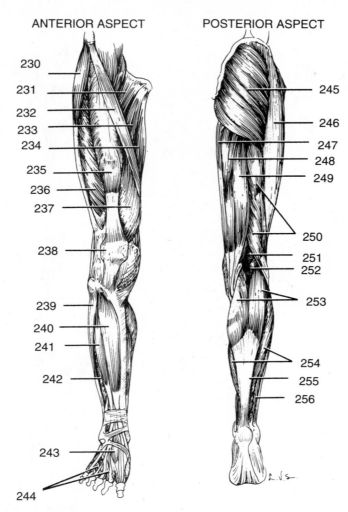

Figure 7–15. The muscles of the right thigh and leg. (Modified and reproduced, with permission, from Lindner HH: *Clinical Anatomy,* Appleton & Lange, p. 598, 1989.)

Directions: With reference to the diagram, match the numbered structures with their corresponding lettered items.

(A) extensor digitorum longus
(B) tibialis anterior
(C) extensor digitorum brevis
(D) peroneus longus
(E) adductor magnus
(F) patella
(G) gluteus maximus
(H) vastus medialis
(I) semitendinosus
(J) biceps femoris
(K) vastus lateralis
(L) peroneus brevis
(M) rectus femoris

(N) plantaris
(O) semimembranous
(P) gracilis
(Q) extensor hallucis brevis
(R) tensor fasciae latae
(S) gastrocnemius
(T) pectineus
(U) soleus
(V) tendo calcaneus
(W) sartorius
(X) peroneus brevis
(Y) adductor longus

LIGAMENTS OF THE KNEE, FULLY FLEXED
(Questions 257 through 266)

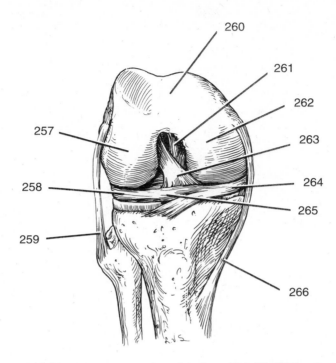

Figure 7–16. The fully flexed right knee. Ligaments of the knee joint. (Modified and reproduced, with permission, from Lindner HH: *Clinical Anatomy,* Appleton & Lange, p. 615, 1989.)

Directions: With reference to the diagram, match the numbered structures with their corresponding lettered items.

(A) posterior cruciate ligament
(B) lateral collateral ligament
(C) medial meniscus
(D) medial femoral condyle
(E) medial collateral ligament

(F) lateral femoral condyle
(G) anterior cruciate ligament
(H) lateral meniscus
(I) transverse genicular ligament
(J) femoral patellar surface

FIBULA AND TIBIA
(Questions 267 through 279)

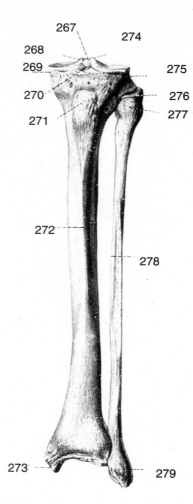

Figure 7–17. Fibula and tibia. (Modified and reproduced, with permission, from Montgomery RL: *Basic Anatomy,* Urban & Schwarzenberg, p. 66, 1980.)

Directions: With reference to the diagram, match the numbered structures with their corresponding lettered items.

(A) lateral intercondylar tubercle

(B) apex of fibular head

(C) fibula

(D) intercondylar fossa

(E) lateral tibial condyle

(F) medial intercondylar tubercle

(G) head of fibula

(H) medial tibial condyle

(I) lateral malleolus

(J) tibial tuberosity

(K) medial malleolus

(L) tibia

CORONAL SECTION THROUGH THE ANKLE JOINT
(Questions 280 through 298)

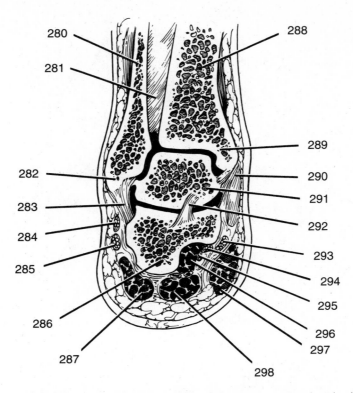

Figure 7–18. Coronal section through the ankle joint. (Modified and reproduced, with permission, from Lindner HH: *Clinical Anatomy,* Appleton & Lange, p. 638, 1989.)

Directions: With reference to the diagram, match the numbered structures with their corresponding lettered items.

(A) calcaneofibular ligament
(B) calcaneus
(C) medial malleolus
(D) interosseous membrane
(E) deltoid ligament
(F) tendon of flexor hallucis longus
(G) tendon of flexor digitorum longus
(H) tendon of peroneus brevis
(I) quadratus plantae
(J) tendon of peroneus longus

(K) talus
(L) flexor digitorum brevis
(M) tendon of tibialis posterior
(N) abductor hallucis
(O) interosseous talocalcaneal ligament
(P) lateral malleolus
(Q) tibia
(R) fibula
(S) abductor digiti minimi

MEDIAL LIGAMENTS OF THE ANKLE JOINT
(Questions 299 through 310)

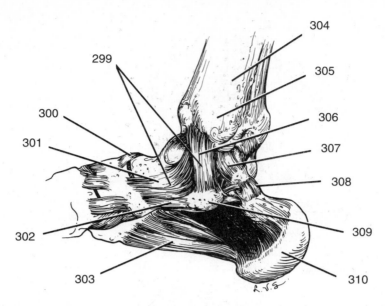

Figure 7–19. Medial ligaments of the ankle joint. (Modified and reproduced, with permission, from Lindner HH: *Clinical Anatomy,* Appleton & Lange, p. 638, 1989.)

Directions: With reference to the diagram, match the numbered structures with their corresponding lettered items.

(A) talonavicular ligament

(B) deltoid ligament

(C) medial malleolus

(D) posterior talotibial ligament

(E) sustentaculum tali

(F) plantar calcaneonavicular ligament

(G) tibionavicular ligament

(H) tibiocalcaneal ligament

(I) calcaneus

(J) posterior talocalcaneal ligament

(K) tibia

(L) long plantar ligament

ANTERIOR VIEW OF THE BONES OF THE FOOT
(Questions 311 through 323)

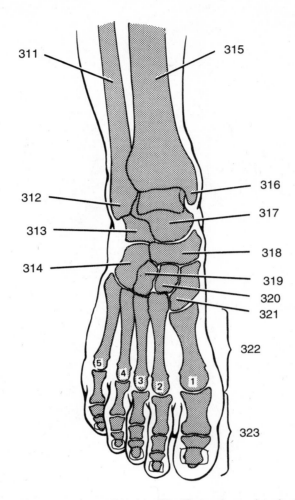

Figure 7–20. Anterior view of the bones of the foot. (Modified and reproduced, with permission, from Lindner HH: *Clinical Anatomy,* Appleton & Lange, p. 643, 1989.)

Directions: With reference to the diagram, match the numbered structures with their corresponding lettered items.

(A) medial malleolus
(B) cuboid
(C) tibia
(D) calcaneus
(E) lateral cuneiform
(F) lateral malleolus
(G) medial cuneiform

(H) metatarsals
(I) fibula
(J) intermediate cuneiform
(K) phalanges
(L) navicular
(M) talus

BONES OF THE FOOT
(Questions 324 through 335)

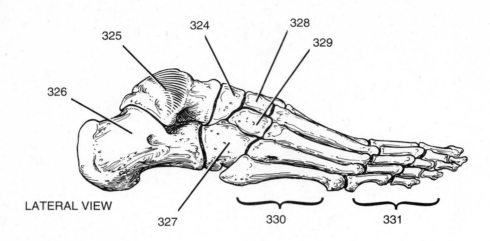

LATERAL VIEW

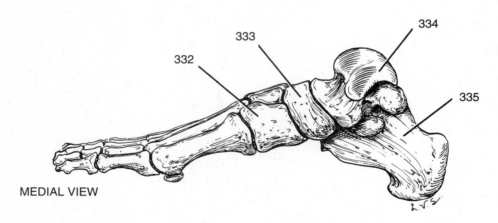

MEDIAL VIEW

Figure 7–21. Bones of the foot. (Modified and reproduced, with permission, from Lindner HH: *Clinical Anatomy,* Appleton & Lange, p. 643, 1989.)

Directions: With reference to the diagram, match the numbered structures with their corresponding lettered items.

(A) navicular

(B) intermediate cuneiform

(C) cuboid

(D) calcaneus

(E) medial cuneiform

(F) talus

(G) lateral cuneiform

(H) metatarsals

(I) phalanges

Lower Limbs—Answers

SACROILIAC, SYMPHYSIS PUBIS, AND HIP ARTICULATION (ANTERIOR VIEW)

170.	(C)	181.	(T)
171.	(F)	182.	(I)
172.	(A)	183.	(L)
173.	(H)	184.	(J)
174.	(B)	185.	(M)
175.	(K)	186.	(M)
176.	(E)	187.	(S)
177.	(M)	188.	(R)
178.	(G)	189.	(N)
179.	(P)	190.	(O)
180.	(R)	191.	(Q)

SACROILIAC, SYMPHYSIS PUBIS, AND HIP ARTICULATION (POSTERIOR VIEW)

192.	(B)	201.	(D)
193.	(E)	202.	(O)
194.	(H)	203.	(M)
195.	(K)	204.	(L)
196.	(N)	205.	(F)
197.	(P)	206.	(J)
198.	(Q)	207.	(G)
199.	(A)	208.	(I)
200.	(C)		

FEMUR

209.	(C)	220.	(J)
210.	(G)	221.	(N)
211.	(A)	222.	(C)
212.	(M)	223.	(G)
213.	(B)	224.	(K)
214.	(H)	225.	(O)
215.	(F)	226.	(P)
216.	(I)	227.	(S)
217.	(D)	228.	(R)
218.	(E)	229.	(Q)
219.	(L)		

MUSCLES OF THE RIGHT THIGH AND LEG

230.	(R)	244.	(C)
231.	(T)	245.	(G)
232.	(W)	246.	(R)
233.	(Y)	247.	(P)
234.	(P)	248.	(E)
235.	(M)	249.	(I)
236.	(K)	250.	(J)
237.	(H)	251.	(O)
238.	(F)	252.	(N)
239.	(D)	253.	(S)
240.	(B)	254.	(U)
241.	(A)	255.	(V)
242.	(L)	256.	(X)
243.	(Q)		

LIGAMENTS OF THE KNEE, FULLY FLEXED

257.	(F)	262.	(D)
258.	(H)	263.	(G)
259.	(B)	264.	(C)
260.	(J)	265.	(I)
261.	(A)	266.	(E)

FIBULA AND TIBIA

267.	(D)	274.	(A)
268.	(F)	275.	(E)
269.	(H)	276.	(B)
270.	(D)	277.	(G)
271.	(J)	278.	(C)
272.	(L)	279.	(I)
273.	(K)		

CORONAL SECTION THROUGH THE ANKLE JOINT

280.	(R)	290.	(E)
281.	(D)	291.	(K)
282.	(P)	292.	(O)
283.	(A)	293.	(M)
284.	(H)	294.	(G)
285.	(J)	295.	(F)
286.	(B)	296.	(I)
287.	(S)	297.	(N)
288.	(Q)	298.	(L)
289.	(C)		

MEDIAL LIGAMENTS OF THE ANKLE JOINT

299.	(B)	305.	(C)
300.	(A)	306.	(H)
301.	(G)	307.	(D)
302.	(F)	308.	(J)
303.	(L)	309.	(E)
304.	(K)	310.	(I)

ANTERIOR VIEW OF THE BONES OF THE FOOT

311.	(I)	318.	(L)
312.	(F)	319.	(E)
313.	(D)	320.	(J)
314.	(B)	321.	(G)
315.	(C)	322.	(H)
316.	(A)	323.	(K)
317.	(M)		

BONES OF THE FOOT

324.	(A)	330.	(H)
325.	(F)	331.	(I)
326.	(D)	332.	(E)
327.	(C)	333.	(A)
328.	(B)	334.	(F)
329.	(G)	335.	(D)

References

1. Basmajian JV: *Grant's Method of Anatomy,* 10th ed. Baltimore, The Williams and Wilkins Company, 1980.
2. Hollinshead WH, Rossee C: *Textbook of Anatomy,* 4th ed. New York, Harper and Row, 1985.
3. Linder HH: *Clinical Anatomy,* Connecticut, Appleton & Lange, 1989.
4. Moore KL: *Clinically Oriented Anatomy,* 3rd ed. Baltimore, The Williams and Wilkins Company, 1992.
5. Woodburne RT, Burkel W: *Essentials of Human Anatomy,* 8th ed. New York, Oxford University Press, 1988.
6. Sadler TW: *Langman's Medical Embryology,* 6th ed. Baltimore, The Williams and Wilkins Company, 1990.

NOTES

NOTES

NOTES

NOTES

NOTES

NOTES